Genetics – Research and Issues

# FORENSIC SCIENCE

# Genetics – Research and Issues

Additional books in this series can be found on Nova's website under the Series tab.

Additional E-books in this series can be found on Nova's website under the E-book tab.

# Law, Crime and Law Enforcement

Additional books in this series can be found on Nova's website under the Series tab.

Additional E-books in this series can be found on Nova's website under the E-book tab.

**Genetics – Research and Issues**

# FORENSIC SCIENCE

**NADIR YACINE
AND
RALPH FELLAG
EDITORS**

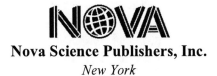

**Nova Science Publishers, Inc.**
*New York*

Copyright © 2012 by Nova Science Publishers, Inc.

**All rights reserved.** No part of this book may be reproduced, stored in a retrieval system or transmitted in any form or by any means: electronic, electrostatic, magnetic, tape, mechanical photocopying, recording or otherwise without the written permission of the Publisher.

For permission to use material from this book please contact us:
Telephone 631-231-7269; Fax 631-231-8175
Web Site: http://www.novapublishers.com

## NOTICE TO THE READER

The Publisher has taken reasonable care in the preparation of this book, but makes no expressed or implied warranty of any kind and assumes no responsibility for any errors or omissions. No liability is assumed for incidental or consequential damages in connection with or arising out of information contained in this book. The Publisher shall not be liable for any special, consequential, or exemplary damages resulting, in whole or in part, from the readers' use of, or reliance upon, this material. Any parts of this book based on government reports are so indicated and copyright is claimed for those parts to the extent applicable to compilations of such works.

Independent verification should be sought for any data, advice or recommendations contained in this book. In addition, no responsibility is assumed by the publisher for any injury and/or damage to persons or property arising from any methods, products, instructions, ideas or otherwise contained in this publication.

This publication is designed to provide accurate and authoritative information with regard to the subject matter covered herein. It is sold with the clear understanding that the Publisher is not engaged in rendering legal or any other professional services. If legal or any other expert assistance is required, the services of a competent person should be sought. FROM A DECLARATION OF PARTICIPANTS JOINTLY ADOPTED BY A COMMITTEE OF THE AMERICAN BAR ASSOCIATION AND A COMMITTEE OF PUBLISHERS.

Additional color graphics may be available in the e-book version of this book.

**Library of Congress Cataloging-in-Publication Data**
Forensic science / editors, Nadir Yacine and Ralph Fellag.
    p. cm.
 Includes index.
 ISBN 978-1-61324-999-4 (hardcover)
 1.  Forensic sciences.  I. Yacine, Nadir. II. Fellag, Ralph.
 HV8073.F5777 2011
 363.25--dc23
                        2011019880

*Published by Nova Science Publishers, Inc. † New York*

# Contents

| | | |
|---|---|---|
| **Preface** | | vii |
| **Chapter 1** | Human and Animal Hair in Forensic Evidence: Problems, Troubleshooting and Workarounds<br>*Elena Pilli* | 1 |
| **Chapter 2** | Forensic Genetics from a Geographic Perspective: Integrating Forensic Genetics and Geostatistics<br>*Amalia N. Díaz-Lacava and Maja Walier* | 59 |
| **Chapter 3** | Human Pigmentation Genes: Forensic Perspectives, General Aspects and Evolution<br>*Caio Cesar Silva de Cerqueira, Carlos Eduardo Guerra Amorim, Francisco Mauro Salzano, Maria Cátira Bortolini* | 85 |
| **Chapter 4** | Bloodstain Investigation: A Review<br>*Ana Castelló, Francesc Francés* | 107 |
| **Chapter 5** | DNA Based Kinship Analysis and Missing Person Identification<br>*Jianye Ge* | 129 |
| **Chapter 6** | Commingled Assemblage from Earthquake 1755 of Lisbon: Forensic Anthropology Study<br>*Cristiana Pereira* | 149 |
| **Chapter 7** | Forensic DNA Databases in Europe: Ethical Challenges<br>*Luciana Caenazzo and Kris Dierickx* | 169 |
| **Chapter 8** | Lip Prints: Past, Present and Future<br>*Ana Castelló and Fernando Verdú* | 179 |
| **Chapter 9** | The Use of Micromanipulation with on Chip LV-PCR System to Isolate Cells from Biological Mixtures<br>*Caixia Li, Lan Hu, Anquan Ji and Junping Han* | 187 |

**Index** 195

# PREFACE

Forensic science is the application of a broad spectrum of sciences to answer questions of interest to a legal system. This may be in relation to a crime or a civil action. This book presents current research from across the globe in the study of forensic science, including integrating forensic genetics and geostatistics; forensic perspectives in human pigmentation genes; bloodstain investigations; forensic DNA typing; forensic anthropology study and the cell separation method as a solution for biological mixtures in forensic science.

Chapter 1- During the course of a criminal investigation, many types of physical and biological evidence are encountered. One of the most common is hair evidence. The identification and comparison of human and animal hairs can be helpful in demonstrating physical contact with a suspect, victim and crime scene. A common forensic approach should proceed from the morphological and microscopic examination to DNA analysis. The non-destructive techniques (morphological and microscopic examination) are a vital step when it is necessary to exclude the synthetic origins of the fibers and to distinguish between human and animal hairs. But the technique is also important to compare the features of the questioned hairs with those of hairs from a known individual. Human hairs are easily distinguishable from those of other animals because they present some typical microscopic characteristics. Today, nuclear and mitochondrial (mtDNA) testing can provide additional information to microscopic examination. In human hairs, routine forensic method for DNA testing (STR analysis of nuclear DNA) is possible when the root and/or adhering tissue are present. However, shed hairs, which are often associated with a crime scene, may harbor no nuclear material. While the nucleus degrades as the hair shaft hardens during keratinization, cellular mitochondria and mtDNA remain relatively intact, making mtDNA analysis of hair shafts possible. Instead the microscopic identification of the species of animal hairs can be complicated because of a general trend of reduced training of and lack of experienced hair examiners. In this case the findings of microscopy may be inconclusive to discriminate one species from the others. When conclusive results about species cannot be performed through microscopic examination, the DNA analysis offers the best opportunity to answer the question: "What species is this?". In this case the mtDNA sequencing analysis has to be not only useful in degraded remains but also in the identification of the species. In this review we report the main applications of human hair analysis to forensic investigations and the recent development in species identification of hairs found at the crime scenes. Moreover the author describes the new prospects offered by the new generation sequencing methods (NGS) and the genome-wide association study applied to hair shaft in forensics science.

Chapter 2- Forensic genetics benefited in the past decades from accelerated advances in molecular genetic technologies. On one side, the quantity of high-quality genotypes increased enormously. And on the other side, principally due to the increasing cooperation of forensic geneticists, standardized high-quality data on various kinds of DNA variation are available in worldwide forensic data sets providing a solid basis for a wide range of population genetics studies relevant to multidisciplinary fields.

Understanding spatial relationships of the extant genetic variation of populations and reconstructing the underlying demographic processes are central topics in forensic genetics. Various statistical methods analyzing spatial genetic variation are implemented in well-established procedures. Forensic genetics studies conducted using such tools have significantly contributed to our understanding of the extant pattern of genetic variation and its underlying history. Nevertheless, plenty of information embedded in the geographical data still remains unexplored, mainly due to methodological restrictions. Integrating the geographic information of forensic genotypes to genetic statistics demands for geostatistical methods. A geographic information system (GIS) offers an appropriated framework to integrate any type of data accounting for a geographic reference and to flexibly address statistical analysis to spatial relationships.

On the basis of concrete examples of widely addressed inquires at population level in forensic genetics, this work shows that combining genetic statistics with geostastistical analysis in a GIS framework opens a wide range of methodological approaches and provides a flexible environment to focus or to adapt the analysis to the phenomena under study and the available data. Results include summary statistics as well as maps displaying precise patterns of genetic variation at the adequate scale and resolution. Inquiries often addressed and related to the distribution and frequency of alleles, haplotypes, or groups of closely related haplotypes are further extended to assess, quantify and map the spatial coverage of the most prevalent alleles or group of closely related haplotypes per tract of land. Advantages and prospects of introducing geostatistics into forensic genetics are discussed.

Chapter 3- Despite the growing number of registered DNA forensic profiles, the rate of profile hits is far below the expected. When a given profile is not found with the standard kits, any available information is important. Ancestry Informative Markers (AIM) have been employed for the identification of the person's ethnicity. However, this is not an adequate approach in certain cases, as, for instance, individuals living in ethnically admixed populations, in which the physical appearance is not necessarily associated with ethnicity. Hence, the use of AIMs in such populations has few or no advantage. The interest in the search for alleles directly linked to physical characteristics is therefore rapidly increasing, resulting in the commercialization of kits for the identification of skin, hair and eye pigmentation phenotypes based on genetic variation of candidate genes such as *ASIP, HERC2, MC1R, OCA2,* and *TYR.* This genetic variation may affect different stages of the pigmentation process, including melanogenesis, the stabilization and transport of enzymes during melanin synthesis, melanosome production and maintenance, and the balance between the synthesis of different types of melanin. In this chapter we examine the most important genes associated to human hair, skin and eye pigmentation, discussing the evolutionary background for the observed variation and their functional relevance for the physiological mechanisms involved with pigmentation, highlighting the forensic application of this knowledge. The authors will also discuss better ways of collecting pigmentation phenotypic data in human populations for forensic and general studies. It is expected that in the near future they may be able to predict with high reliability the externally visible human characteristics based on DNA analyses.

Chapter 4- In criminal investigations, there are three successive stages involved in studying bloodstains: search and orientation, confirmation and individualisation

The first of these tests, called presumptive tests, are responsible for locating latent remains and providing some preliminary information on the possible blood content of the sample.

The second stage consists of establishing the origin of the stain. The question to be answered is: Is this really a human stain?

Confirmatory tests have to be undertaken for two reasons:

To show that the stain contains a human biological fluid. By undertaking this test, a genetic analysis – longer and more costly- on stains that may appear to be blood, but which are not, can sometimes be avoided.

To confirm the type of biological fluid that has been found. Clearly, biological samples are destined for genetic analysis, but to discover the type of fluid under consideration it is also essential to reconstruct and understand the events.

The need to determine the nature of the evidence is reflected in the latest bibliography that includes interesting studies where all these methods have been thoroughly studied. It is necessary to know the possible causes of false positives and negatives as well as the ways of trying to prevent them.

In this chapter, the authors propose to review the methods for search, presumptive and confirmation test of bloodstains, including the most recent works published.

Chapter 5- Over the past two decades, forensic DNA typing has become widely accepted as a powerful tool in criminal and civil investigations. This technology has become invaluable in many missing-person identifications. There are a number of scenarios in which person identification is required: war victims in mass graves, missing soldiers or military personnel from past wars, murdered peoples, remains from mass disasters due to natural catastrophes or terrorism attacks. In attempts to identify these individuals, DNA profiles from unidentified people may be compared with direct reference samples of the missing person, such as buccal swabs collected before their disappearance, or items they have used, such as toothbrushes, hairbrushes or preserved dental casts. In some cases, direct comparisons are not possible because no direct reference is available or the chain of custody may not be established reliably. Alternatively, a missing person may be identified by kinship analysis using family reference samples (e.g., parents, offspring, siblings or cousins) of the person to be identified.

In this chapter, first, the general principle of likelihood ratio (LR) method is explained Second, the pedigree likelihood ratio (PLR) method based on autosomal STR markers is introduced, in which jointly considers the DNA profile data of all available family reference samples with both population substructure and mutation model incorporated. Third, a more sophisticated algorithm for calculating the pedigree likelihood ratio of the lineage markers (i.e., Y chromosome STRs and mitochondrial DNA) is described. Fourth, guidelines are given on which and how many relatives should be selected and typed for missing person identification so that efficiency can be optimized under the constraints of limited resources.

Chapter 6- In this study were analysed 1210 disarticulated teeth, 179 jaws and 65 skulls from a skeletal assemblage of commingled remains belonging to the 1755 Lisbon earthquake victims, excavated in 2004 at the Lisbon Academy of Sciences.

The main objective of this study was to contribute to the paleodemographic and paleopathological characterization of one of the world's biggest catastrophic population by forensic dental and osteological, qualitative and quantitative, methods. Morphological and anthropometric parameters from teeth and cranial bones have been considered.

To attain the authors' purpose, they identified the teeth and jaws. The following main variables have been dealt with: paleodemography, paleopathology, age determination, minimum number of individuals, sex determination, population affinity, trauma, fire and taphonomy.

Sexing was only done on specimens identified as adults except for unidentified cranias and mandibles. There are 39 female and 49 male individuals. It suggests this population is a random sample of the living population present at the time as it is expected that the sex ration of a living population is maintained in a natural disaster context, as death rate is not biased as it is in other contexts such as war and conflict situations.

The age determination, a detailed account of the age of each individual was not possible. Instead, categorical age group were devised and quantified. The majority of individuals were adults from 35 to 50 years old. The second group was sub adults, from 7 moths *in utero* to 6 years old.

The determination of a minimum number of individuals was attempted by counting the most recurrent specimens for each population sample – teeth, jaw and crania: it is n=179.

By investigating the demographic profile of the sample, aspects of the structure and origin of the skeletal series are revealed. Furthermore, the next chapters will deal with pathological, traumatic and taphonomic occurrences in the skeletal sample.

The paleopathological analysis demonstrates that the overall health of the Academy skeletal sample was average for a sample of this time and place.

The presence of abnormally high frequencies of trauma in the Academy skeletal sample further strengthens the argument for the mass disaster hypothesis. Impact fractures best described as blunt force trauma on the skulls were identified in several specimens.

The taphonomic analysis provided further evidence of the main hypothesis. Burnt skulls and teeth affected by low medium and high temperatures constituted the majority of the sample, meaning these people were no doubt trapped when a fire occurred, dying from the direct cause of the fire or were already dead when flames consumed what was left of their homes, churches and palaces. Dog and rodent gnaw marks were also identified. A scenario of bodies scattered around the city for several days, with dogs scavenging whatever they can to survive may not have been far from the truth related. Staining of bones indicates bursting of blood vessels and staining by a iron-containing matter, most likely blood, as a reaction to the exposure to very high temperatures. Further staining resulted from exogenous material and soil.

With this study of the Academy skeletal sample, a contribution was made to increase the knowledge on this 1755 population. It was hypothesised that this collection was part of the victim count of the 1755 earthquake and it is suggested here that this is likely if not indeed certain. Many of pathological and taphonomical indicators suggestive of mass disaster are present in this skeletal series including random sampling, high trauma, burn marks and bite marks, high fragmentation and non-significant differences between the sexes.

However further research on the rest of the skeletal assemblage collection, post cranial sample, is necessary in order to understand the sample further.

Chapter 7- Advances in DNA technology and the discovery of DNA polymorphisms have facilitated the creation of DNA databases of individuals for the purpose of criminal investigation. Therefore, a considerable range of possibilities have been opened up for criminal investigations, and if we compare the DNA profiles of biological evidence found at the crime scene, with the DNA profiles in the database, they can identify the possible perpetrator of the crime. Logically, as the number of citizens whose DNA has been analysed and included in a database increases, the probability of locating suspects also becomes greater. It became obvious that the value of a DNA database is directly related to the number of records that it contains. Depending on legislation in the country, samples and profiles may be stored permanently or for a limited time, routinely searched for matches with crime scene samples and used for familial searching.

The provisions regarding these issues are different among the European Countries and even if in those countries where legal provisions have been established, not everything is completely resolved and some legal implementations that take in account an ethical perspective still seem to be necessary.

Chapter 8- Unquestionably fingerprints are evidences of great value in forensic investigation. Moreover, they are the most known and studied. Nevertheless other prints: palmar, plantar, those of ear or lip prints, also can be useful. The work reviews the possibilities of the lip prints to contribute to solve a criminal event. The way followed for different investigators who have dedicated themselves to study them is revised. Also the methods necessary to find them and to reveal them are described. After knowing its potential it is possible to conclude that lip prints will be an interesting evidence for the criminal investigation, whenever they are evaluated of the suitable form and with the prudence that is demanded in Forensic Sciences.

Chapter 9- Cell separation method proved to be an effective solution for biological mixtures in forensic science. Many of the current platforms adopted laser capture microdissection (LCM) system. Here micromanipulation method was combined with on-chip low volume PCR (LV-PCR) to select and detect single cells. The micromanipulation platform is more economical compared with the LCM system. Three fresh oral epithelial cells could be completely genotyped by two STR kits. Sixty parallel single cell LV-PCRs were performed using Identifiler®; 13 complete profiles (21.7%) were obtained. Seventy single cells were typed by MiniFiler®, showing 48.6% full profiles. The method was successfully utilized in a fatal rape case, where swabs from the victim's nipples were analyzed. Mucosal cells with an intact nucleus were captured by micro capillary resulting in amplification of the suspect's DNA profile, while mixed DNA profile was obtained by routine method. These results showed great promise for biological mixtures

In: Forensic Science
Editors: N. Yacine and R. Fellag

ISBN 978-1-61324-999-4
© 2012 Nova Science Publishers, Inc.

*Chapter 1*

# HUMAN AND ANIMAL HAIR IN FORENSIC EVIDENCE: PROBLEMS, TROUBLESHOOTING AND WORKAROUNDS

## *Elena Pilli*

*Department of Evolutionary Biology "Leo Pardi", University of Florence, Italy*

### ABSTRACT

During the course of a criminal investigation, many types of physical and biological evidence are encountered. One of the most common is hair evidence. The identification and comparison of human and animal hairs can be helpful in demonstrating physical contact with a suspect, victim and crime scene. A common forensic approach should proceed from the morphological and microscopic examination to DNA analysis. The non-destructive techniques (morphological and microscopic examination) are a vital step when it is necessary to exclude the synthetic origins of the fibers and to distinguish between human and animal hairs. But the technique is also important to compare the features of the questioned hairs with those of hairs from a known individual. Human hairs are easily distinguishable from those of other animals because they present some typical microscopic characteristics. Today, nuclear and mitochondrial (mtDNA) testing can provide additional information to microscopic examination. In human hairs, routine forensic method for DNA testing (STR analysis of nuclear DNA) is possible when the root and/or adhering tissue are present. However, shed hairs, which are often associated with a crime scene, may harbor no nuclear material. While the nucleus degrades as the hair shaft hardens during keratinization, cellular mitochondria and mtDNA remain relatively intact, making mtDNA analysis of hair shafts possible. Instead the microscopic identification of the species of animal hairs can be complicated because of a general trend of reduced training of and lack of experienced hair examiners. In this case the findings of microscopy may be inconclusive to discriminate one species from the others. When conclusive results about species cannot be performed through microscopic examination, the DNA analysis offers the best opportunity to answer the question: "What species is this?". In this case the mtDNA sequencing analysis has to be not only useful in degraded remains but also in the identification of the species. In this review we report the main applications of human hair analysis to forensic investigations and the recent development in species identification of hairs found at the crime scenes. Moreover I describe the new prospects offered by the new generation sequencing methods (NGS) and the genome-wide association study applied to hair shaft in forensics science.

# INTRODUCTION

Hair can be considered in all likelihood one of the most common type of trace evidence at the crime scene. In fact during the course of the normal activities of the day, humans and animals shed hair from their bodies, clothes and from other objects or materials with which they make contact. Humans shed an average of 100 hairs daily particularly during physical contact for example between victim and suspect when a crime is being committed. Thus useful information for identification can be determined through the analysis of such findings.

Found exclusively in mammals, hair is one of the defining characteristics of the mammalian class. The hairs are an appendages of the skin and they are horny and thin filaments present on almost all body surface except, in human, for the soles of the feet, the palms of the hands, the lips and the eyelids apart from the eyelashes. The human skin is minimally hairy compared to other mammals, but the fetus to the seventh month is covered by a thick fluff that falls in the last months of pregnancy. The infant is almost completely hairless. Among the animals e.g. one rodent *Heterocephalus glaber* and aquatic mammals are completely hairless. The hairs on the body present differences in number and morphology in relation to both individual factors and sex. In several animals the development of more or less hair in some parts of the body is a secondary sexual character (beard and mustache in human and the lion's mane). But in general this sexual dimorphism in mammals is not as flashy as that of the plumage of many birds; they have in fact a social life dominated by vision, the mammals instead, except primates, by the smell.

# THE BIOLOGY OF HAIR

The hair is an appendage of the skin that grows out of an organ known as the hair follicle. Thus hair growth begins inside the skin of mammals in a hair follicle [Figure 1]. On the macro scale, that is visible without magnification, a single hair has a root, a shaft, and a tip. The root is the only "living" portion of the hair and is found in the follicle, while the hair shaft is considered "dead". At the deep end of the root there is an enlargement called the bulb, which contains the cells that produce the hair shaft. In this hair matrix there are epithelial cells (keratinocytes) often interspersed with the pigment producing cells, melanocytes. They are responsible for hair color. Cell division in the hair matrix produces the cells that will form the major structures of the hair shaft and the inner root sheath. The bulb is hollow at the base to accommodate a structure called dermal papilla.

It is made up mainly of connective tissue and a capillary loop and it has the function to nourish the hair base (the bulb) from which epithelial cells proliferate. The newly formed cells away from the proliferative center become corneas and produce the hair shaft which will gradually become more or less long. The root is surrounded for most of its length by a skin envelope (root sheath) which is composed of three layers: an outer layer (layer of Henle), an intermediate layer (Layer of Huxley) and an inner layer (the cuticle of the root sheath). Also one or more sebaceous glands and a tiny bundle of muscle fiber called the *arrector pili* form the hair follicle. The sebaceous glands have their excretory duct that leads to the follicle. They are microscopic glands in the skin that secrete sebum, an oily matter that is made of fat (lipids), wax to lubricate the skin and hair of mammals. Although it is commonly believed that sebum acts to protect and waterproof hair and skin, scientists have highlighted that: "low levels of sebaceous gland activity are not correlated with dry skin" [1].

The arrector pili muscles is a small muscle attached to each hair follicle in mammals with the exception of the small follicles that produce only fine vellus hairs. They are responsible for causing hairs to stand-up. In fact if this muscle contracts, the hair becomes more erect and the follicle is dragged upward. This creates a protuberance on the skin surface, producing the temporarily condition that is called gooseflesh. The contraction of the muscle is involuntary, stresses such as cold, fear etc., may stimulate the sympathetic nervous system and thus cause contraction. Contraction of the muscles has a number of different purposes. In the majority of mammals the arrector pili muscle has the function to provide insulation. In this way the air becomes trapped between the erect hairs helping the animal retain heat. But also it can help the animals to become more intimidating and scaring predators.

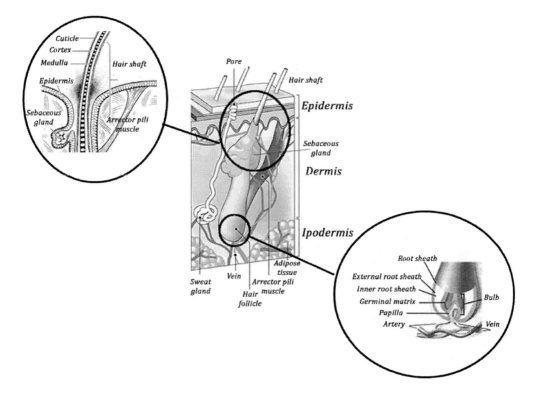

Figure 1. Section of skin showing hair follicle.

In humans some hairs of the face such as, for example, the eyelashes do not have the arrector pili muscle; the effectiveness of muscles' action in humans has been questioned, in fact humans have relatively little body hair to allow for thermal insulation. In humans the thickness of the hair varies between individuals and is influenced by genetic factors. For example in Europe, the hairs of the Nordic countries are much thinner than those of Mediterranean people. For this reason there are two types of hair follicles: 1) the terminal hair follicles are large and lay deep in the skin and they produce long, thick and pigmented hair - an example are the hair, eyelashes and eyebrows-; 2) the follicles of the fleece are small and superficial and they produce short, thin and blond hair of the fleece, which correspond to the hair, often invisible because they lack pigmentation, present in the apparently hairless areas of the body. The terminal hair and the hair of the fleece are not two completely separate structures, in fact the same follicle during one's life can, under the influence of hormones, produce different hair. For example, at puberty the hair of the fleece of the cheeks is transformed in the male in terminal hair forming a beard. The same happens to pubic and underarm hairs. The opposite phenomenon, i.e. the transformation of terminal hair into the hair of the fleece, is characteristic of baldness.

Also in animals there are two different types of hair follicles that produce two different types of hairs: wool hair and guard hair. The wool hairs or down hairs are very thin hairs. They represent the bottom layer made of wool hairs that are short, flattened, curly but denser than the top layer. Its main function is thermal isolation and thus thermoregulation. Instead the guard hairs represent the top layer and consist of long, straight shafts of hair that stick out through the down hairs. They are usually visible for most mammals because they contain most of pigmentation. They protect the down hairs from outside factors, such as rain, and they are often water-repellent. It may also exist an intermediate layer that it has characteristics which are intermediate between the two others.

The term "hair" refers to the body hair of human mammals, while the term "fur" is used more in reference to non-human mammals, particularly to those with extensive body hair coverage. There is an exception when an animal has very coarse or sparse fur, as in the case of pig. In fact in this case we usually call them hair. Animals without fur may be referred to as hairless. At certain stages of life, it is possible that hairs are absent in some of the species.

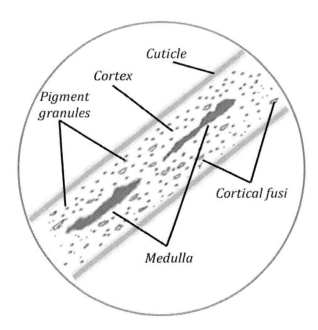

Figure 2. Structure of the hair shaft.

## STRUCTURE OF THE HAIR

The hair shaft can be considered as a slender, thread-like outgrowth composed mainly of keratin (a protein), melanin (a pigment) and traces of metallic elements. These elements are deposited in the hair during its growth and/or absorbed by the hair from an external environment. The hair has a changeable thickness. Internally, hairs have a variable and complex microanatomy. Using microscopy it is possible to observe the three different morphological regions that comprise the hair: the cuticle, the cortex and the medulla [Figure 2].

The structure of the hair root is similar to that of the hair shaft. There is a medulla associated with the cortex, the cuticle and the sheath root, a thin membrane located outside of the cuticle itself.

## Cuticle

The cuticle is the outer covering of the hair shaft consisting of the scales that protect the shaft. The cuticle is made up of overlapping plates or scales of keratin arrayed in characteristic patterns. A single row of transparent and thin cells forms the cuticle. These cells are arranged in a vertical row at the root but rather obliquely like a "flake" with the lower end attached to the cortex and the upper cut off (like ear of corn) at the stem. Because of its position, the cuticle is the first to be damaged when the hair has been abused and gradually the hair grows in length. A single molecular layer of lipid that makes the hair repel water covers the cuticle. There are three basic structures that make up the cuticle: coronal (crown-like), spinous (petal-like) and imbricate (flattened). Very thin hairs can have the *coronal scales*, a structure which resembles a stack of ice-cream cones. Commonly there is this type of makeup in hairs of small rodents and bats but rarely in human hairs. The *spinous scales* have a triangular shape and protrude from the hair shaft. The fur of seals, cats and some other animals have this type of cuticle structure. The *imbricate scales* consist of overlapping scales side by side with narrow margins. They are common in human hairs and in many animal hairs. Much of the shine that makes healthy hair so attractive is due to the cuticle. The figure [Figure 3] shows the three structures of scales and an example of *spinous* scales at the microscope.

## Cortex

The cortex is the main body of the hair and is highly structured and organized. The cortex is composed of elongated and fusiform (spindle-shaped) cells with a pyknotic nucleus and fibrils that they are the primary source of mechanical strength and water uptake. Cortical cells constitute the bulk of a hair, and it is the cortex that gives a hair fiber its eventual shape, resilience, elasticity and curl. The cortex may contain cortical fusi, pigment granules and/or large oval-to-round-shaped structures called ovoid bodies.

The *cortical fusi* [Figure 2] are irregular-shaped and minute air vesicles of varying sizes lying among the cells of the cortex of the shaft. In the human head hair at the base of the follicle the cortex cells are irregular ovoid and ellipsoid not long and fusiform as in the mature hair shaft. During the elongation the cells of the shaft rise toward the follicle mouth and carry upward between some of them irregularly shaped vesicles filled with tissue fluid. But when the hair shaft grows the fusi become increasingly elongate being pressed into this shape by the drying out of the cortex. With this process also comes a loss of their tissue fluid. So they become irregular-shaped airspaces and it is easier to detect among the cortical cells and their elongate nuclei, since they appear darker by transmitted light. The cortical fusi are between and not within the cortical cells. Fusi vary with the region of the hair shaft. They are numerous near the root of a mature hair but they may be present throughout the length of the hair where they become thin and filiform before the tip of the hair.

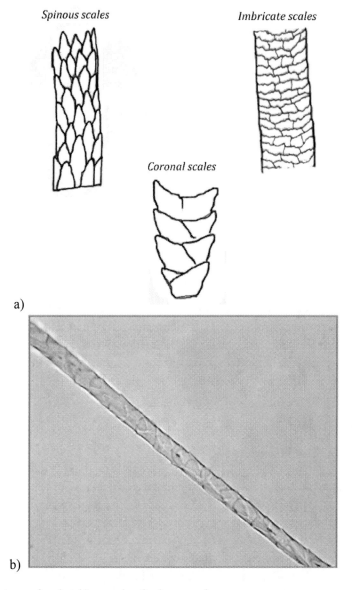

Figure 3. a) Structures of scales; b)example of spinous scales.

*Pigment granules* [Figure 2] are small, dark and solid structures that are granular in appearance and considerably smaller than cortical fusi. The can vary in color, size and distribution in a single hair. Pigments are found in both the cortex and the medulla, but they are absent from the cuticle. The pigment granules themselves, though varying in size from species to species, are commonly of the order of a micron in diameter. The granular pigment found in the epidermal cells is formed exclusively by melanocytes, dendritic cells found scattered among the germinal cells of the skin and those of the hair follicle. Melanocytes are melanin-producing cells. Through a process called *melanogenesis*, these cells produce melanin (Greek μέλας, *black)*, which is a pigment found in the skin, eyes, and hair. So the cortex contains melanin which colors the fiber based on the number, distribution and types of melanin granules. In brown hairs they appear aligned longitudinally, in blond or red hairs they are scattered, while they are absent in white hairs. In humans, pigment granules are commonly distributed toward the cuticle except in red-haired individuals. Animal hairs have the pigment granules commonly distributed toward the medulla. The melanin is responsible of hair coloring. In fact hair has a natural color-producing factory. Simply by varying the proportion of only two melanin pigments, it can produce a surprising diversity of shades. Only two melanin pigments give hair its color: eumelanin and pheomelanin. They are produced inside the hair follicle and packed into granules found in the fibers. In all, there is not more than 1% of melanin in each hair, even in the darkest hair. Pheomelanin colors hair in red. Eumelanin, which has two subtypes of black or brown, determines the darkness of the hair color. A low concentration of brown eumelanin results in blond hair, whereas a higher concentration of brown eumelanin will color the hair in brown. High amounts of black eumelanin result in black hair, while low concentrations give gray hair. All humans have some pheomelanin in their hair.

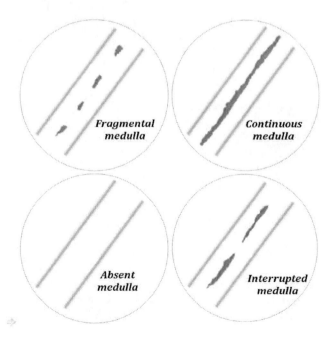

Figure 4. Human hair medulla patterns.

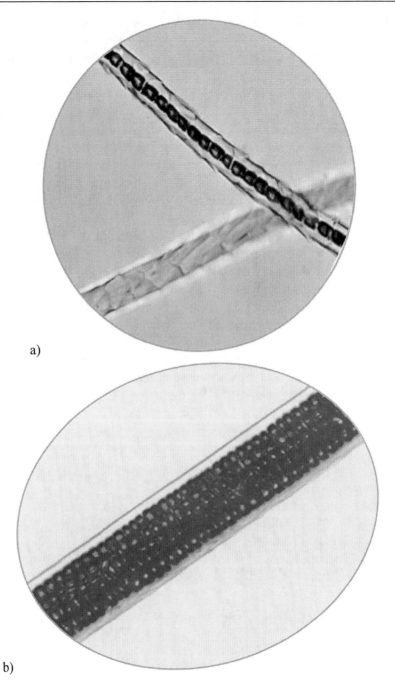

Figure 5. Animal hairs medulla: a) uni-serial ladder medulla; b) multi-serial ladder medulla.

*Ovoides body* are large (larger than pigment granules) solid structures that are spherical to oval in shape with very regular margins. They are abundant in some cattle and dog hair as well as in other animal hairs. To varying degree, they are also found in human hairs.

## Medulla

The medulla is the innermost region of the hair that not always be present. In humans in fact it is an open and unstructured region. It is generally amorphous in appearance and if it is present can be described as fragmental, discontinuous, or continuous [Figure 4]. In coarse hairs it is usually continuous or fragmental, whereas in fine hairs it appears discontinuous or absent.

Instead in animal hairs it has a regular and well-defined structure. It can appear like a uniserial ladder or like a multiserial ladder and exhibits the cellular or vacuolated type [Figure 5].

In some animals the air within the medulla plays a role in the regulation of the body temperature. Some authors think that even though some adult human hairs appear without medulla when observed under the light microscope, all hairs, with the exception of the very fine ones, show a fragmental or discontinuous medulla when viewed under polarized light. The medulla may be only one or two cells in diameter, but it is present nonetheless. The type of medulla present can vary even within the same hair. The medulla is composed of large, loosely connected keratinized cells. Large intra and intercellular air spaces in the medulla determine to a large extent the sheen and color tones of the hair by influencing the reflection of light. This is the reason why hair color looks a lot different in sunlight than it does in the shade.

## HAIR FOLLICLE CYCLING

Hair shows significant differences in the length and diameter in fact there are hairs to limited growth and hairs to prolonged increase. The first ones grows up to a modest length, because soon the dermal papilla retracts from the bulb that is closed. Then the growth stops and the hair falls soon replaced by a new one because the papilla is covered with epithelial elements that come from the follicle wall and so a new hair grows. The eyelashes in human and in general body hair of most mammals are a typical example of a hair with limited growth. The second ones instead continue to grow for a longer period and so stretch considerably. Example are hair and beard in humans, hair of angora cats, the mane of the horse and the lion. Obviously also these hairs grow older, their bulbous ends, they fall and are replaced. The hair with limited increase lives some weeks, while that with prolonged growth can live months or years. In both male and female humans the hairs are very thick and long at the scalp, pubis and armpit. In other parts of the body development of hair is different in relation to sex. For example eyelashes and eyebrows are short and straight hairs of circular cross section; instead, for example, in the genital region, in the armpit and in most of male hair there is a greater length (until a few cm) and the hair section is generally elliptical.

The mammalian hair follicle is a dynamic structure that generates a hair shaft through a tight cycle of birth, growth and dead. In mammals, the cycle of hair growth includes three stages: anagen, catagen and telogen [Figure 6]. Each phase has specific characteristics that determine the length of the hair.

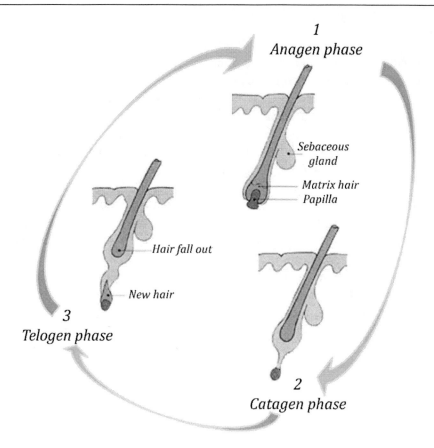

Figure 6. Hair follicle cycling.

## Anagen

Anagen is the growth phase in which the cells of the root are dividing rapidly. During this phase the hair grows about 1 cm every 28 days. Before starting this active phase there is a follicular morphogenesis that leads to the formation of the follicle. Then there is the transition to the growth phase where real growth is an increase of 5-10 times. Finally, the growth remains constant for a long period. The amount of time the hair follicle stays in the anagen phase is genetically determined. Obviously a longer anagen phase will result in a larger growth of the hair. Scalp hair, for example, stays in this active phase from three to six years while the eyebrows only for around 4 months.

## Catagen

Catagen is a transition phase that occurs at the end of the anagen phase. Both the hair growth and the mitotic activity in the matrix stop and it lasts for about 2-3 weeks.

## Telogen

Telogen is the resting phase, it lasts 2-4 months. In this phase the dermal papilla is reduced to a small spherules of cells. The dead and fully keratinized fiber remains in the hair follicle by its club until the end is lost by erosion or expelled by the new hair during the next anagen phase. Shedding is part of the normal replacement process of old hair with new. At the end of the telogen phase the hair follicle restarts the growing phase. The dermal papilla and the base of the follicle join together again and a new hair begins to form. If the old hair has not already been shed, the new hair pushes the old one out and the growth cycle starts all over again.

The length of the hairs depends on the growth rate, which varies by skin area, sex and population membership. In humans the number of hairs can vary from 100 to 150 000 with variations due to age, population membership and color. Both male and female have about 5 million of hair follicles. The hairs are born straight, wavy, or curly depending on the conformation of their follicle. In fact the difference in the shape of the hair between subjects - blacks, whites and Asian- is a consequence of the shape of the hair follicle that is genetically predetermined. The hairs sprout from their follicle with an inclined angle that in the skin of the scalp is about 75 degrees. The African hair follicle has a curved shape and flattened form and this explains the nature of the kinky hair. Instead, the individuals that have a completely straight hairs, also have a hair follicle which is straight and circular. This shape is characteristic of Asian populations. Instead the Europeans have an intermediate form between the other two thus presenting large variations. The figure [figure 7] shows three different conformations of hair follicle and the corresponding cross-sectional shape of hairs.

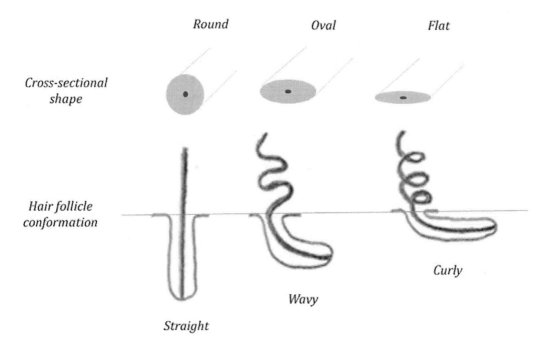

Figure 7. Human hair follicle conformations and cross-sectional shape of the hairs.

## FUNCTION

The fur or other hairs have different functions in mammalians. In fact they provide both excellent insulation from heat and cold, and a protection from rain. Hairs provide thermal regulation and camouflage for many animals. But they can also provide signals to other animals such as warnings, mating or other communicative displays. They can provide defensive functions and they have a sensory function. So it is possible to extend the sense of touch beyond the surface of the skin. Hairs provide the thermal regulation because when the body is too cold, the arrector pili muscles found attached to hair follicles stand up, causing the hair in these follicles to do the same. So the hairs form a heat-trapping layer above the epidermis. In humans this process is known as goose bumps [2]. In other mammals their fur fluffs up to create air pockets between hairs that insulate the body from the cold. In an opposite way when the body is too warm, the arrector pili muscles make the hairs lay flat on the skin so the heat can disperse. In humans, the head hairs are a primary sources of heat insulation and cooling as well as of protection from UV radiation exposure. So the function of hair is to prevent loss of heat by forming an insulating layer near to the skin where the air is trapped. In humans, this function was partially lost and the hairs have become more decorative and protective in significance. The nature of Africans curly hair also allows to the sweat to remain longer in contact with the body increasing the cooling effect. This is a consequence of adaptation to hot and humid climates in which these people live. The hairs can also have the function of protecting some animals from their predators such as the spines of porcupine. Also, the human hairs are used to protect the human body; in fact, even if they cannot protect humans from potential predators, they can help the sense organs to carry out their functions. Other hairs can sense movement of air and are especially sensitive to the presence of insects as well as to the presence of harmful agents, such as the eyelashes [3]. Another important function of the hairs is tactile and sensory. Some hairs called vibrissae (the whiskers) act as touch receptors in carnivores and allow the movement of the animal especially at night. Therefore, they allow the animal to be aware of potential obstacles, making it easier to move around in the dark. They, also provide information on the presence of other living beings in the vicinity, by the perception of air movements caused by them and by the perception of temperature. The vibrissae are hairs at least twice as thick as any other hair on the body of the animals. They have a very thick base and they are inserted up to three times deeper into the dermis in a hair follicle. They have multiple nerve endings and muscle fibers that allow the animal to direct them at will. The hair may also have an aesthetic and sexual appeal.

## HAIR VS FUR: DIFFERENCES AND COMPARISON

Although the human and the animal hair are chemically identical, -in fact they are all made of keratin (a fibrous structural protein produced by keratinocytes)-, but human hairs are distinguishable from hairs of other mammals. Animal hairs are classified into three types: guard hair, wool hair and tactile hairs that are found on the head of animals provide sensory functions. Instead, human hairs are not so differentiated and might be described as a modified combination of the characteristics of guard hairs and wool hairs. Animal hairs exhibit radical color changes in a short distance called banding whereas human hairs have a uniform color and pigmentation throughout the length of the hair shaft or slightly more dense toward the cuticle. Instead the pigmentation of animal hairs is normally distributed toward the medulla. In animal hairs the distribution and density of pigment can also be an identifiable features. Another different between human and animal hairs is the medulla. In human hairs the medulla, if there is, is amorphous whereas the medulla in animal hairs is normally continuous and well structured. In human hairs the width of medulla is generally less than one-third the overall diameter of the hair shaft whereas in animal hairs it is greater than one-third the overall diameter of the hair shaft. In addiction it is important to keep in mind that the cuticle in human hairs is usually imbricate, whereas in animal hairs it may have a different pattern of scales. In animal hairs the shape of the hair shaft is also more variable. Also the root is different between human and animal hairs. In fact the root of human hairs is generally club-shape, while the roots of animal hairs are highly variable [Figure 8].

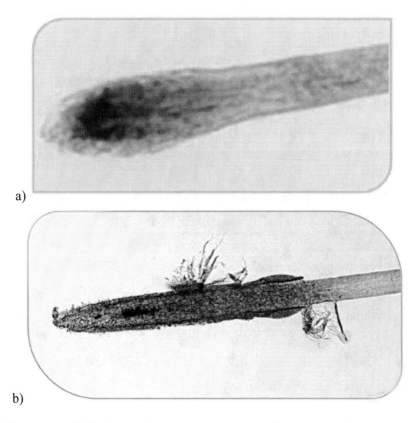

Figure 8. a) human root; b) dog root.

Moreover in some animals such as cats and dogs, it is possible to find a complex follicles in which different hairs can be withdrawn from the same follicle. The diameter of human hairs ranges from 17 to 181 μm whereas fur is much thicker than the human hairs. Another important difference between human and animal hairs is the growth pattern. In humans, the strands of hair tend to grow independently, while in animals the hairs grow more synchronized depending on the weather condition. In fact, for example, a healthy hair of human is made up 82-90% of hairs in the anagen, about 1% of hairs in catagen and at least 10-18% of the hairs in telogen.

## COLLECTION HAIR EVIDENCE

Hair makes good forensic evidence both for its biological nature and the possibility to find it at the crime scene. Hair in fact is one of the most durable materials produced by nature and because of its biological structure it can survive for a long time. Furthermore, as a natural part of his/her life cycle, a person loses an average of 75-100 scalp hairs per day. This process may accelerate during violent crimes in which hair can be pulled and torn. Hair evidence in fact is particularly common during violent crimes such as: homicides, assaults, burglaries, rape etc.. During this type of crimes, whenever such contact occurs there is frequently an inadvertent transfer of microscopic evidence. In the 20$^{th}$ century Edmond Locard, the director of the first crime laboratory in Lyon, France, postulated a theory known as Locard's Theory or Locard Exchange Principle. His principle can be summarized as "every contact leaves a trace". Locard's Principle is applied to crime scenes in which the perpetrator of a crime comes into contact with the scene: so the perpetrator will both bring something into the scene and leave with something from the scene.

> Wherever he steps, whatever he touches, whatever he leaves, even unconsciously, will serve as a silent witness against him. Not only his fingerprints or his footprints, but his hair, the fibers from his clothes, the glass he breaks, the tool mark he leaves, the paint he scratches, the blood or semen he deposits or collects. All of these and more, bear mute witness against him. This is evidence that does not forget. It is not confused by the excitement of the moment. It is not absent because human witnesses are. It is factual evidence. Physical evidence cannot be wrong, it cannot perjure itself, it cannot be wholly absent. Only human failure to find it, study and understand it, can diminish its value". *Paul L. Kirk. 1953. Crime investigation: physical evidence and the police laboratory. Interscience Publishers, Inc.: New York*

So, in summary, the principle states that when two objects come into contact there will always be material that will be transferred from one to another. But sometimes the quantity of material transferred may be too small to detect or it can be lost immediately after the transfer.

### Hair Transfer and Hair Persistance

Hair transfer is a complicated mechanism that can involve many variables. The main types of transfer are two: the direct transfer and the indirect transfer. The first one involves the direct contact between the donor and the receiver: hair that comes directly from the original source, is then transferred to receiver. The second one, instead, involves the presence of one or more objects that act as intermediaries. Hair is transferred from the donor to these object such as clothes or automotive upholstery and then from the latter to the receiver. The likelihood of transfer is dependent on the nature of the contact, the duration thereof, and the nature of the contacting surfaces. The direct transfer of hairs from an individual to another is called a primary transfer. Instead when hairs have already been shed and then are transferred from an object to an individual, it is called secondary transfer.

Several studies have been conducted to try to investigate the hair transfer mechanism and the variables involved. One of these studies highlights the fact that the indirect transfer is more common than direct and that the number of secondarily transferred hairs appears to decrease with time [4]. The results of the experiments also show that the secondary transfer rate is observed with short straight and long straight hair. No clear trend is observed with medium length hair (both straight and curly) and with long curly hair. The extent of the secondary transfer was observed to be very variable and dependent on many different factors such as, for example, the type of materials of clothes or grooming habits of people. In fact, in the study it has been shown that these two factors may increase the probability of secondary transfer. Research has also shown the existence of a secondary transfer with two or more intermediaries, but studies proved this to be less common than secondary transfer involving only one object that acts as intermediary.

Another research published in 1998 [5] measured the frequency of pubic hair transfer between some consenting heterosexual partners. Results show that in 17.3% of cases at least one pubic hair may be transferred. The study also highlights that the transfer from the female to male (23.6%) is more prevalent than from the male to female (10.9%). It is important to note, however, that the assessment of the possibility of secondary transfer should be evaluated case by case and should also be based on the total number of hairs transferred. In fact, in cases where a large number of hair are found, it is easier to think that it was a direct transfer rather than secondary.

Silvana R. Tridico in her case study [6] involving a dog hair found on the bed, on the sweatshirt, and on the front passenger seat of the car of the suspect, concluded that the most likely mode of transfer of hair is the direct contact between the dog and the objects. This view was expressed both in presence of a large number of hairs observed (170 on the bed, 46 on the sweatshirt and about 85 on and around the front passenger seat) and the variety of types of hair (primary and secondary guard hairs and under-hairs). It is important to keep in mind that the trace evidence can be transferred during the commission of the crime but also before, so sometimes the trace may have nothing to do with the crime. In other cases instead the hair evidence may be important to link the suspect to the victim or the presence of a specific person at the crime scene. This type of evidence may be often overlooked by investigators because it is not easily observed. So, during the inspection, it is very important to point out, find, and collect properly trace evidence.

Hairs are ubiquitous in nature and they are very common trace material in a wide range of types of crime. In many instances they are the only trace evidence [7]. In fact, they are very stable to most environmental conditions and they do not deteriorate readily or quickly as other biological evidence. Also, since they are not easily visible to the untrained eye, a criminal will not try to destroy them. So given the presence and persistence for years of trace hair at crime scenes, it is important to be able to obtain information about the factors that influence transfer and persistence of hair under different circumstances. Despite this, however, there are very few studies that analyze the mechanisms of transfer, persistence, and recovery of hair evidence.

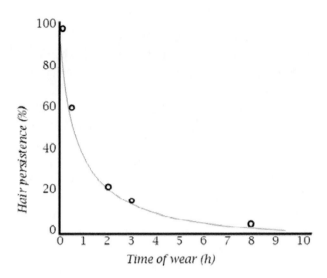

Figure 9. Hair persistence as a function of time of wear.

Gaudette and Tessarolo in their search [8] studied the loss mechanism of hairs from clothing and they found that it was similar to that for fibers. At the beginning during the first 3-4 days it is possible to observe a rapid loss of hairs from clothing but after a few days the decline becomes more gradual and then stabilizes itself and remains constant. In figure [Figure 9] it is possible to observe the typical decay curve of a process like the one just described.

Robertson et al. in their paper show the same decay curve and they highlight the way the movement and loss of hairs are influenced by many variables. Also Mann, in his six-years case study, obtained results about transfer and persistence of scalp hair consistent with those above reported [9]. In a 2002 research Dachs et al. study the persistence behavior of human scalp hairs under a number of different circumstances [10]. The results of their study indicate that different material can lose hairs in different ways. For example, the rate of loss of hairs from non-woolen fabrics during normal wear follows an exponential decay curve, while the rate of loss of hairs from woolen fabrics is quite linear: there is almost a constant loss. This suggests that there is a different mechanism that involves the persistence of hairs on different fabrics. The researchers also show that the speed at which hair is lost from fabrics decreases in the following order polyester, cotton/acrylic, poly-cotton, cotton, smooth wool and rough wool. So the wool can be considered the best material on which it is possible recover hair. Researchers themselves, however, warn using this information with caution before drawing any conclusions.

## Hair Collecting

Methods of collecting hair evidence vary according to the scope and the circumstances of the investigation [11]. In some circumstances more than one method of collection may be utilized. Recovery of hair evidence can be made at the crime scene and in the laboratory. Before starting the collection of evidence, it is important to keep in mind to photograph all evidence prior to removing them. Since the laboratory is a more suitable place than the crime scene for recovering trace evidence, as far as possible hair recovery should be conducted there. So, in the case in which hair is attached to an object, it is always better to not attempt to remove it, but rather leave hair intact on the object. If the object is small, it is necessary to mark it, wrap it, and seal it in an envelope. If the object is large it is necessary to wrap the area containing the hair in paper to prevent loss of hairs during shipment.

One of the methods, the simplest, to collect hair is to pick up only the visually observed hair. The inspection with the naked eyes may be aided by a good natural light sources and a forensic light source such as for example crime-lite® (Forensic light sources -Foster & Freeman USA-). These lights, in fact, enhance the ability of the investigators to visually identify hairs. The investigators may recover the trace by hand or with tweezers. It is important to take care in the use of tweezers because they may cause damage to the structure of the hair. In fact, in some case they can crush the thin root and surrounding tissue which could be used for genetic analysis [11-12].

It is possible to collect hair also by using a clear tape. This method initially used to recover textile fibers, is also useful for collecting hair that is not easily visible to the naked eye. In this way, visible and non-visible hair can be gathered from a variety of surfaces. The clear tape used to collect hair must not be too sticky because it can become filled with fibers of the material on which it is used. The tape is placed on the surface to be treated with the adhesive side down and it is then rubbed on. This process is repeated until the entire area of interest has been taped.

Another technique of collection is the vacuuming method. This is especially used for large crime scenes. The hair is gathered on special filter that can be removed and labeled appropriately. But it is not recommended in most circumstances because it has several drawbacks. One of these is the contamination from hair already lodged in the vacuum cleaner. In fact, hair and debris that were deposited before crime, cannot be distinguished from those associated with the crime. So, after using, it is very important to follow a rigid program of decontamination of the vacuum cleaner. Another problem of the vacuuming method is the non-discriminating nature of collection.

An additional method to collect hair is that of brushing, scraping, and/or shaking the objects on which there can be some of this type of evidence. So, the material is transferred on a white sheet of paper abraded in order to make them adhere to it [12]. Trace evidence on the white paper is then separated into classes such as hair, fiber etc and analyzed. Another method is to put items of interest in a bag and shake. So the evidence is collected at the bottom of the bag rather than dispersed in the air.

## HAIR ANALYSIS

In the seventeenth and eighteenth centuries, scientists such as Robert Hooke, Antony van Leeuwenhoek, and Henry Baker, believed that hair is a ready-made specimen. In the next century however, information about the use of hair as evidence began. In about 1860 the famous detective Francois Goron, head of the French Surete, in his first case found hairs clutched in a dead woman's hand. But unfortunately, because there was no information about the hairs, he could not identified them as human. As a result of this case, attention in scientific world to hair began and for it became important to distinguish between human and animal hair. So in the years that followed research started on studying the structure of both animal and human hairs. In 1899, in a new case, called "L'affaire Gouffe" Goron for the first time used the knowledge obtained in previous years to establish that a murder victim's hair has been dyed. This led to the identification of the victim's body (Gouffe's body) and subsequent arrest of his killer [13]. The success of this case and others led to increase the study of the nature and the structure of hairs and their use in forensic investigations. Today hair evidence can provide investigators with valuable information. Until recently, the microscopic analysis was considered the only reliable tool for the identification and comparison of the microscopic characteristics found in hair. But today, the microscopic analysis is complemented by genetic analysis that can provide additional information useful to investigators. A common forensic approach for studying hair should proceed from the morphological and microscopic examination to DNA analysis. The non-destructive techniques (morphological and microscopic examination) are a vital step when it is necessary to exclude the synthetic origins of the fibers and to distinguish between human and animal hairs. The technique is also important to compare the features of the questioned hairs with those of hairs from a known individual. But it is important to keep in mind that hair must never be used as the single indicator of guilt. In fact, the visual comparison of hair is subjective and it allows for personal interpretations of scientists. But, if genetic analysis and other evidence is added to microscopic analysis, then hair can be considered a good tool for investigators.

## Microscopic Analysis

The forensic hair comparison is a biological discipline that includes several fields such as microscopy, biology, anatomy, histology, and anthropology. The examination and comparison of hair in the forensic laboratory is typically conducted through the use of microscopy. The microscopic analysis of hair provides valuable information, e.g. about the nature of the hair (human or non-human), the macroscopic and microscopic structure (e.g. - root, shaft, tip- -cuticle, cortex, medulla-), the determination of the origin (e.g. pubic or head hair). Furthermore, with this type of analysis it is possible to compare a questioned hair specimen with hair from a known individual. In fact this examination usually involves two steps: 1. the identification of questioned hairs, and 2. the comparison of questioned and known hair. From the beginning forensic hair examiners concentrated their efforts in studying characteristics for both human and animal hair that can be useful for identification but also for comparison. These traits in fact can distinguish one individual from others and one population from another.

### *Identification of Questioned Hair*

In order to identify the characteristics and typical traits of hairs, it is necessary to approach them by describing them from general to specific, from outside to inside. Initially, it is important to look the anatomy at macroscopic level and describe where and how the hair sits on the surface: its shape, length, color etc. Thus hair found at the crime scene is initially inspected by the naked eye simply by viewing it with a suitable light source to describe and photograph the surface on which they are found. Then, the next steps are to observe the surface and describe the micro-traces, changes of the cuticle, the root and the scales. In fact their shape, size and margins may be very important in identifying the nature of hair analyzed. They are observed under the stereomicroscope to highlight the color, length, root, tip and any other characteristic of that hair Finally, in order to also evaluate the inner structure of hair, the representative samples are then examined, after being mounted on a glass slide, by polarized light microscopy, fluorescence microscopy and, if it is possible, by scanning electron microscopy. In this way it is possible to see and describe the medulla, the cortex with its cortical fusi, pigment particles and ovoid bodies. Is the hair human or animal? This is one of the first questions which the researcher has to answer. But it is relatively easy to determine if a hair has a human or non-human origin by a simple microscopic examination. Indeed, animal hair has several macroscopic but also microscopic characteristics that distinguish them from those of humans. Table below shows the features to discriminate between human an non-human hairs.

|  | Color | Pigmentation | Medulla | Width medulla | Root | Cuticle | Diameter |
|---|---|---|---|---|---|---|---|
| **Human Hair** | Uniform color | Uniform or slightly more dense toward cuticle | Amorphous, if presents | <1/3 the overall diameter | Club-shape | Usually imbricate | 17-181 μm |
| **Non-human hair** | Banding color | Distributed toward the medulla | Continuous and well structured | >1/3 the overall diameter | Highly variable | Different pattern of scales | Much thicker |

### *Human Identification*

The macroscopic and microscopic examination of human hair found at the crime scene allows one to describe the morphological and structural characteristics of hairs as well as alterations and abnormalities that, if present, may characterize the hair and may be useful when comparing them with known hair. The table reported in Encyclopedia of Forensic Science [14] shows in detail all human hair characteristics and traits that have to be considered during microscopic examination of hair.

The microscopic analysis is also utilized to identify body area from which the hair has originated, ancestry estimation and damages, treatments, and biological or environmental alterations of hairs.

### *Body Area Determination*

The determination of the body area from which the hair is generated, can have very important consequences for a case, even if sometimes it can be very difficult. Humans exhibit a wide variety of hair on their bodies and the body area from which a hair is originated can be determined by their different morphology. Indeed, hair that comes from different body area has a different characteristics such as length, shape, color, size; and also pigmentation and medullar appearance. The typical body areas from which the hair comes from, are the head, pubic, facial, limb, eyelash and eyebrow, axillary, and chest. The hair that does not fit in these categories can be called, in general, transitional body hair. But because there is a wide range of interpersonal variation in head and pubic hair, the majority of attention in forensics is primarily directed to hair that comes from these body areas. The following table lists some hair characteristics associated with the different body area types.

| Body area type | Diameter /length | Shaft | Tip | Other characteristics |
|---|---|---|---|---|
| **Head hair** (Scalp) | 17-181 μm /100-1000 mm | Straight, wavy or curly | Usually cut | May be artificially treated 0,4 mm/day growth |
| **Pubic hair** | Coarse and prominent variation /10-60 mm | Buckling, sometimes extreme waviness or curly | Usually pointed, may be razor cut | Asymmetrical cross section, broad medulla |
| **Facial hair** (Beard) | Very coarse /50-300 mm | often triangular cross-section | Blunted or razor cut | Complex medullation, 0.40 mm/day growth |
| **Limb hair** (Leg and arm hair) | Fine, tapering /3-6 mm | Slight arc | Usually pointed | Often indistinctly and slightly pigmented |
| **Chest** (Pectoral) | Moderate to considerable diameter variation | Wavy to curly; some more straight | Usually pointed | |
| Axillary (Arm pit) | Some variation /10-50 mm | Less wavy/curly than chest | May be colorless; usually pointed | 0,3 mm/day growth; many cortical fusi |
| **Eyelash** (Ciliary) /Eyebrow (Superciliary) | Tapering /~ 1 cm | Curved; relatively coarse for length | Pointed | 0,16 mm/day growth; large medulla |

It is important to keep in mind that the head hairs, in general, are subject to more alteration than hairs from other body areas. These changes can be due to both chemical modifications such as for example the use of dyes or permanents but also environmental alterations such as exposure to sunlight, wind, or other environmental conditions. For these reasons it is recommended that, when it is necessary to compare the head hair found at the crime scene with those of the suspect, the head hair samples are taken as soon as possible by the suspect. Indeed head hairs obtained years after a crime are generally not suitable for meaningful comparison purposes.

*Ancestry Estimation*

Human hair has a wide range of variation in their morphology and color from one person to another. This fact can give an indication of person's ancestry. In forensic literature, three main ancestral groups are used: Europeans, Asians, and Africans. All these ancestral groups exhibit microscopic characteristics that can distinguish one group from another. The head and pubic hair are the best indicator for ancestry estimation, although hairs from other body areas can be useful. Microscopic examination of hair of infants or individuals with mixed ancestry can be difficult. Indeed hair of individuals with mixed origin may possess characteristics attributed to more than one group. The following table lists the characteristics of different ancestral groups.

| Ancestral Groups | Shaft Diameter | Cross-sectional Shape | Pigment granules | Cuticle | Shaft |
|---|---|---|---|---|---|
| **Europeans** | 70-100 μm | Oval | Evenly distributed | Medium | Undulation uncommon |
| **Africans** | 60-90 μm | Flat | dense, arranged in clumps | Thin | Twist, curl |
| **Asians** | 90-120 μm | Round | Dense to very dense | Thick | Never |

## *Treatments, Damage, and Biological or Environment Alteration*

Human hairs undergo different changes depending on the human culture. They may be dyed, shaved, cut, and removed, or they may suffer from biological or environment alterations. The presence of artificial treatments such as dyes can be identify through microscopic examination. These characteristics can be useful to the investigators because they can be typical of a person. Moreover, since the hair grows at the rate of one centimeter per month, the cosmetic treatments may serve to estimate the point where the coloration was applied i.e. the time interval between treatment and hair loss. The tips of hairs can provide good information about how the hair has been treated. Shaving, for example, is accomplished with a bladed instruments such as razor. The tip of razor-cut hair is angled. While cutting by scissor or clippers develops a straight border. Crushed hair has a enlargement of the shaft and the cortical cells appear separated. Instead broken hair may have a square tip with protruding fragments. Also the roots can help the examiner to determine whether the hair was forcibly removed from the body or shed naturally. Hair that falls out naturally has a club-shaped root, whereas a forcibly removed hair is stretched and may have tissue attached to it. In hair that comes from a body in a state of decomposition it is possible to observe a dark band near the root. The alterations described can be observe not only in head hair but also in the others. Moreover there are some diseases that affect hair morphology and they may characterize a hair from another. Indeed they can be good evidence for identifying the source from where they come. Hair diseases are disorder that may be associated with hairs but primarily with the follicle. The diseases that affect hair shape are rare but when they are present, they may provide a good evidence for identifying a source from which they come from.

*Some hair shaft disease:*

- *Pili annulati* are hair that present colored rings. They have alternating light and dark bands along their length. Also the black hairs may have pili annulati but the hair color masks the disease. The bands are due to the presence of air bubbles that form between cells of the cortex;

- *Pili torti* refers to the rigidly twisted hair. The twisting of the hair fiber occurs at focal points along its length. There may be several twists in one hair fiber;
- *Monilethrix* is characterized by alternating elliptical nodes (of 0.7 to 1 mm in length) and various strictures along the hair shaft. In this way the hair shaft looks similar to a rosary or a necklace (hence the name monilethrix, from the Latin "jewel"). Under the microscope it appears as lack of medullae at the nodes, while at the internodes (those tapered narrowing between node and node) it is easy to see fractures;
- *Trichorrhexis nodosa* is one of the most common of hair diseases as it is one of the most frequent causes of hair shaft abnormalities. It can usually occurs after extensive trauma. Under microscope a large number of fraying and swelling nodes are evident in particular spots along the length of the hair fiber. These defects develop due to the absence of a cuticle layer. If the cuticle is absent the cortex underneath is directly exposed to ultra violet rays, and to harmful synthetic hair care products as well as to harsh hair brushing. The hair is very fragile and breaks more easily.

The diseases of hair shaft can be an important tool in forensic investigation because they may be able to characterize and distinguish one hair from another and to identify the individual from which they come.

### *Non-human Identification*

In the case of animal hair, for its identification it is important to pay attention to the shapes and sizes of the hair, color banding, cuticular patterns, medulla organization, root structure, and scales. The table presented in the Encyclopedia of Forensic Science [14] shows in detail all animal hair characteristics and traits that have to be considered during microscopic examination of hairs. An adequate reference collection is essential for accurate identification of questioned samples. Indeed, the wide variation in characteristics of hair taken from different body areas on the same animal and the large differences from animal to animal that can occur within a species do not allow the identification of species from animal hairs in the absence of a complete and accurate reference collection of hairs. In most cases, the identification can be possible only with the guard hair. When these are not present, only the animal family of origin may be identified. It is important to keep in mind that all questioned hair should be considered singly, unless found in group at the crime scene.

### *Comparison of Questioned and Known Hair*

Most forensic hair may be identify by comparing the questioned hair or the hair found at the crime scene to known hair. For this reason it is important to make, at first, an accurate description separately of the questioned and known hair noting every typical characteristics useful for the next comparison. The origin of questioned hairs, i.e. the body area from which they come from, must be then investigated in order to pick up the known samples from the same area. Indeed, it is fundamental to be able to compare the hair that comes from the same body area. Once the area of the body from which hairs come from is known, there should be a collection of reference samples from the same area of the body of the known person. The collection consists of about 50-100 hairs from all portions of the area of interest, usually the head or pubic area because these are the most common. The reference hairs must present the root both in anagen and telogen phase, so they must be taken by brushing but also torn.

Indeed, they must be representative of the group to which they belong. Then a comparison microscope is used for the examination since it is able to analyze side-by-side specimens. It is composed of two microscopes that are connected by an optical bridge to produce a split view window enabling two separate objects to be viewed simultaneously. This avoids the observer having to rely on memory when comparing two objects under a conventional microscope. This point-by-point comparison represents the strength of a forensic hair comparison since it allows one to confirm or disprove the apparent similarities observed separately with the traditional microscope. The hairs are mounted on glass microscope slides with mounting medium of about 1.5 on the refractive index. Then they are examined from root to tip at magnifications of 40X to 250X. The direct comparison allows one to highlight the area that shows the same features at corresponding points along the length of the hair. Indeed, if the initial examination shows the presence of an area with typical traits, with comparison microscope it is possible to juxtapose these points and confirm the possible presence of the same characteristics in both hair. A single significant difference between the two can be a strong indication that the two hairs come from different sources. It is important to keep in mind that no two hairs are identical in every detail even if they come from the same point on the body. In fact, change is an integral part of the natural hair growth. Hair of two different individuals may be completely dissimilar or very much alike, but not identical. So it is very important that the examiner is experienced and well trained and that, if possible, the conclusion of the analysis should also be checked by another qualified examiner. The second hair examiner must review the hairs microscopically, employing the same methodology used by the first examiner. Obviously the second examiner may agree or disagree with the first, but only if there is agreement, can the result be obtained either negative or positive. There is no criterion for the importance assigned to a particular characteristic. So every consideration is left to the experience of the examiner. Hair has a complicated three-dimensional structure that makes the quantification of the traits very difficult. Consideration must be given to the origin of the samples found at the crime scene. Indeed if many hairs are found together and taken from the same source, they can be regarded as originating from the same source and can be treated as a single sample. However, if the hair is found alone and taken from various sources, may not be considered as a single sample and should be viewed as different evidence. Three are the conclusions which can be reached after a forensic comparison:

1. The questioned hair and the known hair (reference sample) could have come from the same source. In this case, the questioned hair has the same microscopic characteristics of known hair;
2. No conclusion can be made, i.e. it is not possible to say if the hairs come from the same source. For example, the questioned hair exhibits some similarities but also slight differences with the known hair;
3. The questioned hair and the known hair do not come from the same source. The questioned hair exhibits different microscopic traits from the known hair.

Positive hair comparisons are not a means of absolute personal identification but it may support the presence of an individual at the crime scene when hair are properly collected and an adequate number of reference samples are available to the examiner. The probative value of hair comparison may be enhanced today by the DNA analysis.

# Genetic Analysis

DNA technology has opened a new front in forensic science. Until 1985, all biochemical methods available to identify biological samples in criminal cases were of limited applicability. Conventional blood group and enzyme analysis (e.g. typing of ABO, Km, Gm, EsD, PGM1, AcP) had been used for decades, but they would invariably provide modest analytical power. The way to a new course of events was first paved by the introduction of DNA restriction fragment length polymorphism (RFLP) analysis [15-16], which would have soon provided an incomparably higher discrimination power. However, the procedures of molecular typing were too laborious and required too large amounts of intact DNA to be routinely used in the difficult field of DNA sample analysis. The advent of PCR was the turning point in the crucial matter of analytical efficiency [17]. Since then, the field of molecular identification seems to have acquired a virtually unlimited power of analysis, allowing forensic experts to address the most inaccessible sources of DNA evidences. Minute quantities of degraded DNA (such as for cigarette butts, fingerprints, and bone remains) have become, since then, the target of '*DNA profiling*' (molecular analysis of multiple polymorphic sites) with startlingly high rates of success. In mid-1990 the application of new genetic knowledge in the investigation field opened a new era of biological analysis in law enforcement. The analysis of hair also benefited from the advent of genetic testing: the DNA analysis of hair adds information to microscopic hair examination. In fact, once the microscopic examination is completed the hairs undergo genetic analysis in order to have further tests to evaluate the attribution of a hair to an individual. One of the common methods used to clean hair before DNA extraction, foresees washing hair with a detergent, such as Terg-a-zyme 5%, that is capable of removing contamination on its surface. Then the hair is rinsed with water, such as Milli-Q (Millipore Corporation), and finally it is washed with absolute ethanol. Once dried, the hair sample is cut at the level of 5 mm from the root and divided into the shaft and root. The root is immediately incubated over night at 56°C in lysis buffer (SSC 1X, SDS 10%) with added DTT (dithiothreitol) at final concentration of 65 mM and pK (proteinase K) at final concentration of 0.5 mg/ml while the hair shaft is first cut into 5 mm pieces, then placed in a sterile 1,5 ml microcentrifuge tube and incubated in lysis buffer plus DTT and pK. After lysis, the procedure for DNA isolation is the phenol/chloroform extraction.

## *Nature of the Hair Sample*

The hair is an appendage of the skin that grows out of an organ known as the hair follicle and contains DNA. But, when the hair cells that are proliferating in the bulb protruding from the bulb, they undergo the process of keratinization: lose the nucleus and die, thereby turning it into keratin, a horny substance with a particular consistency. Since the production of cells in the array goes on continuously, with new cells pushing outward to escape, the effect is the growth of the hair, which extends about 1 cm per month. The hair shaft is characterized by keratinized cells that have a pyknotic nuclei, fragmented in which the DNA has been digested by specific endonucleases. The root, rich in proliferating cells, is considered a good source of nuclear DNA. But the DNA analysis of the hairs, due to the biological nature of the hair shaft, suffers from a number of experimental problems: (a) the DNA molecules retrieved, if there are any present, and to be copied are often degraded down to 100–300 bases pairs (bp) or less [18]; (b) the amount of molecules per gram of specimen may be critically low (down to thousands and less) [19]; (c) very typical failures in molecular amplification can be met, essentially caused by biochemical modifications and/or the presence of PCR inhibitors; (d) the authenticity of results is often jeopardized by a typical competition between the authentic sample (the one the investigator has an interest in) and a foreign genome (whatever other DNA, in the broadest sense) [19].

## *Size Fragmentation*

The principal type of damage to DNA extracted from hair and fossil remains is its fragmentation to small average size, generally between 100-300bp or less [18,20]. The reduction in size is due to two hydrolytic processes that occur during the keratinisation process and shortly after death: the cleavage of phosphodiester bonds in the phosphate-sugar backbone [21-22] that generate single-stranded nicks, and the cleavage of glycosidic bonds between nitrous bases and the sugar backbone that results in abasic sites [23-25]. Once a nucleotide is released, the abasic site can undergo a chemical rearrangement that promotes occurrence of strand breakage [22,26]. The length of the DNA sequences that can be amplified by the PCR can be limited also by lesions that present blocks to the elongation of DNA strands by the *Taq* polymerase. Many such lesions are induced by free radicals such as peroxide radicals ($O_2$), hydrogen peroxide ($H_2O_2$), and hydroxy radicals (OH), which are created by, among other causes, background radiation. The result of oxidative attacks is the ring fragmentation of both deoxyribose residues and nitrous base [21, 26]. It has been shown that paleontological specimens from a diverse range of environments and ages contain oxidized base residues [27], and no DNA sequences could be amplified via PCR [28] from samples with higher amounts of oxidized pyrimidines which block the *Taq* DNA polymerase.

## *Presence of Inhibitors*

Another important challenge to amplifying DNA samples from this type of source is the fact that the PCR amplification process can be affected by inhibitors present in the samples themselves. Factors that inhibit the amplification of nucleic acids by PCR are present with target DNAs from many sources. More often these substances can be co-extracted with the samples and thus prevent PCR amplification. These molecules are components of body fluids or reagents encountered in forensic science such as melanin, hemoglobin, collagene type I, urea, and heparin, food constituents like organic and phenolic compounds, glycongen, fats and $Ca^{2+}$, or environmental compounds like humic acids, fulvic acids, tannins, porphyrin products (5-10 repeat silica…), heavy metal and phenolic compounds, constituents of bacteria cells, non target DNA or contaminants. In forensic investigation inhibitors can be co-extracted with DNA from bloodstains, feces, buccal swabs, quids, soil, and obviously hair; occasionally substances such as textile dyes from clothing can remain with the DNA throughout the sample preparation process and interfere with the polymerase to prevent successful PCR amplification [29-42]. But although a wide range of inhibitors is reported, the identities and modes of action of many remain unclear.

The inhibitors can act through three main mechanisms:

1. They may bind or degrade to DNA when cells are lysed, so DNA is not available as a template for PCR
2. They can act by chelating metal ions such as $Mg^{2+}$ which are essential for catalytic activity of Taq DNA polymerase

3. They inhibit polymerase activity for amplification of target DNA [43].

The problem of inhibition is less discussed in literature but it is very important when the sample being tested is degraded and in low amount. The presence of PCR inhibitors is often, but not always, indicated by a discoloured DNA extract, usually tinted yellowish-to reddish-brown [30, 44-45]. The inhibition may be total or partial and can manifest itself as complete reaction failure or as reduced sensitivity of detection. In some cases, inhibition may be the cause of false-negative reactions, since few workers incorporate internal controls in each reaction tube [43]. Samples containing PCR inhibitors often produce partial profile results that look similar to a degraded DNA samples. In the absence of amplified target DNA, the presence of inhibitors is also suspected when primer-dimers fail to be produced in PCR reactions [44].

## *Mechanisms of Inhibition*

The inhibition of amplification may be due to a number of factors, none of which has been investigated carefully. It is very difficult to be able to understand the causes of the inhibition because of the complex interactions that are difficult to distinguish. The mechanism of action can be grouped into three broad categories by their point of action in the reaction. These categories are by no means absolute, since an inhibitor may act in more than one way and the relationships between chemical, enzymatic, and physical factors often cannot be distinguished given the poor current knowledge on the subject. It is likely that many inhibitors act through various physical and chemical means by interfering with the interaction between DNA and polymerase [43]. Degradation and capture of target or primers DNA can also be a cause of failed reactions. DNA can be degraded by physical, chemical, or enzymatic process and so it is very difficult to amplify a target. DNA target or primer can also be sequestrated by non-specific blocking that may inhibit amplification. For example bacterial cells or debris, proteins and polysaccharides can sequestrate DNA making the target not available to the polymerase. It was reported [47] that, for example, that milk proteins restrain DNA in high-molecular-weight complexes sequestrating from reaction environment. Lienert *et al.* in 1992 [48] suggested two mechanisms to explain how a forensic sperm genotyping was undermined by inhibition or allele drop-out due to the presence of vaginal microorganisms. Efficient primer extension may be prevented by small, sheared, single-stranded lengths of microbial DNA binding to the target sequence or the primer concentration can be reduced by non-specific binding to non-target microbial DNA. However other studies [49] suggested that high numbers of non-target DNA (organism DNA) were not found to be damaging to PCR. Humic compounds are the most commonly reported group of inhibitors in environmental samples and appear to have deleterious effects on several reaction components and their interactions [50]. It was shown that as little as 1μl of humic-acid-like extract was enough to inhibit a 100μl reaction mix and that this was unlikely to be due to act by chelating of $Mg^{2+}$ by humic compounds [51]. In the extraction of DNA from degraded human bone it was found that 5ng of ancient DNA was inhibitory to the amplification of 1ng of recent DNA, due to co-extraction with humic compounds [52]. These workers found that solvent extraction, ethanol precipitation, the addition of bovine serum albumin (BSA), gelatin, and high concentrations of *Taq* polymerase all failed to facilitate amplification, although ion-exchange chromatography removed inhibitors. Young et al. [53] explained the commonly reported inhibition by soil humic compounds as follows. The phenolic groups of humic compounds denature biological molecules by bonding to amides or oxidize to form a quinone which covalently bonds to DNA or proteins. The addition of polyvinylpolypyrrolidone (PVPP) or polyvinylpyrrolidone (PVP) overcame the inhibition and allowed separation of humic compounds from DNA during agarose gel electrophoresis. PCR yield was reduced by the addition of >0.5% PVP, however. A study on facilitating amplification in the presence of humic acids, and perhaps other inhibitors, in soils involved introducing a component with an affinity for the inhibitor higher than that of the essential reaction component that was inhibited [54]. McGregor et al. consider inhibition to be due to interference in the interaction between polymerase and target DNA. Of nine proteins tested, BSA proved the most effective in overcoming inhibition, as had previously been indicated by other workers. Nucleic acid sequestration and degradation may be overcome by physicochemical separation of target DNA from destructive compounds as soon as possible after cell lysis. Some inhibitors that interfere with PCR amplification are listed in the table.

| Possible Sources | PCR Inhibitor | References |
| --- | --- | --- |
| Blood | Heme (hematin) | Akana *et al.* 1994 |
| Tissue and hair | **Melanin** | **Eckhart *et al.* 2000** |
| Feces | Polysaccharides | Monteiro *et al.* 1997 |
| Soil | Humic compounds | Tsai and Olson 1992 |
| Urine | Urea | Mahony *et al.* 1998 |
| Blue jeans | Textile dyes (denim) | Shutler *et al.* 1999 |

*Melanin and its Mechanism of Inhibition*

Melanin is a pigment that is ubiquitous in nature and is the major pigment in human skin and hair. Melanin is produced and stored by melanocytes in special organelles called melanosomes. Melanocytes are cells located between the dermis and epidermis, in the form of stars, rich in melanin granules which are partly transferred to keratinocytes and hair. The synthetic activity of melanocytes varies among different individuals and between individuals from different populations, while the number of melanocytes is relatively constant even in individuals of different populations. The synthesis of melanin occurs in the cytoplasm forming melanosomes whose size, number, and melanin content, change between individuals and throughout life. The synthesis of melanin is stimulated by the sun and is under the control of pituitary MSH hormone (intermedina). Melanin is composed by a complex and highly heterogeneous polymer consisting of monomeric units of dihydroxyphenyl-alanine (DOPA) and/or cysteinyl-DOPA [55]. In different papers it is reported that the efficiency of PCRs from samples containing melanin was low [56-57]. Different hypothesis are listed on the mechanism of action of melanin but Eckhart et al. in their paper show that the mechanism of inhibition of melanin is against thermostable DNA polymerase rather than DNA. The melanin and DNA polymerase form a complex that can be observed in non-denaturating polyacrylamide gel electrophoresis. The melanin may block PCR at concentrations below 200ng/ml. The study also highlights that large amplicons are more sensitive to melanin than short PCR products.

## Solutions to PCR Inhibition

Given the importance of removing PCR inhibitors from DNA extracts, it is not surprising that a number of techniques have been developed to eliminate this problem. These techniques can be generally divided into two groups: 1. those that subdue the effects of inhibitors by manipulation of template DNA, PCR reagents, or the PCR cycling conditions and 2. those that remove inhibitors during the DNA extraction process prior to PCR amplification. Rådström et al. in 2004 [42] have published a review of strategies to generate PCR-compatible samples. It is possible to dilute the genomic DNA template with DNA-free water in which way the PCR inhibitors are diluted sufficiently to no longer affect the reaction, while at the same time the DNA is not diluted sufficiently to preclude the amplification. Why this technique is effective is uncertain, as the ratio of inhibitors to DNA remains constant. However it is possible that an inhibitor threshold exists, where the concentration of PCR inhibitors is the key factor, regardless of DNA concentration. Diluting inhibitors may not be the best approach when DNA is degraded as the template is already in low concentration [58], indeed McAlpine [59] suggested a three-boost multiphase protocol based on previous reported success in amplifying degraded DNA by "Booster PCR" [60]; this provides an improvement over subduing inhibition by dilution. The protocol consists of three early set of 12 cycles of low annealing temperature PCR. The product of each booster is then used as template for the subsequent rounds of PCR at a low annealing temperature, and finally as a template for a "normal" PCR. This procedure simultaneously dilutes inhibitors while maintaining a high concentration of template DNA. Otherwise more DNA polymerase can be added to reaction to overcome the inhibitors. In this way some Taq polymerase molecules bind to inhibiting substances and remove them from the reaction so the remaining can amplify the DNA template. However, in studies using DNA degraded samples, which often have fewer target molecules to amplify, increased amounts of Taq can be counter-productive as it increases the sensitivity of the PCR reaction to contamination. Another strategy to prevent or minimize the inhibition of PCR is to add to the PCR reaction molecules such as bovine serum albumin (BSA) [61] or betaine [62]. The BSA blocks PCR inhibitors [63] and, thus indirectly promotes polymerase activity. In 1999 Bourke et al. have been shown that sodium hydroxide treatment of DNA neutralize the Taq polymerase inhibitors [64]. The second group of techniques includes those that remove PCR inhibitors from DNA extracts prior to PCR amplification. Ye et al. [65] used cetyltrimethylammonium bromide (CTAB) to increase the yield of DNA extracted from burned bones. Alternatively, the addition of aluminum ammonium sulfate helped to prevent the co-purification of inhibitors with DNA from soil samples [66]. Moreira [67] developed a procedure to remove polysaccharides and humic acids from DNA extraction using DNA in agarose blocks which were subsequently washed with a lysis solution followed by TE buffer. This method takes the advantage of the size difference between DNA macromolecules and smaller sized inhibitor molecules, which readily diffuse out of the agarose. Another advantage to this technique is that DNA embedded in low melting temperature agarose can be used directly as PCR template. This method may remove a wide variety of inhibitors. Hänni et al. [68-69] demonstrated that DNA precipitated with isopropanol during the DNA extraction exhibits significantly less inhibition than DNA precipitated with ethanol or concentrated with centricon 30 columns. He reported that with the use of isopropanol, the brown coloration from DNA extracts disappears. Hypothesizing that the most problematic inhibitors bind to double stranded DNA, Bourke et al. [30] developed a procedure that releases inhibitors into solution by denaturing DNA with 0.4mM

NaOH. When the solution passes though a Microcon-100, the membrane retains the DNA while permitting smaller sized inhibitors to readily pass through. The DNA is then re-natured and used as template in PCR amplification. Bourke et al. [30] attributed their low success rate in casework samples (50%) to the possible hydrostatic shearing of the DNA during the denaturing stage and imperfect re-naturing. Thus, they suggested that this protocol might be inappropriate for extracts containing low quantities of DNA. However, Primorac [70] successfully used the protocol in a study of DNA extracted from bones excavated from mass graves in Croatia, Bosnia, and Herzegovina. Kemp et al. [71] tested this protocol on DNA extracted from Aztec remains (~500 years old) with one slight modification, the substitution of Microcon-30s for Microcon-100s in an effort to control for the fragmented nature of aDNA. As such, it was possible to type the mtDNA of 2 (40%) of 5 samples that previously failed to PCR amplify, presumably due to the presence of inhibitors. A variety of gel-packed columns and affinity beads are also used to remove inhibitors from DNA extracts. Sephadex G-50 chromatography was needed to remove "a reddish brown contaminant" from DNA extracts of 500-800-year-old Chilean human mummies [72]. Tsai and Olson [51] determined that Sephadex G-200 columns were more effective than Bio-Gel P-6, P-30, and Sephadex G-50 columns in removing humic acids from crude bacterial DNA extractions. Consequently, centrifuging extracted DNA through a spin column packed with Sepharose 4B removed humic acids from environmental samples more efficiently than either Sephadex G-200 or G-50 columns [73]. Furthermore, Thiopropyl Sepharose 6B beads have been useful in removing inhibitory textile dyes from DNA extracts [74-75]. Yang et al. [76] demonstrated that a silica-based column (Qiaquick) extraction is more effective than a standard phenol-chloroform extraction in removing inhibition from extracts of human remains dating to 5000 years BP. Yang et al. [77] confirmed the usefulness of the silica-based columns in species identification of ancient salmon bones (dating 2000 and 7000 years BP) from the Namu site in British Columbia. Although many researchers have assumed that PCR inhibitors arise from external sources (e.g. soil), Scholz et al. [78] demonstrated that collagen, which comprises the bulk of the organic portion of bone, is also an inhibitor. They suggested that collagen type I was the principal source of PCR inhibition of aDNA extracted from 1300-1550-year-old human skeletal remains and used collagenase in place of proteinase K to effectively remove this inhibitor during DNA extraction [78]. While most of the techniques cited above have been relatively effective in particular circumstances, it is difficult to predict which types of inhibitors are present in any given sample. As a result, it is desirable to have a generalized technique that can remove as many of them as possible [30]. Kemp et al. 2006 present a novel DNA extraction procedure called "repeat silica extraction" which effectively removes all PCR inhibitors from degraded DNA extracts from two types of archaeological samples from different ages and environments. This technique resulted from a number of initial experiments conducted on Post-Classic Aztec remains and human remains from the Windover archaeological site [79].

*Low Template DNA (LT)*

The conditions in which biological molecules exist in the body are under control. Within the living body, not only are numerous the cells but the DNA is also protected in the nucleus. However, forensic samples are frequently far from ideal. Another problem that often characterize the forensic hair samples is the presence of DNA in low amount. For these samples, in addition to problems discussed above (degradation, contamination and inhibition), there is also another factor that can affect the amplification results. An exciting area of research in many laboratories consists in the ability to obtain DNA profiles from very small amount of sample. Due to the limited nature of biological evidence that may be recovered from some crime scene samples, decisions often have to be made whether or not to proceed with testing low amounts of DNA. However, because of variation in estimates of DNA quantity within and between methods of quantification, LT typing is better defined as the analysis of any results below the stochastic threshold for normal interpretation. When few copies of DNA template are present, stochastic amplification may occur, resulting in either a substantial imbalance of two alleles at a given heterozygous locus or allelic dropout. Many strategies have been used to try to detect low amount of DNA [80-81]. The easiest way to do this is to increase the number of PCR cycles to improve the amplification yield from samples containing extremely low level of DNA template. Anthropologists routinely use an increasing in PCR cycles by to type ancient DNA from samples such as skeletal remains or mummified tissues. Gill et al. [82] employed from 38 to 43 cycles to analyze STR from 70-year-old bones of the Romanov family even if other study has demonstrated the inconsistence of this method [83-84]. Schmerer, Burger and Gerstenberger [85-87] analyzed STR from thousands of years old bone using 60 and 50 PCR cycles. Several other authors used modified PCR methods such as a nested primer PCR strategy [88].

The typical strategy to enable better detection of low template is to increase the number of PCR cycles, for example from 28 to 34 [89-90]. Similarly, Kloosterman and Kersbergen [91] suggested amplifying the DNA using the standard 28 cycles for SGM Plus Kit and typing the samples following standard operating protocols; if a low level result is obtained, then more Taq polymerase is added to the remaining PCR and 6 more cycles of the PCR are performed to carry out LT typing [92]. Other approaches that can be used to detect alleles in the LT range include reducing the PCR volume.

Now with current instrumentation (capillary electrophoresis) it may be possible to obtain reliable results from low levels of DNA without having to boost the PCR cycle number and push the sensitivity of the amplification. Budowle et al. 2001 showed that was possible to achieve results with LT typing without increasing the PCR cycle number and the concomitant increased risk of contamination. The possibilities are: 1. microcon filtration of the amplicons to remove ions that compete with DNA when being injection into the capillary 2. use of a formamide with a lower conductivity, 3. adding more amplified product to the denaturant formamide and 4. increasing injection time. The possibility to obtain DNA profiles from small amounts of biological material has expanded the types of samples available for analysis. For example it is possible to extract and identify human DNA consumed by the insects that can be at crime scenes and so linking a suspect to the crime in question. However, application of LT results should be approached with caution due to the possibilities of allele droup-out, allele droup-in, and increased risk of collection-based and laboratory based contamination [93].

Since the sensitivity of the STR typing assay is turned up so high, it is often not immediately clear if you have a reliable result or even a probative one (Forensic DNA typing). For example Gill [90] in a study shows how DNA profiles recovered at crime scenes may not be associated with the crime itself but rather have been left incidentally before the crime occurred. Also a secondary transfer of skin due to casual contact can occur even in a controlled laboratory settings [94]. Therefore, when analysis for low amount of DNA is performed, at least three type of artefacts can occur: 1. allele drop-in, additional alleles can be observed from sporadic contamination, 2. allele drop-out, can be seen a smaller number of alleles when the reaction fails to amplify low copy number DNA, 3. stutter product amounts are enhanced so that they are often higher than the typical 5-10% of the nominal allele [95]. Another characteristic is the heterozygote peak imbalance due to stochastic PCR amplification, where one of the alleles is amplified by chance during the early rounds of PCR in a preferential fashion. Allele drop-out can be thought of as an extreme form of heterozygote peak imbalance. The allele drop-in phenomenon is usually not reproducible and can be detected through testing the sample multiple times. The probability of obtaining a particular extra allele does not exceed 5% and thus the probability of obtaining the same extra allele in two different PCR reactions is < 1% [96]. So the routine application of LCN analysis involves at least three different PCR from the same sample and an allele cannot be considered unless it is present at least twice in replicate samples [90,95-96]. The consensus or composite STR profile is the one that is reported, this approach has been confirmed when the consensus profiles from separate single cell PCR experiments matching the profile of the cell donor [91, 97] For this reason in a forensic laboratory is essential that LT testing is performed in a sterile environment to prevent contamination from laboratory personnel [90, 98]. It is important that as for "ancient DNA" there are different rooms, one for DNA extraction and another for the PCR reaction, [99]. It is important to keep in mind that many LT profiles are mixtures and difficult to interpret reliably due to the issues of allele drop-out and drop-in and although a DNA profile may be obtained, it is usually not possible to identify the type of cells from which the DNA originated or when the cells were deposited [139]. Furthermore, starting with such little material, it may not possible to preserve the evidence for another confirmatory test by a second laboratory should that be required. For these reasons when LT testing is performed it is important to follow some guidelines described in Forensic DNA typing [93]: 1. multiple tube PCR amplifications with demonstrated duplication of every allele before reporting results, 2. if negative controls associated with a particular batch of samples show duplicated alleles that correspond to any of the samples, then the samples should not be reported and where possible samples should be retested, 3. if there is one allele in a sample that does not match the suspect's STR profile, then further testing may be pursued [89, 100]. Another approach to LT and degraded DNA profiling, yet to be fully examined, is the use of whole genome amplification (WGA). Most WGA methods use random primers and low stringency annealing conditions to amplify large sections of the genome to increase the quantity of the starting DNA template, prior to any downstream analysis. In 2006 Ballantine et al. [101] investigated two commercial available WGA kits for use on LCN and degraded DNA samples. Their results showed that WGA is capable of increasing both the quality and quantity of DNA and has the potential to improve profiling success from difficult samples in forensic casework. Rompler et al. [102] described a method to assemble long, continuous DNA sequences using minimal amounts of fragmented DNA as template. This is achieved by a two-step approach. In the first step, multiple fragments are simultaneously amplified in a single multiplex reaction. Subsequently, each of the generated fragments is amplified individually using a single primer pair, in a standard simplex (monoplex) PCR. The ability to amplify multiple fragments simultaneously in the first step allows the generation of large amounts of sequence from rare template DNA, whereas the second nested step increases specificity and decreases amplification of contaminating DNA. In contrast to current protocols using many template-consuming simplex PCRs, this method allows amplification of several kilobases of sequence in just one reaction. It thus combines optimal template usage with a high specificity and can be performed within a day.

## *The Problem of Contamination*

A further problem in the analysis of degraded and low amount of DNA consists in obtaining a non-endogenous DNA sequence and inability to detect it. There are two different source of contamination: a first type consists in fresh modern human DNA from cells released by personnel of the DNA laboratory or, more frequently, by people who handle the sample prior to analysis; the second type of contamination is due to previously amplified DNA molecules which can be present at high concentration inside a PCR tube. Both samples and reagents used in the analysis can be contaminated. For example, a successful PCR reaction can contain in order to $10^{12}$–$10^{15}$ amplified molecules in a volume of less than 50µl, [103]. Air movement created when opening PCR tubes or transferring liquids create and disperse microscopic aerosol droplets, which can easily contain over a million copies of the template per 0.005 ml. As a consequence, PCR products can quickly become widely distributed across laboratory surfaces, corridors and through entire buildings via personnel movement and air-handling systems. Since one aerosol droplet can easily contain a thousand times the amount of amplifiable DNA found in a forensic sample, DNA laboratories must be completely isolated both physically and logistically, preferably in buildings free from all molecular biological research. Furthermore, daily personnel movement should only proceed from samples to references laboratories, i.e. up the concentration gradient. Such simple precautions can prove as effective as high-tech positive air-pressure and UV irradiation systems, if rigorously enforced. Moreover, human and microbial DNA and cells are ubiquitous in all laboratory settings. It is prudent to assume that all laboratory reagents and tools are contaminated with human and microbial DNA when arriving from the manufacturer. Extensive cleaning of reagents (e.g. ultra filtration) and tools is essential, with complete decontamination requiring prolonged exposure (e.g. UV irradiation (45W, 72h), baking (more than 180°C, 12h), acid (2.5M HCl, 48h) and/or sodium hypochlorite (50%, 48h)).

## Human DNA

### *Nuclear DNA*

The markers that are much more used in forensic DNA laboratories for human identity testing are found in nuclear DNA, in the non-coding regions either between genes or within genes (i.e. introns) and thus do not code for genetic variation. Polymorphic (variable) markers that differ among individuals can be found throughout the non-coding regions of the human genome. A vast majority of our DNA molecules (over 99.7%) is the same between people. Only a small fraction of our DNA (0.3%) differs between people and makes us unique individuals. These variable region of DNA provide the capability of using DNA information for human identity purposes. The types of DNA polymorphisms used in forensic analysis are the length polymorphisms (short tandem repeat -STR-). These are DNA regions with repeat units that are 2-6bp in length. But among the various types of STR system, tetranucleotide repeats have become more popular than di- or trinucleotides. Penta- and hexanucleotide repeats are less common in the human genome but are being examined by some laboratories [104]. The advantages of using tetranucleotide STR loci in forensic DNA typing are: 1. a narrow allele size range that permits multiplexing, 2. a narrow allele size range that reduces allelic droup-out from preferential amplification of smaller alleles and 3. the capability of generating small PCR product sizes that benefit recovery of information from degraded DNA specimens. All these markers have become popular for forensic DNA typing because they are PCR-based and work with low-quantity DNA templates or degraded DNA samples. The number of repeats in STR markers can be highly among individuals, which make these STRs effective for human identification purposes. For this it is important to have DNA markers that exhibit the highest possible variation or a number of less polymorphic markers that can be combined in order to obtain the ability to discriminate between samples.

The selection criteria for candidate STR loci in human identification applications include the following characteristics [105-106]:

- High discrimination power, usually >0.9, with observed heterozygosity >70%,
- Separate chromosomal locations to ensure that closely linked loci are not chosen,
- Robustness and reproducibility of results when multiplexed with other markers,
- Low stutter characteristics,
- Low mutation rate and
- Predicted length of alleles that fall in the range of 90-500bp with smaller size better suited for analysis of degraded DNA samples.

Hair growth phase is an important factor for extracting nuclear DNA from hairs. Hair grows cyclically with alternating periods of growth and quiescence. The anagen phase is that of growth in which the cells proliferate, while the catagen phase is that of transition in which the cells enter a state of quiescence. Finally, in the telogen phase the cells are in a resting state. So, when hair is pulled and the roots are in the anagen phase, it is easier to extract the nuclear DNA because there are many cells that are proliferating. Indeed the genetic material in hair is mainly located in the root and surrounding sheath cells. A single pulled hair may contain as much as 100-500ng of DNA. However most of the hairs found at the crime scene are not suitable for genomic DNA analysis because they are in telogen phase or they do not have the root. Usually they have naturally fallen out. The cells in the root of telogen hairs are dried and inactive. Under these circumstances, when the root is not in anagen phase then the nuclear DNA cannot help the forensic hair examination, but may be used the mitochondrial DNA analysis. While the nucleus degrades as the hair shaft hardens during keratinization, cellular mitochondria and mtDNA remain relatively intact, making mtDNA analysis of hair shafts possible. In some cases, indeed, the mtDNA can be considered the only and last hope to support the hypothesis made by microscopic examination. The mtDNA, due to its characteristics, may survive in large quantity in hairs, bones, and teeth therefore it can be used to solve some forensic case such as e.g. mass disaster.

## *Mitochondrial DNA (mtDNA)*

Samples that have been highly degraded often fail to produce results with nuclear DNA typing system. However, recovery of DNA information from environmentally damage DNA is sometimes possible with mitochondrial DNA (mtDNA). While a nuclear DNA test is usually more valuable, a mtDNA result is better than no result at all. Indeed the probability of obtaining degraded DNA typing result from mtDNA is higher than that of polymorphic markers found in nuclear DNA particularly in cases where the amount of extracted DNA is very small as in hairs but also bones and teeth. A more useful marker in highly degraded DNA studies is the DNA located in the mitochondria. In humans, each mitochondrial genome consists of approximately 16.570bp, coding for 37 genes. Additionally, there are several non-coding sequences, so-called control regions, showing a comparatively high rate of polymorphism. For the regions with the highest mutation rate, the variability is characteristic at the population level or even down to the family level. The mtDNA is inherited only through the females of the previous generation, therefore, in each somatic cell one finds present only a single type of mtDNA sequence. This is due to the fact that oocytes contain a full complement of mitochondria, while sperm cells present most mitochondria located close to the tail. At the moment of fertilizations these mitochondria usually do not penetrate the oocyte because the sperm cells lose their tail. Also, if some mitochondria of sperm cells are able to enter the oocyte, they are destructed after fertilization [107]. Sometimes it happens; the new individual may reveal a mosaic of mitochondria and sequence polymorphisms in the mtDNA called heteroplasmy [108-111]. Through the regular mechanism in which only the female mitochondria contribute to the newly developing individual's genetic composition, all members of a maternal lineage show the same mtDNA. This fact can be helpful in solving missing persons or mass disaster investigations and itcan reduce the significance of a match in forensic cases. Since even distantly related maternal relatives should possess the same mtDNA type, this extends the number of useful reference samples that may be used to confirm the identity of a missing person. Evidence from mtDNA has been helpful in linking families but not in individual identification. From the analysis of isolated chromosomal sperm DNA, a particular type of mutational event is known that may complicate mtDNA analysis. This is the transfer of mtDNA sequences to the nuclear DNA. Since nuclear DNA has significantly lower mutation rates than mtDNA, nuclear insertions that happened early in evolution may represent a kind of mtDNA sequences different and ancestral respect of the effective mtDNA of an individual. To exclude ambiguous results at particular nucleotide positions, it's important that, primers intended to amplify a mtDNA sequence, do not co-amplify the nuclear insertions. The control region located near the nomenclatorial origin of the mitochondrial genome, the so-called D-loop control region, shows a high sequence polymorphism between individuals. This region spans about 1000bp and consists in three hypervariable regions (HVR I-HVR II-HVRIII) that, in total, involve about 750bp. The HVRs reveal about 3% variability between individuals; this means that two randomly selected individuals who are not related show differences in 3 out of 100 nucleotide positions [112]. Moreover, these polymorphic sites are not distributed uniformly but cluster in particular positions called hotspots. The analysis of hypervariable regions enables investigators to identify individuals at the family lineage level [113-117], and, of course, they are elective markers in term of population genetics and phylogenetic studies [118-124]. MtDNA analysis is still the most widely used in forensics when the hairs found at the crime scene are free of root or they have the root in telogen phase. In this way, the genetic results obtained can support or not and add more information to conclusions of microscopic examination. However, when degraded samples are analyzed, the traditional protocol for forensic mtDNA analysis that involves the amplification of the entire region HVRI and HVRII, may not be used. The fragment sizes of 300-400bp are too long and the amplification may fail. So it is necessary to analyze shortened amplicons. For example Eichmann in his work produces ten overlapping fragments (mini-fragments) with size range between 144-237bp to cover the entire human mtDNA control region [125]. The goal of this procedure is also that ten fragments are co-amplified in only two multiplex polymerase chain reactions. But they are sequenced with the individual amplification primers, so, since it is laborious and expensive, if the samples are not highly degraded it is possible to use other primers. These can amplify larger fragments (midi-fragments) and require 10 sequencing reaction instead of 20 [126].

## Non-human DNA

The DNA-based identification of an organism in general is an important tool also in bio-security, ecological monitoring, and wildlife crimes. The type of offences in wildlife crimes may include: the possession of controlled species; the illegal trade in internationally protected species; the poaching, the illegal fur trade, the hunting out of season, horns and tusks used for ornaments etc.. So the forensic expert is forced to deal with several and different wildlife crimes. There are two main issues that he has to face in wildlife crime: 1. he should be able to identify the species; 2. he should determine if the biological sample can belong to a particular member of that species.

### *Nuclear DNA*
In order to identify an individual and to distinguish him from another the genetic marker the STRs are utilized. As human DNA, genetic material of animals contains STR markers that can be useful in differentiating between animals. So, the efforts of researchers are focusing not only on developing a STR tests but also on validating an STR panel for use in forensic casework and on creating a database for forensic animal identification. There also needs to be knowledge of the species present before attempting STR testing. Animal DNA samples have been and are useful evidence in criminal investigations, whether or not a animal is directly involved. For this reason it is necessary that the scientific community may have access to reliable methods for typing animal DNA (least of animals that most frequently can be found at the crime scene) and a DNA database. However, there is currently no commercial kit available and forensically validated for typing animal STR. Actually studies are focusing mainly on developing the nomenclature system of some animal STR such as for examples dogs, cats, and cattle and on setting a multiplex PCR kit [127-168]. Also in this case, when a non-human hair is found at the crime scene, the analysis of nuclear DNA is possible only if the root is present and it is in an anagen phase. But the roots of non-human hair found at the crime scene are mainly in the telogen phase, so the mtDNA analysis is recommended. But in the case of hairs, another problem can be related to the nuclear DNA analysis: a general trend of reduced training of and availability of experienced hair examiners. Indeed in order to analyze the nuclear DNA of hair found at the crime scene it is necessary that the microscopic examiner has acknowledged that hair belongs to certain species. Sometimes, also for skeletal remains, it could be useful to investigate the species through mtDNA analysis.

### *Mitochondrial DNA*
When conclusive results about species cannot be performed through microscopic examination, the DNA analysis offers the best opportunity to answer the question: "What species is this?" [169]. In this case the mtDNA sequencing analysis have to be useful not only in degraded remains but also in the identification of the species. So the mtDNA analysis of

non-human hair supports the microscopic examination with the investigation of hypervariable regions. For several reasons, some loci located on the mitochondrial genome are used in the species identification rather than being nuclear DNA based. The main reason is because there is no recombination of mtDNA. All of the mtDNA molecules of an individual are all equal with the exception of mutations and are inherited through the maternal line [170-171]. In mammals only a little DNA on mtDNA genome is non-coding and there are not introns and pseudo-genes [172]. Then the mtDNA molecules are present in multiple copies per cells [173] and the mitochondria have a protein coat that help to protect the mtDNA from degradation: these characteristics make it more suitable than the nuclear DNA for use in highly degraded samples such as bones, teeth and obviously hair shaft [174-179]. Additionally, enzymes in the mitochondria are not able to read and to correct the DNA bases added incorrectly during the replication [180] so the mutations can be accumulated in mtDNA up to five times more than those that accumulate during nuclear DNA replication. There are a lot of studies about species identification and there are different markers that may be utilized. The choice of markers for forensic species identification derives from taxonomic and phylogenetic studies and exhibits little intra-specific variability, i.e. between members of the same species, but shows sufficient inter-specific variability, i.e. between members of different species, in order to discriminate between individuals of different species. One of these loci is *cytochrome b –cyt b-* [181-183]. Over the years, several forensic and taxonomic studies used the *cyt b* as a marker for identification species [184-196]. But, a little more recently, there has been an increase in the use of an another marker called cytochrome c oxidase I (COI). This is used in DNA barcoding: it has been adopted as a marker in Barcode for Life Consortium - http:www.boldsystems.org- [197-199]. Initially used in the identification of invertebrate species [200-204] then has been exploited as a marker in forensic entomology to identify the beetle larvae on a corpse [205-206]. Now COI has been proposed for identification of many organisms [207-221]. Other mitochondrial genes can be utilized as a marker in forensic species identification: 12S ribosomal RNA [222-224], 16S ribosomal RNA [225-230] and the NDH family [231-232]. The figure [Figure 10] shows the position of each gene in the human mtDNA genome.

While all of these genes have been investigated for species identification, instead, the D-loop analysis was mostly exploited for intra-species identification [233-238] even if sometime can be applied to species identification [239-244]. Usually, the standard analysis of species identification requires the amplification of part of one these genes, the sequencing and the comparison of obtained sequence to that kept on a database such as GenBank. In 2007 Dawnay N. et al. [245] in their study examine the possibility of using the COI in forensic species identification and demonstrate that the COI enables accurate animal species identification if adequate reference sequence data exists. But most of the mitochondrial sequence of these genes is conserved between species and has only a few points variables that can characterize one species from an another. These variable points are termed single nucleotide polymorphism (SNP). So the next development was to analyze only these spots of interest that are species specific. The SNP analysis has the advantage over traditionally sequencing technology that is not necessary to sequence data and it can differentiate between mixture [246]. Currently, one of the most common methods used in species identification is SNaPshot. This process is used in forensic human and non-human identification [247-262]. This techniques is similar to the sequencing reaction but involves the use of fluorescent dye-labeled dideoxynucleotide triphosphates (ddNTPs) to help visualize the results. A single primer is used that bind to the sequence of interest up to SNP to be tested. So, when the DNA polymerase adds one of these modified bases depending on the base in the template, the chain elongation is blocked. These bases are fluorescently tagged and each of the four nucleotides has its own color. So it is possible to distinguish one base from another. Furthermore, the mtDNA analysis can support the microscopic results. In fact when the suspect hair has to be compared with that found at the crime scene, after careful microscopic examination, the mtDNA analysis of *D-loop* region can be set up. The genetic result of compatibility obtained between sample and known hair may provide important genetic data to be associated with results of microscopic investigation. The genetic analysis is an essential tool to be associated with microscopic comparison since there are many factors that impact on the reliability of the hair association in microscopic analysis such as the experience, the training, the adequate instrumentations, and the availability of known hair standards.

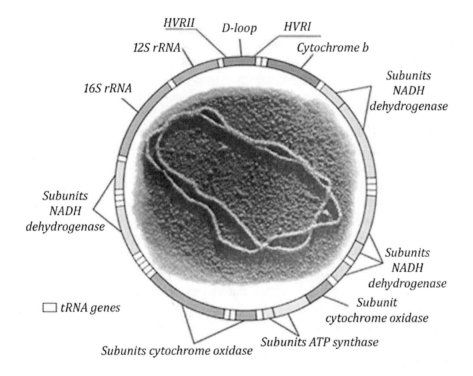

Figure 10. Human mtDNA.

# Conclusion

## Future Prospects

Despite the hair is one of the common biological evidence found at the crime scene, it is one of the more difficult sample to treat. A general forensic approach should proceed from the morphological and microscopic examination to DNA analysis. The microscopic analysis can be complicated because there are many factors that can influence the reliability of the results such as the training and the experience of hair examiners. Because its biological nature, also the genetic analysis can suffer from various problems linked to the extreme degradation of hair DNA, the low amount of DNA present in hair shaft, and the presence of molecules, such as melanin, that can inhibit the amplification reaction. So research is evolving in an attempt to overcome these problems. Currently, the scientific world is focusing on studying of the characteristics of the complex human phenotype from its genotype. Predicting human phenotype from genotype is an important tool especially for medicine: genome information in fact can enable better prognosis, prevention and medical care [263-264] but it could be also successfully applied in forensic applications. The information about the general phenotypic characteristics provided from genotype data could help the investigative intelligence purposes especially in suspect-less cases [265]. The genetic researcher could in the future give a "genetic identikit". However, the genetic understanding of human appearance is still in its infancy even if an exception may be considered the eye color. In fact recent studies show that 15 are the genes involved in eye color [266-274]. The recent progress on predicting genetically of eye color suggests that also the genetic analysis of the hairs could give information about their color and also other traits such as e.g. their structure [275]. Hair morphology is one of the most differentiated traits among human population. However, genetic back-grounds of hair morphological differences among populations have not been clarified yet. Several SNPs have been found with association to human hair color variation such as OCA2, HERC2, SLC24A4, KITLG, TYR, TPCN2, TYRP1, IRF4, EXOC2, KIF26A, OBSCN, SLC45A2, MC1R, ASIP and additional genes such as SLC24A5, MYO5A, MYO7A, MLPH, GPR143, DCT, HPS3, GNAS, PRKARIA, ERCC6, and DTNBP1 [276-280]. Valverde et al. [281] have found that red hair color is associated with the polymorphisms in the MC1R gene and other studies have confirmed it [282-289]. Sulem et al. in their study reveal two SNPs in ASIP gene associated with red hair color [278]. Also, Medland et al. in 2009 [290] have studied the genetic hair morphology (straight, wavy, curly) in three Australian samples of European descent. The results of their study showed that SNPs present in the Trichohyalin gene (TCHH), which is expressed in the developing inner root sheath of the hair follicle, are associated with straight hair in Europeans. The variants in this gene are at their highest frequency in Northern Europeans, like the distribution of the straight-hair EDAR variant in Asian populations [291]. Thus in the next future the hair DNA analysis could help the microscopic comparison in predicting the morpho-structural characteristics of the hairs.

Also, in the recent years new technologies of sequencing DNA have developed that allow to produce huge amounts of sequences if compared to Sanger sequencing. These new techniques are indicated by the acronym NGS, Next Generation Sequencing. One of these is FLX-Titanium Genome Sequencer Roche/454 Life Sciences [292]. The focus of this method has been on the co-development of an emulsion-based PCR [293-295] to isolate and amplify DNA fragments in vitro, and of a fabricated substrate and instrument that performs pyrophosphate-based sequencing "pyrosequencing" [296] in picoliter-sized wells. Initially this techniques involves the construction of genetic library by fragmentation of the whole genomic DNA in the extract. Then two adapters, one specific to the 5' end, the other for the 3' end, bind to each fragments. These fragments are denatured by washing with NaOH and are bound to the nanospheres in a water/oil emulsion. Thus the DNA is used as a template for the PCR reaction [297]. At the end of reaction there is a denaturing step of PCR products. Each nanosphera is then placed in a well of a chip optical fiber whose pores have a diameter of about 44 microns. These allow entry to a single sphere. To the well is then adds a mixture of polymerase sulfurylase, apirase, luciferase and triphosphates to make the pyrosequencing. The advantage of the use of this method is that it is possible to sequence every genetic fragment that is present in the extract. Since this technique is very sensitive, it could be used to try to obtain a complete or partial genetic profile from the analysis of the high degraded nuclear DNA of hair shaft. This method could offer new prospects of the DNA analysis of hair shaft in forensic investigations.

## REFERENCES

[1] Downing, DT; Stewart, ME; Wertz, PW; Colton, SW; Abraham, W; Strauss, JS. "Skin lipids: an update". *The Journal of Investigative Dermatology,* March 1987 88 (3 Suppl), 2s–6s.
[2] Bubenik, GA. "Why do humans get "goosebumps" when they are cold, or under other circumstances?" *Scientific American.* September 1, 2003 available from: http://www.scientificamerican.com/article.cfm?id=why-do-humans-get-goosebu
[3] Sabah, J. Controlled Stimulation of Hair Follicle Receptors. *J Appl Physiol.* 1974 36, 256-257.
[4] Palmer, R; Banks M. The secondary transfer of fibres from head hair. *Sci Justice* 2005 Jul-Sep;45(3), 123-128.
[5] Exline, DL; Smith, FP; Drexler, SG. Frequency of pubic hair transfer during sexual intercourse. *J. Forensic Sci* 1998 May; 43(3), 505-508.
[6] Tridico, SR. Trace evidence analysis more cases in mute witnesses *Edited* by Max M. Houck 2004, Elsevier (USA). Cap 1Hair of the dog : a case study.
[7] Robertson, J; Forensic and microscopic examination of human hair, in: J. Robertson (Ed.), Forensic Examination of Hair, Taylor and Francis, London, 1999, pp. 79–154.
[8] Gaudette, BD and Tessarolo, T; Secondary transfer of human scalp hair. *J. of Forensic Sci. 1987*, 32, 1241-1253.
[9] Mann, M. Hair transfer in sexual assault: a six year case study. *J. of Forensic Sci.* 1990, 35, 951-955.
[10] Dachs, J; McNaught, IJ; Robertson, J. The persistence of human scalp hair on clothing fabrics. *Forensic Sci. Int.* 2003, 138, 27-36.
[11] Greenshields, MR; Scheurman, GD. The Crime Scene: Criminalistics, Science and Common Sense. Toronto: Pearson Education Canada Inc.; 2001.
[12] Bisbing, RE. Finding Trace Evidence. in Mute Witnesses: Trace Evidence Analysis. San Diego California: Houck, Max., (ed.) Academic Press; 2001.
[13] Block, E. Science vs Crime: The Evolution of the Police Lab.San Francisco, California: Cragmont Publications; 1979.
[14] Bisbing, RE. Hair: comparison: microscopic. In: Editor Siegel J, Editor Knupfer G, Editor Saukko P. Encyclopedia of Forensic Science. Elsevier, Academic Press. Aug. 2000. Pages number 1002-1015.
[15] Jeffreys, AJ; Wilson, V; Thein, SL. Hypervariable 'minisatellite' regions in human DNA. *Nature* 1985, 314, 67–73.
[16] Gill, P; Jeffreys, AJ; Werrett, DJ. Forensic application of DNA fingerprints. *Nature,* 1995, 318, 577–579.

[17] Presley, LA; Budowle, B. The application of PCR-based technologies to forensic analysis, in *PCR Technology Current Innovations*, HG Griffin & AM Griffin, Boca Raton, FL, USA.

[18] Pääbo, S. Ancient DNA: extraction, characterization, molecular cloning, and enzymatic amplification. *Proc. Natl. Acad. Sci. U.S.A.* 1989, 86, 1939–1943.

[19] Handt, O; Krings, M; Ward, R.H; Pääbo, S. The retrieval of ancient human DNA sequences. *Am. J. Hum. Genet.* 1996, 59, 368–376.

[20] Hofreiter, M; Serre, D; Poinar, H.N; Kuch, M; Pääbo, S. Ancient DNA. *Nat. Rev. Genet.* 2001b, 2, 353.

[21] Lindahl, T. Instability and decay of the primary structure of DNA. *Nature* 1993, 362, 709–15.

[22] Shapiro, R. *Damage to DNA caused by hydrolysis. In Chromosome Damage and Repair,* ed. E Seeberg, K Kleppe, 3–12. New York: Plenum.

[23] Lindahl, T and Karlstro, O. Heatinduced depyrimidination of deoxyribonucleic acid in neutral solution. *Biochemistry* 1973, 12, 5151–5154.

[24] Lindahl, T; Nyberg, B. Rate of depurination of native deoxyribonucleic acid. *Biochemistry* 1972, 11, 3610.

[25] Schaaper, RM; Kunkel, TA; Loeb LA. Infidelity of DNA-synthesis associatedwith bypass of apurinic sites. *Proc.Natl. Acad. Sci. USA* 1983, 80, 487–491.

[26] Friedberg, EC; Walker, GC; Siede, W. DNA Repair and Mutagenesis. Washington D.C: *ASM Press*. 698.

[27] Höss, M; Jaruga, P; Zastawny, T.H; Dizdaroglu, M; Pääbo, S. DNA damage and DNA sequence retrieval from ancient tissues. *Nucleic Acids Res* 1996, 24, 1304–1307.

[28] Höss, M; Dilling, A; Currant, A; Pääbo, S. Molecular phylogeny of the extinct ground sloth *Mylodon darwinii. Proc. Natl. Acad. Sci. USA* 1996, 93, 181–185.

[29] Akane, A; Matsubara, K; Nakamura, H; Takahashi, S; Kimura, K. Identification of the heme compound copurified with deoxyribonucleic acid (DNA) from bloodstains, a major inhibitor of polymerase chain reaction (PCR) amplification. *Journal of Forensic Sciences* 1994, 39, 362-372.

[30] Bourke, M.T; Scherczinger, CA; Ladd C; Lee HC. NaOH treatment to neutralize inhibitors of Taq polymerase. *J. Forensic Sci.* 1999, 44, 1046-1050.

[31] Bright, JA and Petricevic, SF. Recovery of trace DNA and its application to DNA profiling of shoe insoles, *Forensic Sci. Int.* 2004, 145, 7-12.

[32] Chiou, FS; Pai, CY; Hsu, YPP; Tsai, CW; Yang, CH. Extraction of human DNA for PCR from chewed residues of betel quid using a novel "PVP/CTAB" method. *J. Forensic Sci.* 2001, 46, 1174-1179.

[33] Fisher, DL; Holland, MM; Mitchell, L; Sledzik, PS; Wilcox, AW; Wadhams, M; Weedn, VW. Extraction, evaluation, and amplification of DNA from decalcified and undecalcified United States Civil War Bone. *J. Forensic Sci.* 1993, 38, 60-68.

[34] Holland, MM; Fisher, DL; Mitchell, L; Rodriguez, WC; Canick, JJ; Merril, C.R; Weedn, VW. Mitochondrial DNA sequence analysis of human skeletal remains: Identification of remains from the Vietnam War. *J. Forensic Sci* 1993, 38, 542-553.

[35] Jung, JM; Comey, CT; Baer, DB; Budowle, B. Extraction strategy for obtaining DNA from bloodstains for PCR amplification and typing of the HLA-DQ alpha gene. *Int. J. Legal Med.* 1991, 104, 145-148.

[36] Martin, LR. STR-typing of nuclear DNA from human fecal matter using the Qiagen Qiaamp_ Stool Mini Kit.Twelfth International Symposium on Human Identification, 2001, Promega Corporation, Madison, WI.

[37] Potter, T. Co-amplification of ENFSI-loci WS1358, D8SI179 and D18S51: validation of new primer sequences and allelic distribution among 2874 individuals, *Forensic Sci. Int.* 2003, 138, 104.

[38] Roy, R. To poop or not to poop? That is the question!. Thirteenth International Symposium on Human Identification, 2002, Promega Corporation, Madison, WI.

[39] Salvador, JM; De Ungria, MCA. Isolation of DNA from saliva of betel quid chewers using treated cards. *J. Forensic Sci.* 2003, 48, 794-797.

[40] Shutler, GG; Gagnon, P; Verret, G; Kalyn, H; Korkosh, S; Johnston, E; Halverson, J. Removal of a PCR inhibitor and resolution of DNA STR types in mixed human-canine stains from a five year old case. *J. Forensic Sci.* 1999, 44, 623-626.

[41] De Franchis, R; Cross, NC; Foulkes, NS; Cox, TM. A potent inhibitor of Taq polymerase copurifies with human genomic DNA. *Nucleic Acids Res.* 1988 Nov. 11, 16(21), 10355.

[42] Rädström, P;Knutsson, R; Wolffs, P; Lovenklev, M; Lofstrom, C. Pre-PCR processing: strategies to generate PCR-compatible samples. *Mol. Biotechnology* 2004, 26, 133-146.

[43] Wilson, I.G. Inhibition and facilitation of nucleic acid amplification. *Appl. Environ. Microbiol.* 1997 Oct , 63(10), 3741-51.

[44] Rogan, PK and Salvo, JJ. Molecular genetics of pre-Columbian South American mummies. *Mol. Evol.* 1990, 122, 223-234.

[45] Pääbo, S. Amplifying ancient DNA, in: M.A. Innis (Ed.), PCR Protocols: A Guide to Methods and Applications, Academic Press, San Diego, 1990 159-166.

[46] Fisher, DL; Holland, MM; Mitchell, L; Sledzik, PS; Wilcox, AW; Wadhams, M; Weedn, VW; Extraction, evaluation, and amplification of DNA from decalcified and undecalcified United States Civil War Bone. *J. Forensic Sci.*1993, 38, 60-68.

[47] Rijpens, NP; Jannes, G; Van Asbroeck, M; Rossau, R; Herman, LMF. Direct detection of *Brucella* spp. in raw milk by PCR and reverse hybridization with 16S-23S rRNA spacer probes. *Appl. Environ. Microbiol.* 1996, 62, 1683–1688.

[48] Lienert, K and Fowler, JCS. Analysis of mixed human/microbial DNA samples: a validation study of two PCR AMP-FLP typing methods. *BioTechniques* 1992, 13, 276–281.

[49] Steffan, RJ and Atlas, RM. DNA amplification to enhance detection of genetically engineered bacteria in environmental samples. *Appl. Environ. Microbiol.* 1988, 54, 2185–2191.

[50] Jacobsen, CS and Rasmussen, OF; Development and application of a new method to extract bacterial DNA from soil based on separation of bacteria from soil with cation-exchange resin. *Appl. Environ. Microbiol.* 1992, 58, 2458–2462.

[51] Tsai, Y and Olson, BH. Detection of low numbers of bacterial cells in soils and sediments by polymerase chain reaction. *Appl. Environ. Microbiol* 1992, 58, 754–757.

[52] Goodyear, PD; MacLaughlin-Black, S; Mason, IJ. A reliable method for the removal of co-purifying PCR inhibitors from ancient DNA. *BioTechniques* 1994, 16, 232–235.

[53] Young, C; Burghoff, RL; Keim, LG; Minak-Bernero, V; Lute, JR; Hinton, SM. Polyvinylpyrrolidone-agarose gel electrophoresis purification of polymerase chain reaction-amplifiable DNA from soils. *Appl. Environ. Microbiol* 1993, 59, 1972–1974.

[54] McGregor, DP; Forster S; Steven, J: Adair, J; Leary, SEC: Leslie, DL; Harris, WJ; Titball, RW. Simultaneous detection of microorganisms in soil suspension based on PCR amplification of bacterial 16S rRNA fragments. *BioTechniques* 1996, 21, 463–471.

[55] Prota G; Ischia D; Napolitano A. 1998 in The Pigmentary System (Nordlund J., Boissy R.E., Hearing V.J., King R.A., and ortonne J.-P., Eds), pp.307-332, Oxford Univ. Press, New York.

[56] Yoshii, T; Tamura, K; Taniguchi, T; Akiyama, K; and Ishiyama, I. Water-soluble eumelanin as a PCR-inhibitor and a simple method for its removal. *Jpn. J. Legal Med.* 1993, 47, 323–329.

[57] Giambernardi, TA; Rodeck, U; and Klebe, RJ; Bovine serum albumin reverses inhibition of RT-PCR by melanin. *Bio-Techniques*, 1998, 25, 564–566.

[58] Drake, M; Small, CL; Spence, KD; Swanson, BG. Rapid detection and identification of *Lactobacillus* spp. in dairy products by using the polymerase chain reaction. *J. Food Prot.* 1996, 59, 1031–1036.

[59] Erlich, HA; Gelfand, D; Sninsky, JJ. Recent advances in the polymerase chain reaction. *Science* 1991, 252, 1643–1651.

[60] Ehrlich-Kautzky, E; Shinomiya, N; Marsh, DG. Simplified method for isolation of white cells from whole blood suitable for direct polymerase chain reaction. *BioTechniques* 1991, 10, 39–40.

[61] Comey, CT; Koons, BW; Presley, KW; Smerick, JB; Sobieralski, CA; Stanley, DM; Baechtel, FS. *Journal of forensic Science* 1994, 39, 1254-1269.

[62] Al-Soud, WA and Rådström, P. Purification and characterization of PCR-inhibitory components in blood cells. *Journal of Clinical Microbiology,* 2000, 38, 4463-4470.

[63] Greenwood, AD; Lee, F; Capelli, C; DeSalle, R; Tikhonov, A; Marx, PA; MacPhee, RD. Evolution of endogenous retrovirus-like elements of the woolly mammoth (*Mammuthus primigenius*) and its relatives. *Mol. Biol. Evol.* 2001, 18, 840–847.

[64] Bourke, MT; Scherczinger, CA; Ladd, C; Lee, HC. NaOH treatment to neutralize inhibitors of Taq polymerase. *J. of Forensic Sci* 1999, 44, 1046-1050.

[65] Ye, J; Ji, A; Parra, EJ; Zheng, X; Jiang, C; Zhao, X; Hu, L; Tu, Z. A simple and efficient method for extracting DNA from old and burned bone. *J. Forensic Sci.* 2004 Jul., 49(4), 754-9.

[66] Braid, MD; Daniels, LM; Kitts, CL. Removal of PCR inhibitors from soil DNA by chemical flocculation. *Journal of Microbiological Methods* 2003, 52:389-393.

[67] Moreira, D. Efficient removal of PCR inhibitors using agarose-embedded DNA preparations, *Nucleic Acids Research* 1998, 26, 3309 -310.

[68] Hänni, C; Begue, A; Laudet, V; Stehelin, D; Brousseau, T; Amouyel, P; Duday, H. Molecular typing of neolithic human bones. *J. Archaeol. Sci.* 1995, 22, 649-658.

[69] Hänni, C; Brousseau, T; Laudet, V; Stehelin, D. Isopropanol precipitation removes PCR inhibitors from ancient bone extracts. *Nucleic Acids Res.* 1995, 23, 881-882.

[70] Primorac, D. Identification of human remains from mass graves found in Croatia and Bosnia and Herzegovina, Tenth International Symposium on Human Identification, Promega Corporation, Madison, WI 1999.

[71] Kemp, BM; Resendez, A; Roman Berrelleza, JA; Malhi, RS; Smith, DG. An analysis of ancient Aztec mtDNA from Tlatelolco: Pre-Columbian relations and the spread of

Uto-Aztecan, in: D.M. Reed (Ed.), Biomolecular Archaeology: Genetic Approaches to the Past, Southern Illinois University, Carbondale, IL 2005, 22-46.

[72] Rogan, PK and Salvo, JJ. Molecular genetics of pre-Columbian South American mummies. *Mol. Evol.* 1990, 122, 223-234.

[73] Jackson, CR; Harper, JP; Willoughby, D; Roden, EE; Churchill, PF. A simple, efficient method for the separation of humic substances and DNA from environmental samples. *Appl. Environ. Microbiol.* 1997, 63, 4993-4995.

[74] Shutler, GG; Gagnon, P; Verret, G; Kalyn, H; Korkosh, S; Johnston, E; Halverson, J. Removal of a PCR inhibitor and resolution of DNA STR types in mixed human-canine stains from a five year old case. *J. Forensic Sci.* 1999, 44, 623-626.

[75] Williamson, J; Waye, J; Newall, P; Bing, D; Blake, E. The use of comprehensive approach for neutralization of PCR inhibitors found in forensic samples and its use in a homicide/sexual assault case, Sixth International Symposium on Human Identification, Promega Corporation, Madison, WI, 1996, 186-187.

[76] Yang, DY; Eng, B; Waye, JS; Dudar, JC; Saunders, SR. Technical note: Improved DNA extraction from ancient bones using silica-based spin columns. *Am. J. Phys. Anthropol.* 1998, 105, 539-543.

[77] Yang, DY; Cannon, A; Saunders, SR. DNA species identification of archaeological salmon bone from the Pacific Northwest coast of North America. *J. Archaeol. Sci.* 2004, 31, 619-631.

[78] Scholz, M; Giddings, I; Pusch, CM. A polymerase chain reaction inhibitor of ancient hard and soft tissue DNA extracts is determined as human collagen type I. *Anal. Biochem.* 1998, 259, 283-286.

[79] Kemp, BM; Monroe, C; Smith, DG. Repeat silica extraction: a simple technique for the removal of PCR inhibitors from DNA extracts. *J. Archeol. Sci.* 2006, 33(12), 1680-89.

[80] Moretti, T; Koons, B; Budowle, B. Enhancement of PCR amplification yield and specificity using AmpliTaq Gold DNA polymerase, *Biotechniques,* 1998 Oct., 25(4), 716-22.

[81] Leclair, B; Sgueglia, JB; Wojtowicz, PC; Juston, AC; Fregeau, CJ; Fourney, RM. STR DNA typing: increased sensitivity and efficient sample consumption using reduced PCR reaction volumes. *J. Forensic Sci.*, 2003 Sep, 48(5), 1001-13.

[82] Gill, P; Ivanov, PL; Kimpton, C; Piercy, R; Benson, N; Tully, G; Evett, I; Hagelberg, E; Sullivan, K. Identification of the remains of the Romanov family by DNA analysis. *Nat. Genet.,* 1994, 6, 130-5.

[83] Knight, A; Zhivotovsky, LA; Kass, DH; Litwin, DE; Green. LD; White, PS. Ongoing controversy over Romanov remains. *Science,* 2004 Oct. 15, 306(5695), 407-10.

[84] Knight, A; Zhivotovsky, LA; Kass, DH; Litwin, DE; Green, LD; White, PS; Mountain, JL. Molecular, forensic and haplotypic inconsistencies regarding the identity of the Ekaterinburg remains. *Ann. Hum. Biol.,* 2004 Mar-Apr, 31(2), 129-38.

[85] Schmerer, WM; Hummel, S; Herrmann, B. Optimized DNA extraction to improve reproducibility of short tandem repeat genotyping with highly degraded DNA as target. *Electrophoresis,* 1999, 20, 1712-6.

[86] Burger, J; Hummel, S; Hermann, B; Henke, W. DNA preservation: a microsatellite-DNA study on ancient skeletal remains. *Electrophoresis,* 1999, 20, 1722-8.

[87] Gerstenberger, J; Hummel, S; Schultes, T; Hack, B; Herrmann, B. Reconstruction of a historical genealogy by means of STR analysis and Y-haplotyping of ancient DNA. Eur. *J. Hum. Genet.*, 1999 May-Jun., 7(4), 469-77.

[88] Strom, CM; Rechitsky, S. Use of nested PCR to identify charred human remains and minute amounts of blood. *J. Forensic Sci.*, 1998, 43, 696-700.

[89] Gill, P; Whitaker, J; Flaxam, C; Brown, N; and Buckleton, J. An investigation of the rigor of interpretation rules for STRs derived from less than 100 pg of DNA. *Forensic Sci. Int.*, 2000,112, 17-40.

[90] Gill, P. Application of low copy number DNA profiling. *Croat. Med. J.*, 2001 Jun 42(3), 229-32.

[91] Kloosterman, A; and Kersbergen, P. Efficiency and limits of genotyping low copy number (LCN) DNA samples by multiplex PCR STR loci. Presented at 19th Congress of the International Society of Forensic Genetics, Munster, Germany. 2001,

[92] Budowle, B; Hobson, DL; Smerick, JB; and Smith, JAL. Proceeding of the Twelfth International Symposium on Human Identification. Madison, Wisconsin; Promega Corporation. 2001, Available at: http://www.promega.com/geneticidproc/ussymp 12proc/contents/budowle.pdf.

[93] Butler, JM. Forensic DNA Typing, Biology, Technology, and Genetics of STR Markers. Elsevier Academic Press USA -Second Edition-. 2005,

[94] Lowe, A; Murray, C; Whitaker, J; Tully, G; and Gill, P. The propensity of individuals to deposit DNA and secondary transfer of low level DNA from individuals to inert surfaces. *Forensic Sci. Int.*, 2002, 129, 25-34.

[95] Whitaker, JP; Cotton, EA; Gill, P. A comparison of the characteristics of profiles produced with the AMPFlSTR SGM Plus multiplex system for both standard and low copy number (LCN) STR DNA analysis. *Forensic Sci Int.*, 2001 Dec 1, 123(2-3), 215-23.

[96] Taberlet, P; Griffin, S; Goossens, B; Questiau, S; Manceau, V; Escaravage, N; Waits, LP and Bouvet, J. Reliable genotyping of samples with very low DNA quantities using PCR. *Nucleic Acids Res.*, 1996, 24, 3189-3194.

[97] Butler, JM and Hill, CR. Scientific issues with analysis of low amounts of DNA. *Profiles in DNA (Promega)*, 13(1), 2010 Available at http://www.promega.com/profiles/.

[98] Rutty, GN; Hopwood, A and Tucker, V. The effectiveness of protective clothing in the reduction of potential DNA contamination of the scene of crime. *Int. J. Legal Med.*, 2003, 117, 170-174.

[99] Capelli, C; Tschentscher, F; Pascali, VL. "Ancient" protocols for the crime scene? Similarities and differences between forensic genetics and ancient DNA analysis. *Forensic Sci. Int.*, 2003 Jan 9, 131(1), 59-64.

[100] Caragine, T; Mikulasovich, R; Tamariz, J; Bajda, E; Sebestyen, J; Baum, H; Prinz, M. Validation of testing and interpretation protocols for low template DNA samples using AmpFlSTR Identifiler. *Croatian Med. J.* 2009, 50: 250-267

[101] Ballantyne, KN; van Oorschot, RA; Mitchell, RJ. Comparison of two whole genome amplification methods for STR genotyping of LCN and degraded DNA samples. *Forensic Sci. Int.*, 2007 Feb 14, 166(1), 35-41.

[102] Rompler, H; Dear, PH; Krause, J; Meyer, M; Rohland, N; Schoneberg, T; Spriggs, H; Stiller, M; Hofreiter, M. Multiplex amplification of ancient DNA. *Nat. Protoc.*, 2006, 1(2), 720-8.

[103] Kwok, S; Higuchi, R. Avoiding false positives with PCR. *Nature,* 1989 May 18, 339(6221), 237-8.

[104] Bacher, JW; Hennes, LF; Gu, T; Tereba, A; Micka, KA; Sprecher, CJ; Lins, AM; Amiott, EA; Rabbach, DR; Taylor, JA; Helms, C; Donis-Keller, H; Schumm, JW. Proceedings of the Ninth International Symposium on Human Identification. 1999, 24-37. Madison, Wisconsin: Promega Corporation.

[105] Gill, P; Kimpton, CP; Urquhart, A; Oldroyd, N; Millican, ES; Watson, SK; Downes, TJ. Automated short tandem repeat (STR) analysis in forensic casework -a strategy for the future. *Electrophoresis* 1995 Sep., 16(9), 1543-52.

[106] Carracedo, A and Lareu, MV. Proceedings from the NinthInternational Symposium on Human Identification 1998, 89-107. Madison, Wisconsin: Promega Corporation.

[107] Sutovsky, P; Moreno, RD; Ramalho-Santos, J; Dominko, T; Simerly, C; Schatten G. Development: Ubiquitin tag for sperm mitochondria. *Nature* 25 November 1999 402, 371-372.

[108] Gill, P; Ivanov, PL; Kimpton, C; Piercy, R; Benson, N; Tully, G; Evett, I; Hagelberg, E; Sullivan, K. Identification of the remains of the Romanov family by DNA analysis. *Nat. Genet.* 1994, 6, 130–135.

[109] Ivanov, P; Parsons, T; Wadhams, M; Holland, M; Rhoby, R; Weedn, V. Mitochondrial DNA variations in the Hessian lineage: heteroplasmy found in Grand Duke of Russia Georgij Romanov and disputes over authenticity of the remains of Tzar Nicholas II. In: Proceedings of the ISFH, Hakone Simposium on DNA polymorphism. 1996, Hakone, Japan.

[110] Hühne, J; Pfeiffer, H; Brinkmann, B. Heteroplasmic substitutions in the mitochondrial DNA control region in mother and child samples. *Int. J. Legal Med.* 1999, 112, 27-30.

[111] Pfeiffer, H; Hühne, J; Ortmann, C; Waterkamp, K; Brinkmann, B. Mitochondrial DNA typing from human axillary, pubic and head hair shafts – success rates and sequence comparisons. *Int. J. Legal Med.* 1999, 112, 287-290.

[112] Stoneking, M. Hypervariable sites in the mtDNA control region are mutational hotspots. *Am. J. Hum. Genet.* 2000, 67, 1029-1032.

[113] Ginther, C; Issel-Tarver, L; King, MC. Identifying individuals by sequencing mitochondrial DNA from teeth. *Nat. Genet.* 1992, 2, 135-138.

[114] Holland, M; Fisher, DL; Mitchell, LG; Rodriquez, WC; Canik, JJ; Merril, CR; Weedn, VW. Mitochondrial DNA sequence analysis skeletal remains: identification of remains from the Vietnam war. *J. Forensic Sci.* 1993, 38, 542-553.

[115] Butler, JM and Lewin, BC. Forensic applications of mitochondrial DNA. *Focus* 1998, 16, 158-162.

[116] Jehaes, E; Decorte, R; Peneau, A; Petrie, JH; Boiry, PA; Gilissen, A; Moisan, JP; Van den Berghe, H; Pascal, O; Cassiman, JJ. Mitochondrial DNA analysis on remains of a Putative son of Louis XVII, King of France and Marie- Antoniette. *Eur. J. Hum. Genet.* 1998, 6, 383-395.

[117] Caramelli, D; Lalueza-Fox, C; Capelli, C; Lari, M; Sampietro, ML; Gigli, E; Milani, L; Pilli, E; Guimaraes, S; Chiarelli, B; Marin, VT; Casoli, A; Stanyon, R; Bertranpetit, J;

Barbujani, G. Genetic analysis of the skeletal remains attributed to Francesco Petrarca. *Forensic Sci. Int.* 2007 Nov 15;173(1):36-40. Epub 2007 Feb 22.

[118] Cann, RL; Brown, WM; Wilson, AC. Polymorphic sites and the mechanism of evolution in human mitochondrial DNA. *Genetics* 1984, 106, 479-499.

[119] Richards, M; Corte-Real, H; Forster, P; Macaulay, V; Wilkinson, H; Demaine, A; Papiha, S; Hedges, R; Bandelt, HJ; Sykes, B. Paleolithic and Neolithic lineages in the European mitochondrial gene pool. *Am. J. Hum. Genet.* 1996, 59, 185-203.

[120] Stoneking, M and Soodyall, H. Human evolution and the mitochondrial genome. *Curr. Opin. Genet .Dev.* 1996,6, 731-736.

[121] Cavalli-Sforza, LL. The DNA revolution in population genetics. *Trends Genet.* 1998, 14, 60-65.

[122] Stone, A and Stoneking, M. mtDNA analysis of a prehistoric Oneota population: implications for the peopling of the New World. *Am. J. Hum. Genet.* 1998,62, 1153-1170.

[123] Caramelli, D; Lalueza-Fox, C; Vernesi, C; Lari, M; Casoli, A; Mallegni, F; Chiarelli, B; Dupanloup, I; Bertranpetit, J; Barbujani, G; Bertorelle, G. Evidence for a genetic discontinuity between Neandertals and 24,000-year-old anatomically modern Europeans. *Proc Natl Acad Sci U S A.* 2003 May 27, 100(11), 6593-7.

[124] Vernesi, C, Caramelli, ., Dupanloup, ., Bertorelle, ., Lari, ., Cappellini, ., Moggi-Cecchi, Chiarelli, B; Castri, L; Casoli, A; Mallegni, F; Lalueza-Fox, C; Barbujani, G. The Etruscans: a population-genetic study. *Am. J. Hum. Genet* 2004 Apr, 74(4), 694-704.

[125] Eichmann, C and Parson, W. "Mitominis": multiplex PCR analysis of reduced size amplicons for compound sequence analysis of the entire mtDNA control region in highly degraded samples. *Int. J. Legal Med.*, 2008 Sep, 122(5):385-8. Epub 2008 Mar 28.

[126] Berger, C and Parson, W. Mini-midi-mito: adapting the amplification and sequencing strategy of mtDNA to the degradation state of crime scene samples. *Forensic Sci Int Genet.*, 2009 Jun, 3(3):149-53. Epub 2009 Feb 27.

[127] Berger, B, et al. Forensic canine STR analysis. In Coyle, H.M. (ed.) Nonhuman DNA Typing: Theory and Casework Applications. Boca Raton: CRC Press; Chapter 4 2008,. pp. 45-68.

[128] Brauner, P; Reshef, A; Gorsky, A. DNA profiling of trace evidence —mitigating evidence in a dog biting case. *Journal of Forensic Sciences* 2001, 46, 1232-1234.

[129] Clarke, M and Vandenberg, N. Dog attack: the application of canine DNA profiling in forensic casework. *Forensic Science, Medicine, and Pathology* 2010, 6, 151-157.

[130] Dayton, M; Koskinen, MT; Tom, BK; Mattila AM; Johnston, E; Halverson, J; Fantin, D; DeNise, S; Budowle, B; Smith, DG; Kanthaswamy, S. Developmental validation of short tandem repeat reagent kit for forensic DNA profiling of canine biological material. *Croatian Medical Journal* 2009,50, 268-285.

[131] DeNise, S; Johnston, E; Halverson, J; Marshall, K; Rosenfeld, D; McKenna, S; Sharp, T; Edwards, J. Power of exclusion for parentage verification and probability of match for identity in American Kennel Club breeds using 17 canine microsatellite markers. *Animal Genetics* 2004,35, 14-17.

[132] Eichmann, C; Berger, B; Parson, W. A proposed nomenclature for 15 canine-specific polymorphic STR loci for forensic purposes. *International Journal of Legal Medicine* 2004,*118*, 249-266.

[133] Eichmann, C; Berger, B; Reinhold, M; Lutz, M; Parson, W. Canine-specific STR typing of saliva traces on dog bite wounds. *International Journal of Legal Medicine* 2004,*118*, 337-342.

[134] Eichmann, C; Berger, B, Steinlechner, M; Parson, W. Estimating the probability of identity in a random dog population using 15 highly polymorphic canine STR markers. *Forensic Science International* 2005,*151*, 37-44.

[135] Halverson, J, et al. Microsatellite sequences for canine genotyping. U.S. Patent 1999, 5, 874, 217.

[136] Halverson, J and Basten, C. A PCR multiplex and database for forensic DNA identification of dogs. *Journal of Forensic Sciences* 2005, *50*, 352-363.

[137] Hellmann, AP; Rohleder, U; Eichmann, C; Pfeiffer, I; Parson, W; Schleenbecker, U. A proposal for standardization in forensic canine DNA typing: allele nomenclature of six canine-specific STR loci. *Journal of Forensic Sciences* 2006,*51*, 274-281.

[138] Ichikawa, Y; Takagi, K, Tsumagari, S; Ishihama, K; Morita, M; Kanemaki, M; Takeishi, M; Takahashi, H. Canine parentage testing based on microsatellite polymorphisms. *Journal of Veterinary Medicine and Science* 2001,*63*, 1209-1213.

[139] Kanthaswamy, S. Development and validation of a standardized canine STR panel for use in forensic casework. Final report for NIJ Grant 2009, 2004-DN-BX-K007. Available at http://www.ncjrs.gov/pdffiles1/nij/grants/226639.pdf.

[140] Kanthaswamy, S; Tom, BK; Mattila, AM; Johnston, E; Dayton, M; Erickson, BJ, Halverson, J; Fantin, D; DeNise, S; Kou, A; Malladi, V; Satkoski, J; Budowle, B; Smith, DG; Koskinen, MT. Canine population data generated from a multiplex STR kit for use in forensic casework. *Journal of Forensic Sciences* 2009, *54*, 829-840.

[141] Koskinen, MT and Bredbacka, P. A convenient and efficient microsatellite-based assay for resolving parentages in dogs. *Animal Genetics* 1999,*30*, 148-149.

[142] Muller, S; Flekna, G; Muller, M; Brem, G. Use of canine microsatellite polymorphisms in forensic examinations. *Journal of Heredity* 1999,*90*, 55-56.

[143] Pádár, Z; Angayal, M; Egyed, B; Füredi, S; Woller, J; Zöldág, L; Fekete, S. Canine microsatellite polymorphisms as the resolution of an illegal animal death case in a Hungarian zoological gardens. *International Journal of Legal Medicine* 2001,*115*, 79-81.

[144] Pádár, Z; Egyed, B; Kontadakis, K; Füredi, S; Woller, J; Zöldág, L; Fekete, S. Canine STR analyses in forensic practice: observation of a possible mutation in a dog hair. *International Journal of Legal Medicine* 2002, *116*, 286-288.

[145] Shutler, GG; Gagnon, P; Verret, G; Kalyn, H; Korkosh, S; Johnston, E; Halverson, J. Removal of a PCR inhibitor and resolution of DNA STR types in mixed human-canine stains from a five year old case. *Journal of Forensic Sciences* 1999, *44*, 623-626.

[146] Sundqvist, AK; Ellegren, H; Vilà, C. Wolf or dog? Genetic identification of predators from saliva collected around bite wounds on prey. *Conservation Genetics* 2008,*9*, 1275-1279.

[147] Sutter, NB and Ostrander, EA. Dog star rising: the canine genetic system. *Nature Reviews Genetics* 2004,*5*, 900-910.

[148] Tom, BK; Koskinen, MT; Dayton, M; Mattila, AM; Johnston, E; Fantin, D; Denise, S; Spear, T; Smith, DG; Satkoski, J; Budowle, B. Development of a nomenclature system for a canine STR multiplex reagent kit. *Journal of Forensic Sciences* 2010, *55,* 597-604.

[149] van Asch, B; Alves, C; Gusmão, L; Pereira, V; Pereira, F; Amorim, A. A new autosomal STR nineplex for canine identification and parentage testing. *Electrophoresis* 2009,*30,* 417-423.

[150] van Asch, B; Alves, C; Santos, L; Pinheiro, R; Pereira, F; Gusmão, L; Amorim, A. Genetic profiles and sex identification of found-dead wolves determined by the use of an 11-loci PCR multiplex. *Forensic Science International: Genetics* 2010, *4,* 68–72.

[151] van Asch, B; Pinheiro, R; Pereira, R; Alves, C; Pereira, V; Pereira, F; Gusmão, L; Amorim, A. A framework for the development of STR genotyping in domestic animal species: characterization and population study of 12 canine X-chromosome loci. *Electrophoresis* 2010, *31,* 303-308.

[152] Zenke, P; Egyed, B; Zöldág, L; Pádár, Z. Population genetic study in Hungarian canine populations using forensically informative STR loci. *Forensic Science International: Genetics* 2011, *5,* e31-e3.

[153] Menotti-Raymond, MA; David, VA; Wachter, LA; Butler, JM; O'Brien, SJ. An STR forensic typing system for genetic individualization of domestic cat (*Felis catus*) samples. *J. Forensic Sci* 2005,50(5): 1061-1070.

[154] Butler, JM; David, VA; O'Brien, SJ; Menotti-Raymond, M. The MeowPlex: a new DNA test using tetranucleotide STR markers for the domestic cat. *Profiles in DNA* 2002, Promega Corporation, Volume 5, No. 2, pp. 7–10.

[155] Barendse, W; Armitage, SM; Kossarek, LM; Kirkpatrick, BW; Ryan, AM; Clayton, D; Li, L; Neibergs, HL; Zhang, N, et al. A genetic linkage map of the bovine genome. *Nature Genetics* 1994, 6: 227-35.

[156] Baylor College of Medicine Human Genome Sequencing Center. (2006) Bovine Whole Genome Assembly release Btau_3.1.

[157] Bishop, MD; Kappes, SM, Keele, JW; Stone, RT; Sunden, SL, Hawkins, GA; Toldo, SS; Fries, R; Grosz, MD; Yoo, J, et al. A genetic linkage map for cattle. *Genetics* 1994,136: 619-639.

[158] Brezinsky, L; Kemp, SJ; Teale, AJ. ILSTS006: a polymorphic bovine microsatellite. *Animal Genetics* 1993,24: 73.

[159] Budowle, B; Garofano, P; Hellman, A; Ketchum, M; Kanthaswamy, S; Parson W; van Haeringen, W; Fain, S; Broad, T. Recommendations for animal DNA forensic and identity testing. *Int. J. Legal Med* 2005, 119: 295-302.

[160] Georges, M and Massey, J. Polymorphic DNA markers in Bovidae. World Intellectual Property Organization. Geneva (Patent application WO PUBL NO 92/13102) 1992.

[161] Solinas-Toldo, S; Fries, R; Steffen, P; Neibergs, HL; Barendse, W; Womack, JE; Hetzel, DJ; Stranzinger, G. Physically mapped, cosmid-derived microsatellite markers as anchor loci on bovine chromosomes. *Mammalian Genome* 1993,4: 720-727.

[162] Steffen, P; Eggen, A; Dietz, AB; Womack, JE; Stranzinger, G; Fries, R. Isolation and mapping of polymorphic microsatellites in cattle. *Animal Genetics* 1993,24: 121.

[163] Sunden, SLF; Stone, RT; Bishop, MD; Kappes, SM; Keele, JW; Beattie, CW. A highly polymorphic bovine microsatellite locus: BM2113. *Animal Genetics* 1993,24: 69.

[164] Thieven, U; Solinas-Toldo, S; Friedl, R; Masabanda, J; Fries, R; Barendse, W; Simon, D; Harlizius, B. Polymorphic CA-microsatellites for the integration of the bovine genetic and physical map. *Mammalian Genome* 1997, 8: 52.

[165] Vaiman, D; Mercier, D; Moazami-Goudarzi, K, Eggen, A; Ciampolini, R, Lépingle, A; Velmala, R; Kaukinen, J; Varvio, SL; Martin, P; et al. A set of 99 cattle microsatellites: characterization, synteny mapping, and polymorphism. *Mammalian Genome* 1994, 5: 288-297.

[166] van de Goor, LHP and van Haeringen, WA. Identification of stolen cattle using 22 microsatellite markers. *Nonhuman DNA Typing: Theory and Casework Applications* (edited by Heather Miller Coyle). CRC Press: Boca Raton, FL 2007, pp 122-123.

[167] van de Goor, LHP; Panneman, H; van Haeringen, WA. A proposal for standardization in forensic bovine DNA typing: allele nomenclature of 16 cattle-specific short tandem repeat loci. *Animal Genetics* 2009, 40: 630-636.

[168] van de Goor, LHP; Koskinen, MT; van Haeringen, WA. Population studies of 16 bovine STR loci for forensic purposes. *Int J Legal Med* 2011 Jan;125(1):111-9. Epub 2009 Jun 9.

[169] Tobe SS and Linacre A. DNA typing in wildlife crime: recent developments in species identification. *Forensic Sci Med Pathol*, 2010 6:195-206.

[170] Clayton DA. Replication of animal mitochondrial-DNA. *Cell* 1982, 28(4):693-705.

[171] Hayashi, JI; Tagashira, Y; Yoshida, MC. Absence of extensive recombination between interspecies and intraspecies mitochondrial-dna in mammalian-cells. *Expl Cell Res* 1985, 160(2):387-395.

[172] Pereira SL. Mitochondrial genome organization and vertebrate phylogenetics. *Genetics Molec Biol* 2000, 23:745-752.

[173] Robin, ED and Wong, R. Mitochondrial-DNA molecules and virtual number of mitochondria per cell in mammalian-cells. *J Cell Physiol* 1988, 136(3):507-513.

[174] Pfeiffer, H; Benthaus, S; Rolf, B; Brnkmann, B. The Kaiser's tooth. *Int J Legal Med* 2003, 117(2):118-120.

[175] Ginther, C; Isseltarvern, L; King, MC. Identifying individuals by sequencing mitochondrial-DNA from teeth. *Nature Genetics* 1992, 2(2):135-138.

[176] Loreille, OM; Degoli, TM; Irwin, JA; Coble, MD; Parsons, TJ. High efficiency DNA extraction from bone by total demineralization. *Forensic Sci Int-Genetics* 2007, 1(2):191-195.

[177] Anslinger, K; Weichhold, G; Keil, W; Bayer, B; Eisenmeger, W. Identification of the skeletal remains of Martin Bormann by mtDNA analysis. *Int J Legal Med* 2001, 114(3):194-196.

[178] Parson, W. Relevance of mtDNA analysis for forensic applications. *Rechtsmedizin* 2009, 19(3):183-192.

[179] Allen, M; Saldeen, T; Pettersson, U; Gyllensten, U. Mitochondrial DNA sequencing of shed hairs and saliva on robbery caps: Sensitivity and matching probabilities. *J Forensic Sci* 1998, 43(3):453-464).

[180] Brown, WM; George, M; Wilson, AC. Rapid evolution of animal mitochondrial-DNA. *Proc Natl Acad Sci USA* 1979, 76(4):1967-1971.

[181] Kuwayama, R; Ozawa, T. Phylogenetic relationships among European Red Deer, Wapiti, and Sika Deer inferred from mitochondrial DNA sequences. *Molec Phylogenetics Evolution* 2000, 15(1):115-123.

[182] Irwin, D; Kocher, T; Wilson, A. Evolution of the cytochrome b gene of mammals. *J Molec Evolution* 1991, 32(2):128-144.

[183] Kocher, TD; Thomas, WK; Meyer, A; Edwards, SV; Pääbo, S; Villablanca, FX; Wilson, AC. Dynamics of mitochondrial DNA evolution in animals: amplification and sequencing with conserved primers. *Proc Natl Acad Sci USA* 1989, 86(16):6196-6200.

[184] Tobe, SS and Linacre, A. A method to identify a large number of mammalian species in the UK from trace samples and mixtures without the use of sequencing. *Forensic Sci Int: Genetics Suppl Series* 2008, 1(1):625-627.

[185] An, J; Lee, MY; Min, MS; Lee, MH; Lee, H. A molecular genetic approach for species identification of mammals and sex determination of birds in a forensic case of poaching from South Korea. *Forensic Sci Int* 2007, 167(1):59-61.

[186] Tobe, SS and Linacre, A. Species identification of human and deer from mixed biological material. *Forensic Sci Int* 2007, 169(2-3):278-279.

[187] de Pancorbo, MM; Castro, A; Fernandez-Fernandez, I; Gonzalez-Fernandez, MC; Martnez-Bouzas, C; Cuevas, N. Cytochrome b and HVI sequences of mitochondrial DNA to identify domestic animal hair in forensic casework. *Int Congress Series* 2003, 1239:841-845.

[188] Wan, QH and Fang, SG. Application of species-specific polymerase chain reaction in the forensic identification of tiger species. *Forensic Sci Int* 2003, 131(1):75-78.

[189] Wetton, JH; Tsang, CS; Roney, CA; Spriggs, AC. An extremely sensitive species-specific ARMs PCR test for the presence of tiger bone DNA. *Forensic Sci Int* 2004, 140(1):139-145.

[190] Tobe, SS and Linacre, A. Identifying endangered species from degraded mixtures at low levels. *Forensic Sci Int: Genetics Suppl Series* 2009, 2(1):304-305.

[191] Moore, MK; Bemss, JA; Rce, SM; Quattro, JM; Woodley, CM. Use of restriction fragment length polymorphisms to identify sea turtle eggs and cooked meats to species. *Conservation Genetics* 2003, 4(1):95-103.

[192] Hsieh, HM; Huang, LH; Tsai, LC; Liu, CL; Kuo, YC; Hsiao, CT; Linacre, A; Lee, JC. Species identification of Kachuga tecta using the cytochrome b gene. *J Forensic Sci* 2006, 51(1):52-56.

[193] Rohilla, MS and Tiwari, PK. Restriction fragment length polymorphism of mitochondrial DNA and phylogenetic relationships among five species of Indian freshwater turtles. *J Appl Genetics* 2008, 49(2):167-182.

[194] Meganathan, PR; Dubey, B; Haque, I. Molecular identification of crocodile species using novel primers for forensic analysis. *Conservation Genetics* 2009, 10(3):767-770.

[195] Hsieh, HM; Huang, LH; Tsai, LC; Kuo, YC; Meng, HH; Linacre, A; Lee, JC. Species identification of rhinoceros horns using the cytochrome b gene. *Forensic Sci Int* 2003, 136(1-3):1-11.

[196] Gupta, SK; Verma, SK; Singh, L. Molecular insight into a wildlife crime: the case of a peafowl slaughter. *Forensic Sci Int* 2005, 154(2-3):214-217).

[197] Hebert, PD; Cywinska, A; Ball, S; deWaard, JR. Biological identifications through DNA barcodes. *Proc Roy Soc B: Biolog Sci* 2003, 270(1512):313-321.

[198] Borisenko, AV; Lim, BK; Ivanova, NV; Hanner, RH; Herbert, PDN. DNA barcoding in surveys of small mammal communities: a field study in Suriname. *Molec Ecol Res* 2008, 8(3):471-479).

[199] Hebert, PDN; Ratnasingham, S; deWaard, JR. Barcoding animal life: cytochrome c oxidase subunit 1 divergences among closely related species. Proc. R. Soc. Lond. B (Suppl.) 2003, 270: S96-S99.

[200] Meier, R; Shiyang, K; Vaidya, G; Ng, PK. DNA barcoding and taxonomy in diptera: A tale of high intraspecific variability and low identification success. *Systematic Biology* 2006, 55(5):715-728.

[201] Janzen, DH; Hajibabaei, M; Burns, JM; Hallwachs, W; Remigio, E; Hebert, PD. Wedding biodiversity inventory of a large and complex Lepidoptera fauna with DNA barcoding. *Phil Trans Roy Soc B-Biolog Sci* 2005, 360(1462):1835-1845.

[201] Hajibabaei, M; Janzen, DH; Burns, JM; Hallwachs, W; Hebert, PD. DNA barcodes distinguish species of tropical Lepidoptera. *Proc Natl Acad Sci USA* 2006, 103(4):968-971.

[202] Rojo Velsco, S; Ståhls, G; Pérez Baňón, C; Marcos Garcia, MA. Testing molecular barcodes: Invariant mitochondrial DNA sequences vs the larval and adult morphology of West Palaearctic Pandasyopthalmus species (Diptera : Syrphidae : Paragini). *Eur J Entomol* 2006, 103(2):443-458.

[203] Smith, MA; Woodley, NE; Janzen, DH; Hallwachs, W; Hebert, PD. DNA barcodes reveal cryptic host-specificity within the presumed polyphagous members of a genus of parasitoid flies (Diptera : Tachinidae). *Proc Natl Acad Sci USA* 2006, 103(10):3657-3662.

[204] Cywinska, A; Hunter, FF; Hebert, PDN. Identifying Canadian mosquito species through DNA barcodes. *Med Vet Entomol* 2006, 20(4):413-424.

[205] Nelson, LA; Wallman, JF; Dowton, M. Using COI barcodes to identify forensically and medically important blowflies. *Med Vet Entomol* 2007, 21(1):44-52.

[206] Mitchell, A. DNA barcoding demystified. *Australian J Entomol* 2008, 47:169-173).

[207] Smith, MA; Poyarkov, NA; Hebert, PDN. CO1 DNA barcoding amphibians: take the chance, meet the challenge. *Molec Ecol Res* 2008, 8(2):235-246.

[208] Holmes, BH; Steinke, D; Ward RD. Identification of shark and ray fins using DNA barcoding. *Fisheries Res* 2009, 95(2-3):280-288.

[209] Hebert, PDN; Stoeckle, MY; Zemlak, TS; Francis, CM. Identification of birds through DNA barcodes. *Plos Biol* 2004, 2(10):1657-1663.

[210] Yoo, HS; Eah, JY; Kim, JS; Kim, YJ; Min, MS; Paek, WK; Lee, H; Kim, CB. DNA barcoding Korean birds. *Molec Cells* 2006, 22(3):323-327.

[211] Tavares, ES and Baker, AJ. Single mitochondrial gene barcodes reliably identify sister-species in diverse clades of birds. *BMC Evolutionary Biol* 2008, 8:81.

[212] Lohman, DJ; Prawiradilaga, DM; Meier, R. Improved COI barcoding primers for Southeast Asian perching birds (Aves: Passeriformes). *Molec Ecol Res* 2009, 9(1):37-40.

[213] Wong, EHK; Shivji, MS; Hanner, RH. Identifying sharks with DNA barcodes: assessing the utility of a nucleotide diagnostic approach. *Molec Ecol Res* 2009, 9:243-256.

[214] Huang, J; Qin Xu; Zhen Jun Sun, Gui Lau Tang. Identifying earthworms through DNA barcodes. *Pedobiologia* 2007, 51(4):301-309.

[215] Dalton, DL; Kotze, A. DNA barcoding as a tool for species identification in three forensic wildlife cases in South Africa. Forensic Sci Int. 2011 Apr 15;207(1-3):e51-4. Epub 2011 Jan 28.

[216] Guo, H; Wang, W; Yang, N; Guo, B; Zhang, S; Yang, R; Yuan, Y; Yu, J; Hu, S; Sun, Q; Yu J. DNA barcoding provides distinction between Radix Astragali and its adulterants. *Sci China Life Sci* 2010 Aug;53(8):992-9. Epub 2010 Sep 7.

[217] Tyagi, A; Bag, SK; Shukla, V; Roy, S; Tuli, R. Oligonucleotide frequencies of barcoding loci can discriminate species across kingdoms. *PLoS One* 2010 Aug 20;5(8):e12330.

[218] Botti, S and Giuffra, E. Oligonucleotide indexing of DNA barcodes: identification of tuna and other scombrid species in food products. *BMC Biotechnol* 2010 Aug 23;10:60.

[219] Bruni, I; De Mattia, F; Galimberti, A; Galasso, G; Banfi, E; Casiraghi, M; Labra, M. Identification of poisonous plants by DNA barcoding approach. *Int J Legal Med* 2010 Nov;124(6):595-603. Epub 2010 Mar 31

[220] Boehme, P; Amendt, J, Disney, RH; Zehner, R. . Molecular identification of carrion-breeding scuttle flies (Diptera: Phoridae) using COI barcodes. *Int J Legal Med* 2010 Nov;124(6):577-81. Epub 2010 Mar 2.

[221] Ferri, G; Alù, M; Corradini, B; Beduschi, G. Forensic botany: species identification of botanical trace evidence using a multigene barcoding approach. *Int J Legal Med* 2009 Sep;123(5):395-401. Epub 2009 Jun 7.

[222] Balitzki-Korte, B; Anslinger, K; Bartsch, C; Rolf, B. Species identification by means of pyrosequencing the mitochondrial 12S rRNA gene. *Int J Legal Med* 2005;119(5):291–294. 200.

[223] Melton, T and Holland, C. Routine forensic use of the mitochondrial 12S ribosomal RNA gene for species identification. *J Forensic Sci* 2007;52(6):1305–1307.

[224] Kitano, T; Umetsu, K; Tian, W, Osawa, M. Two universal primer sets for species identification among vertebrates. *Int J Legal Med* 2007 Sep;121(5):423-7. Epub 2006 Jul 15.

[225] Mitani, T; Akane, A; Tokiyasu, T; Yoshimura, S; Okii, Y, Yoshida, M. Identification of animal species using the partial sequences in the mitochondrial 16S rRNA gene. *Leg Med (Tokyo)* 2009;11(Suppl 1):S449–S450.

[226] Imaizumi, K; Akutsu, T, Miyasaka, S; Yoshino, M. Development of species identification tests targeting the 16S ribosomal RNA coding region in mitochondrial DNA. *Int J Legal Med* 2007 May;121(3):184-91. Epub 2006 Nov 16.

[227] Gurdeep, R, Mahesh, SD; Sandeep, W; Ashutosh, K; Milind, SP; Yogesh, S. Shouche Species identification and authentication of tissues of animal origin using mitochondrial and nuclear markers. *Meat Science* Volume 76, Issue 4, August 2007, Pages 666-674.

[228] Mitani, T, Akane, A, Tokiyasu, T; Yoshimura, S, Okii, Y; Yoshida, M. Identification of animal species using the partial sequences in the mitochondrial 16S rRNA gene. *Leg Med (Tokyo)* 2009, 11(Suppl 1):S449–S450.

[229] Imaizumi, K; Akutsu, T; Miyasaka, S; Yoshino, M. Development of species identification tests targeting the 16S ribosomal RNA coding region in mitochondrial DNA. *Int J Legal Med* 2007 May;121(3):184-91. Epub 2006 Nov 16.

[230] Gurdeep R; Mahesh, SD; Sandeep, W; Ashutosh, K; Milind SP; Yogesh, S. Shouche Species identification and authentication of tissues of animal origin using mitochondrial and nuclear markers. *Meat Science* Volume 76, Issue 4, August 2007, Pages 666-674.

[231] Schwenke, PL; Rhydderch, JG; Ford, MJ; Marshall, AR; Park, LK. Forensic identification of endangered Chinook Salmon (Oncorhynchus tshawytscha) using a multilocus SNP assay. *Conservation Genetics* 2006;7(6):983–989.

[232] Junqueira, AC; Lessinger, AC; Torres, TT; da Silva, FR; Vettore, AL, Arruda, P; Azeredo Espin, AM. The mitochondrial genome of the blowfly Chrysomya chloropyga (Diptera: Calliphoridae). *Gene* 2004;339:7–15.

[233] Mayer, F; Dietz, C; Kiefer, A. Molecular species identification boosts bat diversity. *Frontiers Zoology* 2007;4(1):4.

[234] Clifford, SL; Anthony, NM, Bawe-Johnson, M; Abernethy, KA; Tutin, CE; White, LJ; Bermejo, M; Goldsmith, ML; McFarland, K; Jeffery, KJ; et al. Mitochondrial DNA phylogeography of western lowland gorillas (Gorilla gorilla gorilla). *Molec Ecol* 2004;13(6):1551–1565.

[235] Zhang, W; Zhang, Z; Shen, F; Hou, R, Lv, X; Yue, B. Highly conserved D-loop-like nuclear mitochondrial sequences (Numts) in tiger (Panthera tigris). *J Genetics* 2006;85(2):107–116.

[236] Himmelberger, AL; Spear, TF; Satkoski, JA, George, DA; Garnica, WT; Malladi, VS, Smith, DG; Webb, KM; Allard, MW; Kanthaswamy, S. Forensic utility of the mitochondrial hypervariable region 1 of domestic dogs, in conjunction with breed and geographic information. *J Forensic Sci* 2008 Jan;53(1):81-9.

[237] Eichmann, C and Parson, W. Molecular characterization of the canine mitochondrial DNA control region for forensic applications. *Int J Legal Med* 2007 Sep;121(5):411-6. Epub 2007 Jan 12.

[238] Schneider, PM; Seo, Y; Rittner, C. Forensic mtDNA hair analysis excludes a dog from having caused a traffic incident. *Int. J. Legal Med* 1999, 112:315-316.

[239] Pun, K-M; Albrecht, C; Castella, V; Fumagalli, L. Species identification in mammals from mixed biological samples based on mitochondrial DNA control region length polymorphism. *Electrophoresis* 2009;30(6):1008–14.

[240] Gupta, SK; Thangaraj, K; Singh, L. A simple and inexpensive molecular method for sexing and identification of the forensic samples of elephant origin. *J Forensic Sci* 2006;51(4):805–7.

[241] Kitano, T; Umetsu, K; Tian, W; Osawa, M. Two universal primer sets for species identification among vertebrates. *Int J Leg Med* 2007;121(5):423–7.

[242] Kocher, TD; Thomas, WK; Meyer, A; Edwards, SV; Paabo, S; Villablanca, FX; et al. Dynamics of mitochondrial DNA evolution in animals: amplification and sequencing with conserved primers. *Proc Natl Acad Sci USA* 1989;86(16):6196–200.

[243] Nussbaumer, C and Korschineck, I. Non-human mtDNA helps to exculpate a suspect in a homicide case. *Int Congr Ser* 2006;1288:136–8.

[244] Fumagalli, L; Cabrita, CJ; Castella, V. Simultaneous identification of multiple mammalian species from mixed forensic samples based on mtDNA control region length polymorphism. *Forensic Sci Int Genet Sup* 2009;2(1):302–3.

[245] Dawnay, N; Ogden, R; McEwing, R; Carvalho, GR; Thorpe, RS. Validation of the barcoding gene COI for use in forensic genetic species identification. *Forensic Sci Int* 2007 Nov 15;173(1):1-6. Epub 2007 Feb 14.

[246] Tobe, SS and Linacre, AMT. A multiplex assay to identify 18 European mammal species from mixtures using the mitochondrial *cytochrome b* gene. *Electrophoresis* 2008, 29(2)::340-7.

[247] Alvarez-Iglesias, V; Jaime, JC; Carracedo, A; Salas, A. Coding region mitochondrial DNA SNPs: Targeting East Asian and Native American haplogroups. *Forensic Sci Int Genet* 2007; 1(1):44–55.94.
[248] Sanchez, JJ; Børsting, C; Balogh, K; Berger, B; Bogus, M; Butler, JM; et al. Forensic typing of autosomal SNPs with a 29 SNPmultiplex—Results of a collaborative EDNAP exercise. *Forensic Sci Int Genet* 2008;2(3):176–83. 95.
[249] Volgyi, A; Zalan, A; Szvetnik, E; Pamjav, H. Hungarian population data for 11 Y-STR and 49 Y-SNP markers. *Forensic Sci Int Genet* 2009;3(2):e27–8. 96.
[250] Westen, AA; Matai, AS; Laros, JFJ; Meiland, HC; Jasper, M; de Leeuw, WJF; et al. Tri-allelic SNP markers enable analysis of mixed and degraded DNA samples. *Forensic Sci Int Genet* 2009;3(4):233–41. 97.
[251] Mosquera-Miguel, A; Alvarez-Iglesias, V; Cerezo, M; Lareu, MV; Carracedo, A; Salas, A. Testing the performance of mtSNP minisequencing in forensic samples. *Forensic Sci Int Genet* 2009;3(4):261–4. 98.
[252] Grignani, P; Turchi, C; Achilli, A; Peloso, G; Alù, M; Ricci, U; et al. Multiplex mtDNA coding region SNP assays for molecular dissection of haplogroups U/K and J/T. *Forensic Sci Int Genet* 2009;4(1):21–5. 99.
[253] Børsting, C; Rockenbauer, E; Morling, N. Validation of a single nucleotide polymorphism (SNP) typing assay with 49 SNPs for forensic genetic testing in a laboratory accredited according to the ISO 17025 standard. *Forensic Sci Int Genet* 2009;4(1):34–42. 100.
[254] Krjutskov, K; Viltrop, T; Palta, P; Metspalu, E; Tamm, E; Suvi, S; et al. Evaluation of the 124-plex SNP typing microarray for forensic testing. *Forensic Sci Int Genet* 2009;4(1):43–8. 101.
[255] Dixon, LA; Murray, CM; Archer, EJ; Dobbins, AE; Koumi, P; Gill, P. Validation of a 21-locus autosomal SNP multiplex for forensic identification purposes. *Forensic Sci Int* 2005;154(1): 62–77. 102.
[256] Heaton, MP; Harhay, GP; Bennett, GL; Stone, RT; Grosse, WM; Casas, E. Selection and use of SNP markers for animal identification and paternity analysis in U.S. beef cattle. *Mamm Genome* 2002;13(5):272–81. 103.
[257] Andreassen, R; Hagen-Larsen, H; Sanchez-Ramos, I; Lunner, S; Høyheim, B. STR and bi-allelic polymorphisms in Atlantic salmon: Tools for tracing large scale escapees from salmon farms. *Forensic Sci Int Genet Sup* 2008;1(1):586–8. 104.
[258] Sato, I; Nakaki, S; Murata, K; Takeshita, H; Mukai, T. Forensic hair analysis to identify animal species on a case of pet animal abuse. *Int J Leg Med* 2010;124(3):249–56. 105.
[259] Martinsohn, JT; Ogden, R. FishPopTrace—Developing SNP based population genetic assignment methods to investigate illegal fishing. *Forensic Sci Int Genet Sup* 2009;2(1):294–6.
[260] Shin-ichi, N; Daiki, H; Miki, M; Hideki, N; Hiroyuki, M; Toshio, M; Koji, I. Study of animal species (human, dog and cat) identification using a multiplex single-base primer extension reaction in the cytochrome *b* gene. *Forensic Sci. Int* Volume 173, Issues 2-3, 20 December 2007, Pages 97-102.
[261] Sato, I; Nakaki, S; Murata, K; Takeshita, H; Mukai, T. Forensic hair analysis to identify animal species on a case of pet animal abuse. *Int J Legal Med* 2010 May;124(3):249-56. Epub 2009 Nov 18.

[262] Köhnemann, S and Pfeiffer, H. Application of mtDNA SNP analysis in forensic casework. *Forensic Sci Int Genet* 2010 Feb 18. [Epub ahead of print]).

[263] Brand, A; Brand, H; Schulte in den Baumen, T. The impact of genetics and genomics on public health. *Eur J Hum Genet* 2008; 16:5–13.

[264] Janssens, AC and van Duijn, CM. Genome-based prediction of common diseases: advances and prospects. *Hum Mol Genet* 2008; 17:166–173).

[265] Kayser, M and Schneider, PM. DNA-based prediction of human externally visible characteristics in forensics: motivations, scientific challenges, and ethical considerations. *Forensic Sci Int Genet* 2009; 3:154–161.

[266] Eiberg, H; Troelsen, J, Nielsen, M; Mikkelsen, A; Mengel-From, J; Kjaer, KW; Hansen, L. Blue eye color in humans may be caused by a perfectly associated founder mutation in a regulatory element located within the HERC2 gene inhibiting OCA2 expression. *Hum Genet* 2008; 123:177–187.

[267] Frudakis, T; Thomas, M; Gaskin, Z; Venkateswarlu, K, Chandra, KS, Ginjupalli, S; Gunturi, S; Natrajan, S; Ponnuswamy, VK; Ponnuswamy, KN. Sequences associated with human iris pigmentation. *Genetics* 2003; 165:2071–2083

[268] Graf, J; Hodgson, R; van Daal, A. Single nucleotide polymorphisms in the MATP gene are associated with normal human pigmentation variation. *Hum Mutat* 2005; 25:278–284.

[269] Han, J; Kraft, P; Nan, H; Guo, Q; Chen, C; Qureshi, A; Hankinson, SE; Hu, FB; Duffy, DL; Zhao, ZZ; Martin, NG; Montgomery, GW; Hayward, NK; Thomas, G; Hoover, RN; Chanock, S, Hunter, DJ. A genome-wide association study identifies novel alleles associated with hair color and skin pigmentation. *PLoS Genet* 2008 May 16;4(5):e1000074.

[270] Kanetsky, PA; Swoyer, J; Panossian, S; Holmes, R; Guerry, D; Rebbeck, TR. A polymorphism in the agouti signaling protein gene is associated with human pigmentation. *Am J Hum Genet* 2002; 70:770–775.

[271] Kayser, M; Liu, F; Janssens, AC; Rivadeneira, F; Lao, O; van Duijn, K; Vermeulen, M; Arp, P; Jhamai, MM; van Ijcken, WF; et al. Three genome-wide association studies and a linkage analysis identify HERC2 as a human iris color gene. *Am J Hum Genet* 2008; 82:411–423.

[272] Liu, F, Wollstein, A; Hysi, PG; Ankra-Badu, GA; Spector, TD; Park, D; Zhu, G; Larsson, M; Duffy, DL, Montgomery, GW; et al. Digital quantification of human eye color highlights genetic association of three new loci. *PLoS Genet* 2010; 6:e1000934.

[273] Rebbeck, TR; Kanetsky, PA; Walker, AH; Holmes, R; Halpern, AC; Schuchter, LM; Elder, DE; Guerry, D. P gene as an inherited biomarker of human eye color. *Cancer Epidemiol Biomarkers Prev* 2002; 11:782–784.

[274] Sulem ,P; Gudbjartsson, DF; Stacey, SN; Helgason, A; Rafnar, T; Magnusson, KP; Manolescu, A; Karason, A; Palsson, A; Thorleifsson, G; et al. Genetic determinants of hair, eye and skin pigmentation in Europeans. *Nat Genet* 2007; 39:1443–1452)

[275] Wojciech Branicki, Fan Liu, Kate van Duijn, Jolanta Draus-Barini, Ewelina Pospiech, Susan Walsh, Tomasz Kupiec, Anna Wojas-Pelc, Manfred Kayser. Model-based prediction of human hair color using DNA variants. *Hum Genet* 2011 Apr;129(4):443-54. Epub 2011 Jan 4.

[276] Han, J; Kraft, P; Nan, H; Guo, Q; Chen, C; Qureshi, A; Hankinson, SE; Hu, FB; Duffy, DL; Zhao, ZZ; Martin, NG; Montgomery, GW; Hayward, NK; Thomas, G; Hoover,

RN; Chanock, S; Hunter, DJ. A genome-wide association study identifies novel alleles associated with hair color and skin pigmentation. *PLoS Genet* 2008; 4:e1000074.

[277] Sulem, P; Gudbjartsson, DF; Stacey, SN; Helgason, A; Rafnar, T; Magnusson, KP; Manolescu, A; Karason, A; Palsson, A; Thorleifsson, G; et al. Genetic determinants of hair, eye and skin pigmentation in Europeans. Nat Genet 2007; 39:1443–1452

[278] Sulem, P; Gudbjartsson, DF; Stacey, SN; Helgason, A; Rafnar, T; Jakobsdottir, M; Steinberg, S; Gudjonsson, SA; Palsson, A; Thorleifsson, G; et al. Two newly identified genetic determinants of pigmentation in Europeans. *Nat Genet* 2008; 40:835–837.

[279] Valenzuela, RK; Henderson, MS; Walsh, MH; Garrison, NA; Kelch, JT; Cohen-Barak, O; Erickson, DT; John Meaney, F; Bruce Walsh, J; Cheng, KC; Ito, S; Wakamatsu, K; Frudakis, T; Thomas, M; Brilliant, MH. Predicting phenotype from genotype: normal pigmentation. *J Forensic Sci* 2010; 55(2):315–322.

[280] Mengel-From, J, Wong, TH, Morling, N; Rees, JL; Jackson, IJ. Genetic determinants of hair, eye colours in the Scottish, Danish populations. *BMC Genet* 2009; 10:88.

[281] Valverde, P; Healy, E; Jackson, I; Rees, JL; Thody, AJ. Variants of the melanocyte-stimulating hormone receptor gene are associated with red hair and fair skin in humans. *Nat Genet* 1995; 11:328–330.

[282] Box, NF; Wyeth, JR; O'Gorman, LE; Martin, NG; Sturm, RA. Characterization of melanocyte stimulating hormone receptor variant alleles in twins with red hair. *Hum. Mol. Genet.,*1997, 6:1891-1897.

[283] Han, J; Kraft, P; Nan, H; Guo, Q; Chen, C; Qureshi, A; Hankinson, SE; Hu, FB; Duffy, DL; Zhao, ZZ; Martin, NG; Montgomery, GW; Hayward, NK; Thomas, G; Hoover, RN; Chanock, S; Hunter, DJ. A genome-wide association study identifies novel alleles associated with hair color and skin pigmentation. *PLoS Genet.* 2008;4:e1000074.

[284] Harding, RM; Healy, E; Ray, AJ; Ellis, NS; Flanagan, N; Todd, C; Dixon, C; Sajantila, A; Jackson, IJ; Birch-Machin, MA; Rees, JL. Evidence for variable selective pressures at *MC1R*. *Am J Hum Genet.* 2000;66:1351–1361.

[285] Flanagan, N; Healy, E; Ray, A; Philips, S; Todd, C; Jackson, IJ; Birch-Machin, MA; Rees, JL. Pleiotropic effects of the melanocortin 1 receptor (*MC1R*) gene on human pigmentation. *Hum Mol Genet.* 2000;9:2531–2537.

[286] Kanetsky, PA; Ge, F; Najarian, D; Swoyer, J; Panossian, S; Schuchter, L; Holmes, R; Guerry, D; Rebbeck, TR. Assessment of polymorphic variants in the melanocortin-1 receptor gene with cutaneous pigmentation using an evolutionary approach. *Cancer Epidemiol Biomarkers Prev.* 2004;13:808–819.

[287] Pastorino, L; Cusano, R; Bruno, W; Lantieri, F; Origone, P; Barile, M; Gliori, S; Shepherd, GA; Sturm, RA; Bianchi-Scarra, G. Novel *MC1R* variants in Ligurian melanoma patients and controls. *Hum Mutat.* 2004;24:103.

[288] Rana, BK; Hewett-Emmett, D; Jin, L; Chang, BH; Sambuughin, N; Lin, M; Watkins, S; Bamshad, M; Jorde, LB; Ramsay, M; Jenkins, T; Li, WH. High polymorphism at the human melanocortin 1 receptor locus. *Genetics.* 1999;151:1547–1557.

[289] Sulem, P; Gudbjartsson, DF; Stacey, SN; Helgason, A; Rafnar, T; Magnusson, KP; Manolescu, A; Karason, A; Palsson, A; Thorleifsson, G; et al. Genetic determinants of hair, eye and skin pigmentation in Europeans. *Nat Genet.* 2007;39:1443–1452.

[290] Medland SE, Nyholt DR, Painter JN, McEvoy BP, McRae AF, Zhu G, Gordon SD, Ferreira MA, Wright MJ, Henders AK, Campbell MJ, Duffy DL, Hansell NK, Macgregor S, Slutske WS, Heath AC, Montgomery GW, Martin NG. Common variants

in the trichohyalin gene are associated with straight hair in Europeans. *Am J Hum Genet.* 2009 Nov;85(5):750-5. Epub 2009 Nov 5.

[291] Fujimoto, A; Kimura, R; Ohashi, J; Omi, K; Yuliwulandari, R; Batubara, L; Mustofa, MS; Samakkarn, U; Settheetham-Ishida, W; Ishida, T; Morishita, Y; Furusawa, T; Nakazawa, M; Ohtsuka, R; Tokunaga, K. A scan for genetic determinants of human hair morphology: EDAR is associated with Asian hair thickness. *Hum Mol Genet.* 2008 Mar 15;17(6):835-43.

[292] Margulies, M; Egholm, M; Altman, Attiya, S; Bader, JS; Bemben, LA; Berka, J; Braverman, MS; Chen, YJ; Chen, Z; Dewell, SB; Du, L; Fierro, JM; Gomes, XV; Goodwin, BC; He, W; Helgesen, S; Ho, CH; Irzyk, GP; Jando, SC; Alenquer, MLI; Jarvie, TP; Jirage, KB; Kim, JB; Knight, JR; Lanza, JR; Leamon, JH; Lefkowitz, SM; Lei, M; Li, J; Lohman, KL; Lu, H; Makhijani, VB; McDade, KE; McKenna, MP; Myers, EW; Nickerson, E; Nobile, JR; Plant, R; Puc, BP; Ronan, MT; Roth, GP; Sarkis, GJ; Simons, JF; Simpson, JW; Srinivasan, M; Tartaro, KR; Tomasz, A; Vogt, KA; Volkmer, GA; Wang, SH; Wang, Y; Weiner, MP; Yu, P; Begley, RF and Rothberg, JM. Genome Sequencing in Open Micro fabricated High Density Picoliter Reactors. *Nature.* 2005 September 15; 437(7057): 376–380.

[293] Tawfik, DS; Griffiths, AD. Man-made cell-like compartments for molecular evolution. *Nat Biotechnology,* 1998, 16:652.

[294] Ghadessy, FJ; Ong, JL; Holliger, P. Directed evolution of polymerase function by compartmentalized self-replication. *Proc Nat Acad Sci* USA 2001;98:4552.

[295] Dressman, D; Yan, H; Traverso, G; Kinzler, KW; Vogelstein, B. Transforming single DNA molecules into fluorescent magnetic particles for detection and enumeration of genetic variations. *Proc Nat Acad Sci* USA 2003;100:8817.

[296] Ronaghi, M; Uhlen, M; Nyren, P. A sequencing method based on real-time pyrophosphate. *Science* 1998, 281:363.

[297] Dressman, D; Yan, H; Traverso, G; Kinzler, KW; Vogelstein, B. Transforming single DNA molecules into fluorescent magnetic particles for detection and enumeration of genetic variations. *Proc Natl Acad Sci U S A.* 2003 Jul 22;100(15):8817-22.

In: Forensic Science
Editors: N. Yacine and R. Fellag

ISBN 978-1-61324-999-4
© 2012 Nova Science Publishers, Inc.

*Chapter 2*

# FORENSIC GENETICS FROM A GEOGRAPHIC PERSPECTIVE: INTEGRATING FORENSIC GENETICS AND GEOSTATISTICS

*Amalia N. Díaz-Lacava*[1,2,3,*] *and Maja Walier*[3]

[1]Cologne Center for Genomics, University of Cologne, Germany
[2]DNA Analysis Unit, Official College of Pharmacists and Biochemists, Buenos Aires, Argentina
[3]Institute of Medical Biometry, Informatics and Epidemiology, University of Bonn, Germany

## ABSTRACT

Forensic genetics benefited in the past decades from accelerated advances in molecular genetic technologies. On one side, the quantity of high-quality genotypes increased enormously. And on the other side, principally due to the increasing cooperation of forensic geneticists, standardized high-quality data on various kinds of DNA variation are available in worldwide forensic data sets providing a solid basis for a wide range of population genetics studies relevant to multidisciplinary fields.

Understanding spatial relationships of the extant genetic variation of populations and reconstructing the underlying demographic processes are central topics in forensic genetics. Various statistical methods analyzing spatial genetic variation are implemented in well-established procedures. Forensic genetics studies conducted using such tools have significantly contributed to our understanding of the extant pattern of genetic variation and its underlying history. Nevertheless, plenty of information embedded in the geographical data still remains unexplored, mainly due to methodological restrictions. Integrating the geographic information of forensic genotypes to genetic statistics demands for geostatistical methods. A geographic information system (GIS) offers an

---

[*] Correspondence: PhD Amalia N. Díaz-Lacava. CCG - Cologne Center for Genomics, University of Cologne, Germany. Weyertal 115b, 50931 Cologne, Germany, Phone: (++ 49) 221 - 478 96844; Fax: (++ 49) 221 - 478 96866; E-mail: a.diaz-lacava@uni-koeln.de.

appropriated framework to integrate any type of data accounting for a geographic reference and to flexibly address statistical analysis to spatial relationships.

On the basis of concrete examples of widely addressed inquires at population level in forensic genetics, this work shows that combining genetic statistics with geostastistical analysis in a GIS framework opens a wide range of methodological approaches and provides a flexible environment to focus or to adapt the analysis to the phenomena under study and the available data. Results include summary statistics as well as maps displaying precise patterns of genetic variation at the adequate scale and resolution. Inquiries often addressed and related to the distribution and frequency of alleles, haplotypes, or groups of closely related haplotypes are further extended to assess, quantify and map the spatial coverage of the most prevalent alleles or group of closely related haplotypes per tract of land. Advantages and prospects of introducing geostatistics into forensic genetics are discussed.

# 1. INTRODUCTION

Forensic genetics relays on good knowledge of the genetic structure of the sampled population. A long tradition of population genetics studies provides substantial evidence of geographical genetic structure of continuously populated territories at broader scales (e.g. Barbujani & Sokal, 1990; Cavalli-Sforza, Menozzi, & Piazza, 1994; Roewer et al., 2005; Rosser et al., 2000; Zerjal et al., 2001). For instance, studies based on whole genome genotypes clearly demonstrated a spatial correspondence of major human groups to main socio-demographic regions in West Europe (Lao et al., 2008; Novembre et al., 2008). Among the most cited methods used to disclose spatial patterns of genetic structure are: assignment procedures, ordination methods, analysis of spatial variation in polymorphism frequency on the basis of visualization tools or population genetics summary statistics, summary maps, and the search of genetic boundaries -areas of abrupt change in genetic frequencies, also known as genetic discontinuities (reviewed in e.g. Barbujani, 2000; Epperson, 2003; Manel, Schwartz, Luikart, & Taberlet, 2003; Storfer et al., 2007). Several of these methods were frequently applied to forensic data in order to detect and to demonstrate spatial patterns of genetic variation (e.g. Gusmão et al., 2003; Roewer et al., 2005; Zerjal et al., 2001). Well-established implementations of these methods search for a specific overall type of pattern fitting the data. Accordingly, different types of spatial patterns were reported for certain populations depending on the method used. While on one hand several studies on population structure of Europe demonstrated patterns of clinal variation (e.g. Gusmão et al., 2003; Rosser et al., 2000), others verified spatial genetic discontinuities (e.g. Barbujani & Sokal, 1990; Kayser et al., 2005; Zerjal et al., 2001). These results indicate that spatial genetic structures may include complex patterns, combining clines, discontinuities and even gaps (e.g. Fechner et al., 2008). A more appropriate strategy to detect complex spatial genetic structures may include: (a) increasing the information gained from the sample, and (b) assessing the patterns of genetic variation without setting a prior on the overall type of expected spatial structure.

Methods successfully increasing the amount of information extracted from population genetics data were presented in recent years in the fields of molecular biology and ecology (e.g. Guillot, Estoup, Mortier, & Cosson, 2005; Hardy & Vekemans, 2002; Manel et al., 2007). These methods make use of individual geographical references of samples and jointly analyze inter-individual genetic and spatial information. An individual-based georeference of genetic data may not necessarily be a possible or suitable choice for studies of modern human populations due to at least two main reasons: restrictions related to guaranteeing sample anonymity and admixture of modern societies.

In the scope of population genetics studies of modern human populations, sample characterization must exclude any possibility of personal identification. A precise geographical reference, which would allow to assign a unique geographical coordinate to each human sample (e.g. postal address), may be in conflict with most ethical restrictions holding anywhere. If the geographical reference is not precise at local scale, many samples will probably aggregate into one location. This situation arises because sampling design of genetic studies on modern humans usually involves a considerably low number of sampling locations in relation to the number of samples. Consequently, more than one sample will be referenced to one site, e.g. urban center, hospital, or postal area. Since most modern localities would present a certain degree of admixture, simply aggregating data geographically would reduce the potentials of the method to detect spatial patterns of genetic heterogeneity.

An alternative approach to overcome this drawback could be to group the samples according to genetic similarities and then to evaluate the spatial distribution of such groups. Studies in the field of forensic genetics using such an approach showed genetic clines and differences in frequencies among regions at continental and country scales (e.g. Brion *et al.*, 2004; Gusmão *et al.*, 2003). Basically these patterns were detected and analyzed on the basis of visualization methods. Either spatial differences in group frequency were jointly compared, e.g., using pie or bar charts of group frequencies per location (e.g. Brion *et al.*, 2004; Gusmão *et al.*, 2003; Rosser *et al.*, 2000), or the spatial distribution of frequencies was evaluated separately for each group, e.g. on the basis of visual examination of interpolated surfaces estimating the spatial frequency, separately for each group (e.g. Lao *et al.*, 2008; Roewer *et al.*, 2005). The first type of visualization methods, pie or bar charts, facilitates the comparison of frequencies among groups at each sampling location. However, estimating the spatial patterns of variation in frequencies becomes more difficult with an increase in the number of compared groups, the number of observed locations, or pattern complexity. An interpolated surface of frequencies is indeed an estimation of how frequencies of one group are spatially distributed. Several interpolation methods as well as stand-alone software are available to create interpolated surfaces. However, in order to assess the spatial pattern of genetic heterogeneity, the information contained in these surfaces must be somehow summarized (e.g. Barbujani, 2000). To make full use of spatial information gained from the data requires to go beyond visual evaluation of spatial relationships and to perform deep geostatistical analysis. A geographic information system (GIS) provides the most adequate platform for geostatistical analysis. Integrating genetic statistics with geostatistical analysis provides a solid basis to detect spatial genetic patterns of admixed populations. Furthermore, once genetic data has been framed within a GIS, a wide range of geostatistical computations may be conducted to generate and, eventually, to test hypotheses for the influence of the geographical relationships on the genetic pattern.

Forensic Y-chromosome short tandem repeat (Y-STR) markers, also known as Y microsatellites, are extremely polymorphic. Also, Y-STR loci are very likely selection-neutral. Non-recombinant Y-chromosomal loci are jointly inherited. Consequently, these loci may be combined into unambiguous haplotypes. Y-STR haplotypes offer an even more polymorphic data set. Forensic Y-STR loci and haplotypes provide outstanding data for the analysis of population heterogeneity (e.g. Bosch *et al.*, 2001; Brion *et al.*, 2004; Diaz-Lacava,

Walier, Penacino, Wienker, & Baur, 2011a; Diaz-Lacava et al., 2011b; Gusmão et al., 2003; Kayser et al., 2005; Roewer et al., 2005; Zerjal et al., 2001). Moreover, several studies confirmed the suitability of forensic Y-STR loci and haplotypes for genetic studies of spatially contiguous, admixed populations (e.g. Brion et al., 2004; Diaz-Lacava et al., 2011a; Diaz-Lacava et al., 2011b; Kayser et al., 2005). Grouping samples according to genetic similarity which are estimated on the basis of forensic Y-chromosomal data and examining their geographical distribution by means of geostatistical analysis is best suited for elucidating spatial patterns of genetic variation in continuously populated regions. The aim of this chapter is to describe and to illustrate a GIS-based approach for assessing the spatial distribution of groups of genetically similar individuals and quantifying the spatial coverage of the groups with the highest frequency per tract of land on the basis of forensic genetic data.

## 2. ASSESSING THE REGIONAL DISTRIBUTION OF MOST FREQUENT GROUPS OF GENETICALLY SIMILAR INDIVIDUALS

A scenario of a continuously populated, admixed region is presumed. In such a region a complex spatial pattern of genetic composition is expected. This region includes individuals of several genetic backgrounds (Figure 1a). A main assumption of this scenario is that individuals do not populate an area randomly; rather, genetically similar individuals, related to each other by familiar, cultural or just lingual bounds, tend to reside in geographically adjacent areas (Figure 1b). Considering a group of genetically similar individuals, this assumption implies a spatial dependence of the probability to find one of its individuals at a certain location. This probability is conditional on the frequency of this group at that location or in its neighborhood (within-group spatial dependence). It is further assumed that the spatial distribution of a group of genetically similar individuals is independent of the location of other groups (no spatial interference among groups). This implies that such groups present an overlapping spatial coverage. The spatial frequency of each group varies across the region, presenting areas with higher and lower frequencies (Figure 1b). Based on these two assumptions and from a methodological point of view it follows that the geographical distribution of each group must be first explored independently from other groups. The regional distribution of the most frequent groups per tract of land can thus be assessed by jointly analyzing the distribution of all groups (Figure 1c).

This search begins with the identification of groups of similar individuals. Individuals are grouped according to a single attribute (e.g. STR allele) or according to a set of attributes (e.g. genetically similar haplotypes). Following, the spatial distribution of each group is estimated. Separately for each group, a geographical *raster layer* (i.e. spatially continuous surface or grid) is created. Each cell or pixel of this raster layer stores the estimated spatial frequency of one group (Figure 1d-i). For this purpose, point or areal data (i.e. group frequency per location or areal unit) must be transformed into continuous spatial data (i.e. continuous group frequency distribution). Frequencies per location or areal unit can be transformed into continuous spatial data using surface interpolation methods. The number of computed interpolated surfaces, or raster layers, equals the number of groups. The spatial distribution per group is regarded as one of the total number of "genetic layers" into which the genetic admixture could be decomposed. Based on these "genetic layers" the most frequent groups per tract of land can be identified. Such a query is performed on the basis of a pixel-wise screening through all layers. Results are stored in two new layers, also called *composite maps* (Figure 1d-ii). The first layer stores at each pixel the maximum frequency value of all layers. The second layer stores at each pixel the label of the group accounting for the maximum frequency. Composite maps may be used for further geostatistical computations. For example, coverage and frequency of the most frequent groups per tract of land may be jointly examined by overlapping data of both composite maps (Figure 1d-iii). A pixel-wise screening of the second highest frequency values may be performed in order to assess the spatial pattern of genetic heterogeneity remaining after excluding the groups with the highest spatial frequency.

## 3. GEOSTATISTICAL ANALYSIS OF THE ARGENTINEAN GENETIC ADMIXTURE

The approach described above will be illustrated in this chapter on the basis of forensic Y-STR Argentinean data. In recent years there has been much attention to Argentinean population stratification (e.g. Alfaro, Dipierri, Gutiérrez, & Vullo, 2005; Corach *et al.*, 2010; Diaz-Lacava *et al.*, 2011a; Dipierri *et al.*, 2005; Marino, Sala, Bobillo, & Corach, 2008; Toscanini *et al.*, 2007). In a rather short historical period the Argentinean population went through massive demographic changes. Overwhelmingly large immigration waves populating Argentina since the 1850s introduced a strong male European component (e.g. Avena *et al.*, 2001; Corach *et al.*, 2010; Levene, 1992; Rock, 1987). This relatively recent immigration largely diluted the previous admixture and played a major role in modulating the extant Argentinean genetic background (Avena *et al.*, 2001; Corach *et al.*, 2010). As a result of almost two hundred years of admixture among worldwide incoming lineages and the previously settled population, a complex spatial pattern of genetic variation is expected. Questions related to the history, extent, and geographical structure of admixture and the characteristics of nowadays genetic composition were addressed under several perspectives (e.g. Alfaro *et al.*, 2005; Avena *et al.*, 2001; Corach *et al.*, 2010; Diaz-Lacava *et al.*, 2011a; Dipierri *et al.*, 2005; Marino *et al.*, 2008; Sala, Penacino, & Corach, 1998; Toscanini *et al.*, 2007). From a methodological point of view, two main factors contribute to make the study of this population interesting. On one hand, the expected complex admixture poses a methodological challenge. On the other hand, since most influencing socio-demographic processes affecting contemporary Argentinean genetic background took place in a relatively recent and short historical period, there are enough historical, ethnological, and census data available to analyze and validate the results.

In this chapter two evaluations regarding the spatial pattern of genetic admixture of the contemporary Argentinean population were addressed: (a) regional distribution of the most frequent alleles per Y-STR locus, and (b) regional distribution of the most frequent groups of genetically similar Y-STR haplotypes. In each case, composite maps were created showing the estimated spatial coverage of the most frequent groups. Transects were constructed displaying the spatial distribution of group frequencies across the study region. The worldwide provenance of most frequent haplotypes was inspected.

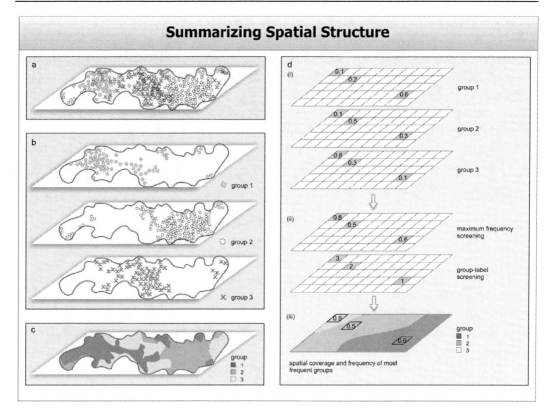

Figure 1. Schematic view of a geostatistical approach to delimit the spatial coverage of the most frequent groups in an area. (a) the basic scenario: an admixed area is assumed, in this scenario individuals with a certain degree of similarity are clustered into 3 groups indicated in the figure by squares (group 1), dots (group 2), and crosses (group 3); (b) spatial distribution of groups of similar individuals; (c) schematic view of the spatial coverage of the most frequent groups; (d) geostatistical assessment of the spatial coverage of the most frequent groups: (i) independently for each group, spatial frequency is estimated and represented in a georeferenced raster layer; each pixel stores the estimated spatial frequency of the group at that geographical position; (ii) for each pixel, the maximum frequency value of all layers is screened and two composite maps (raster layer) are created; maximum frequency values are stored in one layer, label of the group accounting for the maximum frequency value at each pixel is stored in a second layer; (iii) juxtaposing these two composite maps a new composite map is created, which describes the spatial coverage and frequency of the most frequent groups in an area.

## 3.1. Argentinean Population from a Historical Perspective

Present-day Argentinean population is highly admixed (e.g. Alfaro *et al.*, 2005; Avena *et al.*, 2001; Corach *et al.*, 2010; Diaz-Lacava *et al.*, 2011a; Marino, Sala, & Corach, 2007; Toscanini *et al.*, 2007). In the territory of the contemporary Argentina admixture between Amerindians and not Amerindians began with the European arrival in the 16th century (Levene, 1992). Since then, immigration from all over the world populated this territory, in particular since the 1850s. Originally, aboriginal tribes were not large in comparison with other American territories; during the first three centuries, until the revolution of 1810, admixture took place mainly among few sedentary native groups, a small number of

Spaniards and an even much smaller number of Africans (Rock, 1987; Sanchez-Albornoz, 1994). The River Plate colonies extended over relatively circumscribed regions of the present Argentinean territory, along the routes to more profitable Spanish territories -located in Peru, Paraguay and Chile. Settlements were small, poor hamlets, with not more than a few hundred inhabitants (Levene, 1992; Rock, 1987). Since only Spanish ships were allowed to approach these coasts, besides a few possible smugglers, only Spaniards and few Africans settled in the River Plate viceroyalty. Most Africans were further delivered to the modern territory of Bolivia and northern regions (Rock, 1987). Although Spain encouraged the arrival of Spanish matrimonies, few Spanish women arrived to this viceroyalty; most patrician families were created by the union of Spaniards and Indian chief daughters (Levene, 1951).

Since the 1850s population grew at accelerated rates as a consequence of immigration. Between 1871 and 1914 an immense number of immigrants arrived, largely outnumbering the local population. The majority of immigrants settled in main urban centers. Until the end of the nineteenth century the largest extension of the present-day Argentinean territory still remained unexplored and inhabited by nomadic native tribes. Most of these individuals eluded conquerors for generations, even centuries. Rural settlements were attacked from time to time by nomadic tribes. Cattle and white population were taken captive. But in 1879 the "conquest of the wilderness" (la conquista del desierto), the largest military expedition across the central and southern territories, subdued, drove out or exterminated the left nomadic tribes. As a result of this extermination, 85,000 $km^2$, a surface comparable in size to the Austrian territory, passed into the hands of 381 people. The few surviving individuals were constrained to reservations. By 1914 around one-third of the country's population was foreign-born, and around 80 percent of the population comprised immigrants and those descended from immigrants since 1850: mainly Spaniards and Italians, followed by Russians and Poles, French, and Ottoman Turks, including Lebanese and Syrians (reviewed in Rock, 1987). Over-sea immigration decreased in the 1930s and 1940s, and fell steeply soon after, subsequently followed by domestic rural migrants settling in heavily urbanized areas and by migrants from neighboring countries. As a result, in the 1960s-1970s three-quarters of resident foreigners were displaced migrant peasants from neighboring countries (Rock, 1987; Sanchez-Albornoz, 1994). This last demographic movement towards main metropolitan centers, primarily to Buenos Aires, Santa Fe, Cordoba, and the triangle between these cities (Rock, 1987), may have reintroduced a strong Amerindian component in the genetic structure of the littoral and central urban Argentina (e.g. Avena *et al.*, 2001).

Nowadays, self-identifying Amerindian groups or individuals, contributing only to an exiguous portion of the total population, are practically restricted to scanty, marginal areas (Bartolome, 1976; INDEC, 2005; Sanchez-Albornoz, 1994). The largest contemporary Amerindian population, the Kollas, inhabits the extreme northwestern region of Argentina (INDEC, 2005). In the Argentinean northeast, a region indicated as Mesopotamia, including Misiones, Corrientes, and Entre Rios provinces, the local Amerindian language "Guarani" survived, but the autochthonous Guaranies did not. Urban as well as rural population, predominantly small holders, overwhelmingly consists of descendants of over-sea immigrants. According to Bartolome (1976), the left Amerindian populations living in the northeast of Argentina are scattered, isolated groups of very small size and deprived socio-economic condition. Their ancestors immigrated to this region for some generations, presumably from Paraguay and Brazil (Bartolome, 1976).

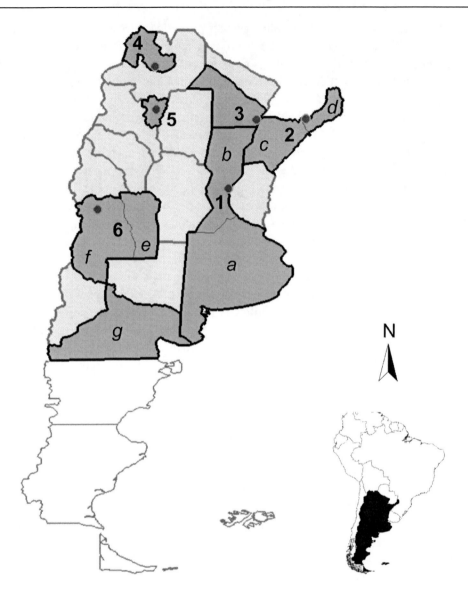

Figure 2. Map of Argentina indicating the study region (thicker contour). The study region included 20 of the 24 Argentinean provinces. Six sampling units were delimited out of 10 sampled provinces (1*a*: Buenos Aires; 1*b*: Santa Fe; 2*c*: Corrientes; 2*d*: Misiones; 3: Chaco; 4: Jujuy; 5: Tucuman; 6*e*: San Luis; 6*f*: Mendoza; 6*g*: Rio Negro). Grey circles show capital cities used as geographical reference of genetic frequencies. The inset shows the Argentinean location in South America.

Table 1. Description of the sampling units (SID sampling-unit identification (see Fig. 2), *n* number of samples, Cov. spatial coverage in percentage in relation to the study region, Georeference capital city used as geographical reference of point data, Province provinces (federal state) included in the sampling unit)

| SID | Sampling Unit | n | Cov. | Georeference | Province |
|---|---|---|---|---|---|
| 1 | Santa Fe | 20 | 15.9 | Santa Fe | Santa Fe |
|   |          |    |      |          | Buenos Aires |
| 2 | Misiones | 8 | 4.3 | Posadas | Misiones |
|   |          |   |     |         | Corrientes |
| 3 | Chaco | 7 | 3.5 | Resistencia | Chaco |
| 4 | Jujuy | 18 | 2.0 | Jujuy | Jujuy |
| 5 | Tucuman | 33 | 0.8 | Tucuman | Tucuman |
| 6 | Mendoza | 59 | 15.3 | Mendoza | Mendoza |
|   |         |    |      |         | San Luis |
|   |         |    |      |         | Rio Negro |

## 3.2. Materials and Methods

### 3.2.1. Study Region and Sampling Units

The study region covers central and northern Argentina. It includes 10 sampled provinces and 10 further provinces within the area circumscribed by the sampled provinces (Figure 2). These 20 provinces (out of a total of 24 Argentinean provinces) represent 80 percent of the total Argentinean area. It is worth noting that the sampled area contains the absolute majority of the total population. Argentina is an extremely centralized and highly urbanized country. While the 10 sampled provinces include 75 percent of the total population, the study region includes 98 percent (INDEC, 2010).

Sampling units were primarily defined by sampled provinces. Sampled provinces with small number of samples were aggregated to neighboring sampled provinces. As a result, out of 10 sampled provinces 6 sampling units were defined (Figure 2, Table 1). Provincial capital cities were used to georeference point data to sampling units (see section "Geostatistical Analysis"). In case of sampling units containing more than one provincial capital city (i.e. aggregated sampled provinces) the capital city of the province with the largest number of samples was defined as the geographical reference of point data.

### 3.2.2. Subjects and Genotypes

DNA material was obtained from 145 unrelated male Argentinean citizens in year 2007. Donors were recruited in the framework of legal paternity testing. No sampling bias may be assumed due to socio-economic condition of donors; depending on the socio-economic situation of the donor paternity-testing costs were either privately or publicly financed. Sampling did not include any restriction related to the donor's ethnic background. Care was taken that neither closely related individuals nor non-Argentinean citizens were included in the sample. Since sampling did not include any further restrictions, this data set may be regarded as a random sample of the extant male Argentinean population in the study region. Samples and genotypes were treated anonymously, following local ethical restrictions.

Samples were solely referenced to the sampled province (federal state), thus guaranteeing donor anonymity.

DNA was extracted from blood stains or buccal swab specimens by conventional organic extraction methods. DNA was prepared and genotyped at the DNA Analysis Unit, Official College of Pharmacists and Biochemists, Buenos Aires, using the commercial typing kit PowerPlex Y System (Promega Corp.) - DYS19, DYS385a/b, DYS389I/II, DYS390, DYS391, DYS392, DYS393, DYS437, DYS438, and DYS439- in a 25 µl reaction volume, as specified by the manufacturer (Promega, Madison, Wisconsin, http://www.promega.com/). Detection of the amplified fragments was done using the ABI Prism 377 (Applied Biosystems, Foster City, California). PowerTyper Y Macro (Promega) was used to assign the alleles. DYS385 was excluded from the analysis since it is not possible to unequivocally assign one allele to a specific locus (e.g. Gusmão *et al.*, 2003).

Alleles were coded in terms of the number of variable repeats, in agreement with the freely-accessible worldwide YHRD database (http://www.yhrd.org/). Y-STR loci -DYS19, DYS389I/II, DYS390, DYS391, DYS392, and DYS393- were combined to define haplotypes. Haplotypes were denoted by listing the seven alleles in the same order as in YHRD, concatenated by a dash (i.e., DYS19 _ 389I _ 389II _ 390 _ 391 _ 392 _ 393).

Most probable worldwide provenance of frequent haplotypes was investigated. Historical and ethnological data (Bartolome, 1976; Rock, 1987; Sanchez-Albornoz, 1994) indicate that the contemporary Argentinean population to the greatest extent is the result of modern admixture arisen from major immigration processes, officially promoted since the 1850s. This relatively new and long-lasting immigration arrived from all over the world. It largely outnumbered the colonial population and most probably diluted a previous admixture among a reduced group of sedentary Amerindian populations, Spaniards, and some other minor ethnicities (Levene, 1951; Levene, 1992; Rock, 1987; Sanchez-Albornoz, 1994). Since Y-STR haplotypes are paternally inherited as a block, without recombination, it was assumed that the worldwide distribution of a haplotype would provide a good clue about the region where that haplotype came from before it integrated into the Argentinean population. All different haplotypes identified in the sample were ranked according to their absolute frequency. The worldwide geographical distribution of the most frequent haplotypes was inspected. Relative frequency and worldwide geographical distribution were searched in the YHRD database (http://www.yhrd.org/).

### 3.2.3. Genetic Frequencies

Allele frequencies of each of the seven Y-STR loci were scored by single-gene counting procedures. Bar plots of each Y microsatellite showing the allele frequencies were created with the basic module *barplot* of the R software package, version 2.11.1 (R : A Language and Environment for Statistical Computing; http://www.r-project.org/; R Development Core Team, 2010-05-31). Independently for each Y-STR locus, allele frequencies per sampling unit were calculated.

Different haplotypes were identified and grouped into 4 clusters according to molecular distance following the stepwise mutation model. Clustering was performed with the statistical software package SAS v. 9.1. (SAS Institute Inc., Cary, NC, USA; http://www.sas.com/; clustering method: Ward; Euclidean distance). The cluster frequency per sampling unit was computed as the number of samples corresponding to one cluster in relation to the total number of samples per sampling unit. The number of clusters was chosen on the basis of geostatistical results, the composite maps, displaying the spatial distribution of the haplotype clusters with the highest spatial frequencies (see section "Composite Maps"). Explorative runs were performed by varying the number of clusters, with $n=3, 4, 5$, and 7 clusters. Composite maps were evaluated pursuing a regionalization of the study region into a maximal number of differentiated regions and a minimum of interpolation artifacts (e.g. patterns including multiple neighboring stripes as well as extremely small or unexpected patches).

Allele frequencies as well as cluster frequencies were transformed in order to spread frequency values in the spectrum of small and large values. Frequencies ($q$) were transformed by an *arc sine* transformation (Barbujani, 1985) and weighted in order to obtain a percentage scale:

$$f' = 100 \cdot arcsin\left(\sqrt{q}\right) / arcsin(1)$$

where $f'$ is the transformed frequency in percentage.

### 3.2.4. Geostatistical Analysis

Geostatistical analysis was performed with the open-source geographic information system GRASS GIS v. 6.4. (Geographic Resources Analysis Support System, http://grass.itc.it/).

The assessment of the regional distribution of frequent groups involved the same steps for both types of inquires defined above, which included the geostatistical analysis of spatial patterns of genetic structure at the Y-STR level and at the haplotype level (see section "Genetic Frequencies"). At each level of analysis a different type of parameter was used to define groups, i.e. alleles at the Y-STR level, and cluster membership at the haplotype level.

Each of the seven Y-STR loci was evaluated separately from each other. For each single STR, alleles identified in the sample were used as grouping parameters. Consequently, different numbers of groups were defined for each of the seven Y-STR loci. At the haplotype level, cluster membership was used as grouping parameter. In each case, frequencies per sampling unit, i.e. Y-STR-allele frequency or haplotype-cluster frequency (see section "Genetic Frequencies") were imported into GRASS as point-data layers. Geographical coordinates of capital cities were used to georeference point data to the sampling unit (Figure 2, Table 1). Further geostatistical computations were performed on continuous spatial data represented in GRASS as raster layers. Surface interpolation was conducted in order to transform point data into raster data: $f' \rightarrow f$, where $f$ is the estimated frequency per pixel.

Separately for each group, one interpolated surface (i.e. raster layer) was created. Surface interpolation was performed using the function "regularized spline with tension", implemented in the package *v.surf.rst* (Mitasova & Mitas, 1993). This method computes the values of the interpolated surface using a function which simulates a thin flexible plate passing through or close to the points (Mitasova & Mitas, 1993). Splines are flexible to model differential local patterns based on change of elastic properties of the interpolation function. Splines proved to be rather successful for cases where the phenomena have a less random component (uncertainty) and are more driven by processes which minimize energy (Neteler & Mitasova, 2004). Since it seemed intuitive to assume that the genetic admixture of a region may be more influenced by local socio-demographic processes than by random processes (uncertainty), the spline function was selected as the best choice to model genetic layers representing the spatial distribution of groups of genetically similar individuals by means of surface interpolation. One interpolated surface was created for each group, i.e. the groups were defined according to either Y-STR alleles or cluster membership. Interpolation parameters, smooth and tension, were selected in each case by tuning, attempting to achieve minimal statistical error (also called predictive error) defined by root mean squared deviation (*rms*) (Neteler & Mitasova, 2004). Tuning was performed independently for each set of groups of each of the seven Y-STR loci and for each haplotype cluster. At the same time, tuning attempted to reduce interpolation artifacts (e.g. several neighboring stripes, extremely small or unexpected patches) and to increase the number of regions detected with the final composite maps (see section "Composite Maps"). Surface interpolation was performed with the default tension value of the GRASS module *v.surf.rst* (tension=40) for both sets of frequency data, the allele frequencies per sampling unit and the cluster frequencies per sampling unit. Table 2 lists the selected smooth-parameter value and minimal and maximal root mean square deviation (*rms*) of all interpolated surfaces per Y-STR locus (estimated spatial distribution of allele frequencies). Smooth-parameter value, minimum and maximum values of the interpolated surfaces, minimum and maximum values of the sampled data, and the root mean square deviation (*rms*) per cluster layer are shown in table 3.

Table 2. Root mean square deviation (*rms*) per Y-STR locus (*n* number of interpolated surfaces, corresponding to the total number of alleles per locus, *smooth* smooth-parameter value used for the interpolation procedure, *min* and *max* minimum and maximum *rms* values of all *n* interpolated surfaces)

| Y-STR | n | smooth | rms min | rms max |
|---|---|---|---|---|
| DYS19 | 5 | 0.5 | 1.01 | 6.88 |
| DYS389I | 4 | 0.2 | 0.63 | 2.56 |
| DYS389II | 7 | 1.0 | 1.32 | 6.35 |
| DYS390 | 5 | 0.5 | 1.04 | 4.88 |
| DYS391 | 3 | 0.2 | 1.78 | 2.17 |
| DYS392 | 8 | 0.5 | 1.00 | 5.43 |
| DYS393 | 4 | 0.5 | 1.82 | 3.86 |

Table 3. Root mean square deviation (*rms*) and minimum and maximum values (in percent) obtained by surface interpolation of $f'$, where $f'$ is the cluster frequency per sampling unit (see section "Genetic Frequencies"; *smooth* smooth-parameter value used to perform surface interpolation, *min* and *max* minimum and maximum interpolated values, [ $f'$ ] minimum and maximum $f'$ values, respectively)

| Cluster | smooth | min [$f'$] | max [$f'$] | rms |
|---|---|---|---|---|
| 1 | 0.5 | 33.6 [ 32.8 ] | 44.9 [ 46.8 ] | 1.78 |
| 2 | 1.5 | 21.3 [ 18.8 ] | 47.1 [ 60.8 ] | 7.45 |
| 3 | 2.0 | 15.7 [ 0.0 ] | 39.8 [ 58.0 ] | 16.71 |
| 4 | 2.0 | 13.3 [ 0.0 ] | 37.3 [ 54.6 ] | 14.58 |

As described above an interpolated surface (i.e. raster layer) estimates the spatial distribution of frequencies of one group. In the present context, this raster layer represents the estimated probability of sampling an individual belonging to one group at a certain sampling point, conditioned to the geographical location of the sampling point. A sampling point within a raster layer is represented in GRASS by a raster pixel. From this stage onwards a separate analysis was conducted for each spatial query. In total, eight independent geostatistical queries were addressed, one for each of the seven Y-STR loci and the last one for the spatial analysis of haplotype clusters.

## 3.2.4.1. Screening Algorithms

Considering one query $l$, $l = 1, ..., Q$, where $Q = 7$ at the single-locus level and $Q = 1$ at the haplotype level, the $k$th group (i.e. groups are defined by alleles at the single-locus level and by clusters at the haplotype level) is assumed to be present at the $r$th raster pixel, where $r$ represents one of the total $R$ pixels of the study region, with a certain probability estimated by $f$ (see section "Geostatistical Analysis"), where $k$ represents one of the $n$ groups, and

$$\sum_{k=1}^{n} f_k = 100 \pm RMS$$

. RMS is the root mean squared deviation (*rms*) in relation to all $n$ raster layers at the $r$th pixel. At each pixel the maximal $f$ of all $n$ groups as well as $k$, label of the corresponding group, were screened and stored in two separated layers: MAX_1_freq and MAX_1_group.

Pixel-wise screening over all $n$ groups, run independently for each one of the $Q$ queries:

$l$ = 1 to $Q$          ## independent run for each query
    $r$ = 1 to $R$          ## screening across the study region

        max_1_freq $_{l,r}$ = max($f_{l,r,1}, ... f_{l,r,n}$)
        max_1_group $_{l,r}$ = k $_{l,r}$ ( max($f_{l,r,1}, ... f_{l,r,n}$) )

    done
    >> array: MAX_1_freq $_l$
    >> array: MAX_1_group $_l$
done

This procedure was repeated searching for the 2nd maximum value at each pixel and results were stored in two further sets of layers: MAX_2_freq $_l$ and MAX_2_group $_l$.

## 3.2.4.2. Composite Maps

Two types of layers, also called composite maps, were created with the basic GRASS module *r.mapcalc* using the screening procedure described above: one type displayed the spatial distribution of the maximum (and 2nd maximum) frequency values among groups and the second showed the spatial distribution of groups accounting for the maximum (and 2nd maximum) frequency (where groups were defined by Y-STR alleles or by haplotype-cluster membership).

In case of the analysis at the locus level (Y STR), the composite maps storing frequency values, MAX_1_freq $_l$ and MAX_2_freq $_l$, were used for tuning and visual evaluation of result consistency. The composite maps MAX_1_group $_l$ and MAX_2_group $_l$ were exported and saved as graphics for result presentation. The exported graphics separately showed for each Y STR the regions where one allele presented the maximum (as well as the 2$^{nd}$ maximum) frequency per tract of land in relation to the other alleles.

At the haplotype level, composite maps storing frequency values, MAX_1_freq and MAX_2_freq, were used for tuning and visual evaluation of result consistency as well as for further analysis. Contour-line layers were created based on these frequency maps. Contour lines were set along points of equal $f$, where $f$ is the estimated frequency per pixel (in percent) of a certain group (see section "Geostatistical Analysis"), with a step of 0.5 percent difference. A second set of contour-line layers was created with larger steps. On the basis of the map MAX_1_freq, contour lines were delineated along the values: 35, 37.5, 40, 42.5, and 45 percent. For the map MAX_2_freq contour lines were constructed along the values: 30, 32.5, 35, and 36.5 percent. Final graphics were exported showing the regional distribution of the clusters with the maximum (as well as the 2$^{nd}$ maximum) frequency per tract of land and the respective spatial distribution of frequencies. The spatial distribution of frequencies was displayed juxtaposing contour lines to the regional maps, MAX_1_group and MAX_2_group.

The spatial pattern of frequencies was further inspected on the basis of transects. For each frequency map, MAX_1_freq and MAX_2_freq, one transect was set up between the local maximum value in the central region and the local maximum value in the northwest region. Frequencies (in percent) were measured along transects and profile charts were created with the interactive GRASS tool *profile*.

## 3.3. Results and Discussion

### 3.3.1. Allele Frequencies

All seven Y-STR loci -DYS19, DYS389I/II, DYS390, DYS391, DYS392, and DYS393- were polymorphic and presented from 3 to 8 alleles. Allele frequency distributions of the seven loci are shown in Figure 3. All loci presented a unimodal distribution except for DYS392, clearly showing a bimodal allele-frequency distribution. With the exception of DYS389II, unimodal loci presented one frequent allele and less-frequent alleles differentiated from the next most-frequent allele by a single repeat unit. By DYS389II, allele 27 was not detected in the sample. Allele frequency distribution of all seven loci is in good accordance with the results of a global survey of 986 males including a large number of European samples ($n$=470) (Kayser et al., 2001). In every case, the most-frequent allele as well as the shape of the allele frequency distribution in relation to the less-frequent alleles matches to the global allele-frequency distribution, as described by Kayser et al. (2001). A less-frequent allele of DYS392 (allele 17) was found in the Argentinean sample and not in the global survey (Kayser et al., 2001). This result is consistent with a higher genetic variance of DYS392 in the Argentinean population in relation to globally distributed populations, as reported by Kayser et al. (2001). On the other hand, a less-frequent allele of DYS389II (allele 27) detected in the global survey (Kayser et al., 2001) was absent in this sample (see above).

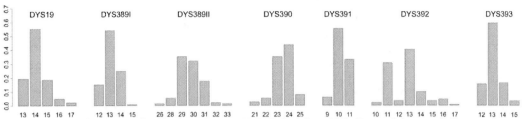

Figure 3. Allele frequency distribution of seven Y-STR loci ($n = 145$). For each locus, allelic notation (designated in number of repeats) is indicated on the x-axis, observed frequencies are shown on the y-axis.

Regional-specific allelic differences were indicated by the composite maps (Figure 4). Allelic differentiation of the northwest region was observed for the loci DSY19, DSY389I, DSY389II, and DSY390. In every case, one allele presented the highest frequency almost everywhere in the study region and the second highest frequency in the northwest, where a second allele showed the highest frequency. DSY19 and DSY389I presented a third allele, which had the second highest frequency in central Argentina. DSY389I presented as well an allelic differentiation of the Misiones Province, located in northeastern Argentina. DSY389II was the only locus in the MAX_1_group map which presented three areas of allelic differentiation: central, northwest, and northeast. The MAX_2_group map showed in the northwest a transition zone, evidenced by a stripe pattern. This stripe pattern arose due to very similar frequencies of all three alleles in the same region. This result is in good agreement with the expected high genetic variance of DSY389II (Kayser *et al.*, 2001). DSY389II composite maps indicate that (a) this microsatellite may allow a differentiation of the male Argentinean population among three main socio-demographic regions, and (b) the highest variance of this locus may be primarily centered in the northwest of Argentina. Further deeper analysis will be necessary to confirm these observations.

DSY391 and DSY392 presented a quite similar spatial pattern to the previously described loci but differed in the geographical area where a second allele showed the highest frequency. While one allele had the highest frequency over the largest portion of the study region, another had the highest frequency in the central northern area, a region known as the "Argentinean Chaco" (Figure 4).

A single allele of DSY393 had the highest frequency all over the study region. The two next most-frequent alleles (Figure 3) had the second highest frequency, one in the northern and the other in the southern portion of the study region (Figure 4).

The observed spatial patterns of allelic differentiation of all seven Y-STR loci considered as a whole indicate a strong regional differentiation of the northwest in relation to the rest of the Argentinean territory as well as a lower differentiation of two other regions: the Argentinean Chaco and the central and littoral Argentina. The spatial patterns observed at the Y-STR level corroborate prior expectations of a regional genetic differentiation of the contemporary male Argentinean population (e.g. Alfaro *et al.*, 2005; Corach *et al.*, 2010; Marino *et al.*, 2007; Marino *et al.*, 2008; Toscanini *et al.*, 2007).

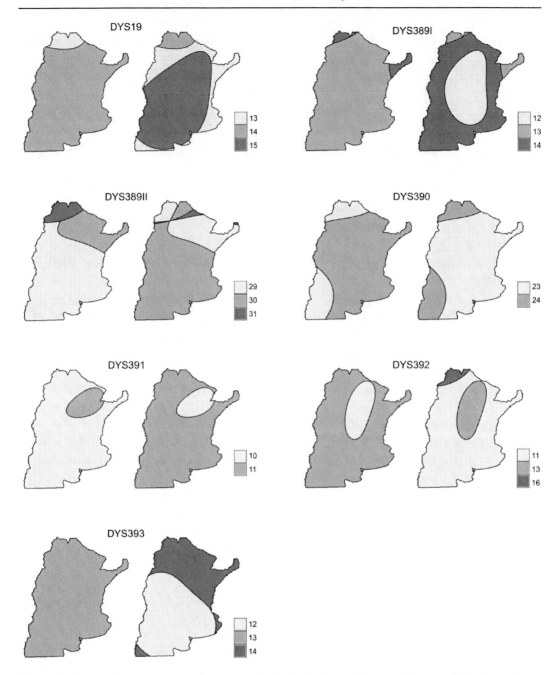

Figure 4. Composite maps showing the geographical distribution of the most frequent alleles for each of the seven Y-STR loci. Gray coding indicates the allelic designation (in number of repeats). Each region in the composite maps delimits an area where one allele presented: (a) the highest frequency (left map), and (b) the 2nd highest frequency (right map).

## 3.3.2. Haplotype Clusters

Out of a total of 145 males 97 different haplotypes were identified. Out of these, 72 haplotypes were detected only once and 18 haplotypes twice. About 75 percent of the sample corresponded to haplotypes with an absolute frequency equal or smaller than two. The rest 25 percent of the sample carried one of seven different haplotypes (Table 4). These figures are in agreement with the expected strong admixture of the Argentinean population (Alfaro *et al.*, 2005; Avena *et al.*, 2001; Corach *et al.*, 2010; Diaz-Lacava *et al.*, 2011a; Marino *et al.*, 2007; Toscanini *et al.*, 2007).

According to the worldwide YHRD database (http://www.yhrd.org/) the most frequent haplotype (14_13_29_24_10_13_13; $n = 9$) shows higher frequencies in Western Europe, and only one frequent haplotype of this sample (13_14_31_23_10_16_14; $n = 5$) shows higher frequencies in South America.

The clustering procedure sorted different haplotypes into relatively similar clusters with respect to both total count of different haplotypes and total count of samples per cluster (Table 5). Haplotypes with an absolute frequency larger than two were assigned to the first three clusters (Table 4).

According to the YHRD database (http://www.yhrd.org/) the most frequent haplotypes ($n \geq 3$) of cluster 1 and of cluster 3 (Table 4) throughout the world are most frequently registered in Western Europe and with considerable frequency in North and South America. One of these haplotypes (14_13_30_23_10_11_12; $n=3$; cluster 3) also shows higher frequencies in the Middle East and in Southern Asia. The most frequent haplotypes ($n \geq 3$) included in cluster 2 present higher frequencies of matches in Latin America and in North Africa. Non-unique cluster-4 haplotypes ($n = 2$) are scarcely distributed throughout the world, with higher frequency of matches either in South America, Africa or Southeastern Asia (http://www.yhrd.org/). These figures indicate that haplotypes grouped into cluster 1 and cluster 3 were introduced most probably by immigrants or immigrant descendants from West European countries. Haplotypes grouped into cluster 2 correspond most probably to descendants from local Amerindian populations and those grouped into cluster 4 are of admixed origin.

**Table 4. Absolute frequency ($n$) and cluster assignment of haplotypes found in three or more individuals**

| Haplotype | n | (%) | Cluster | (%) |
|---|---|---|---|---|
| 14_13_29_24_10_13_13 | 9 | ( 6.2 ) | 1 | ( 20.9 ) |
| 14_13_29_24_11_13_13 | 6 | ( 4.1 ) | 1 | ( 14.0 ) |
| 14_14_30_24_11_13_13 | 6 | ( 4.1 ) | 3 | ( 15.8 ) |
| 14_13_30_24_11_13_13 | 5 | ( 3.4 ) | 3 | ( 13.2 ) |
| 13_14_31_23_10_16_14 | 5 | ( 3.4 ) | 2 | ( 18.5 ) |
| 14_13_29_23_11_13_13 | 3 | ( 2.1 ) | 1 | ( 7.0 ) |
| 14_13_30_23_10_11_12 | 3 | ( 2.1 ) | 3 | ( 7.9 ) |
| **Total** | 37 | ( 25.5 ) | | |

The percentage of samples carrying the haplotype in relation to the total sample ($n = 145$) and to the number of samples per cluster are indicated in parentheses.

**Table 5. Distribution of different haplotypes (*hap*) and samples (*n*) per cluster**

| Cluster | *hap* | (%) | *n* | (%) |
|---|---|---|---|---|
| 1 | 24 | ( 24.7 ) | 43 | ( 29.7 ) |
| 2 | 19 | ( 19.6 ) | 27 | ( 18.6 ) |
| 3 | 23 | ( 23.7 ) | 38 | ( 26.2 ) |
| 4 | 31 | ( 32.0 ) | 37 | ( 25.5 ) |
| Total | 97 | ( 100.0 ) | 145 | ( 100.0 ) |

The percentage of different haplotypes and samples in relation to total figures are indicated in parentheses.

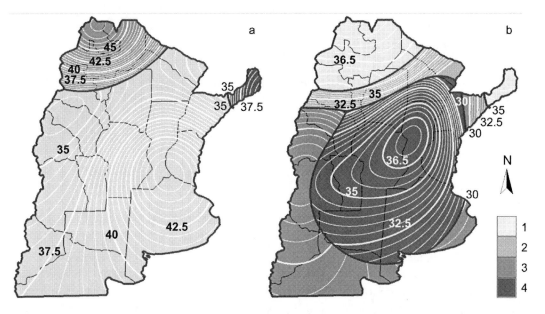

Figure 5. Regional coverage of the most frequent haplotype clusters quantified and presented in the form of composite maps: (a) regional coverage of clusters accounting for the highest frequencies, (b) regional coverage of clusters accounting for the 2$^{nd}$ highest frequencies. Contour lines (white lines) of cluster frequencies (in percent) have been drawn (thinner line: step=0.5 %; frequency values corresponding to the thicker lines are shown in the map).

Cluster 1 was found to be present with the highest frequency in 86 percent of the study region (Figure 5a) and second highest frequency in the rest (Figure 5b). In the northwest, cluster 2 accounted for the highest frequencies (Figure 5a). This region covered 13 percent of the study region and included the provinces of Jujuy and Salta. In the northeast, in the region corresponding to the Misiones Province, cluster 3 was higher in frequency (one percent of the study region) (Figure 5a). In the littoral area cluster 4 had the second highest frequency after cluster 1 in 52 percent of the area (Figure 5b).

The highest frequencies of cluster 1 were measured in the Argentinean littoral, centered in Santa Fe and surroundings. Although cluster 1 presented the highest frequencies over the largest area, these values were much lower than frequencies measured in the northwestern region (Figure 5a). Contour lines drawn in Figure 5a show the spatial distribution of frequencies in the study region. Comparing frequencies among regions, the highest values were registered in the northwest, in the Jujuy Province, where cluster 2 was the most frequent cluster. Figure 6a shows a profile of frequencies (in percent) along a transect running between the geographical positions accounting for the maximum frequency values of cluster 1 and cluster 2. While cluster-1 frequencies vary smoothly, cluster-2 frequencies show an abrupt decline towards the south.

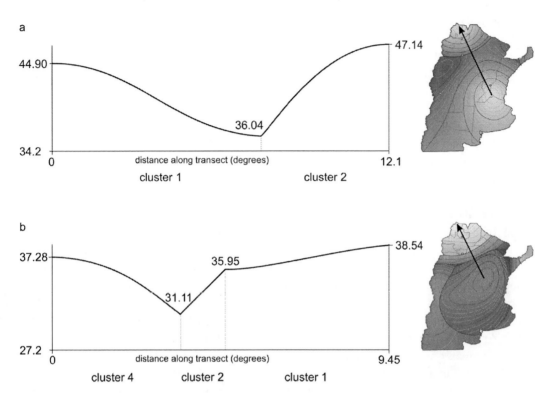

Figure 6. Profile of frequency values of the most frequent clusters along a transect measured in the composite maps of (a) regional coverage of clusters accounting for the maximum frequency values, (b) regional coverage of clusters accounting for the 2$^{nd}$ maximum frequency values. Transects, indicated with an arrow in the composite map on the right side (see Figure 5), have been set between the local maximum value in the central region and the local maximum value in the northwestern region. Frequencies (in percent) are indicated on the y-axis. The relative portion of the transect corresponding to each cluster and the transect length in degrees are indicated on the x-axis.

Figure 5b shows on the basis of contour lines the spatial distribution of frequencies of the clusters second in frequency in the study region. Similar maximal values were registered in all four regions. Frequencies (in percent), measured along a transect set up between the littoral and the northwestern area, show a similar smooth pattern of spatial variation of frequencies of cluster 1 and cluster 4 in the corresponding regions (Figure 6b).

As mentioned above, the worldwide distribution of the most frequent haplotypes of cluster 1 (http://www.yhrd.org/) supports an expected European origin. The regional coverage of cluster 1 is in good agreement with previous studies and literature, indicating a major male European component (e.g. Avena *et al.*, 2001; Corach *et al.*, 2010; Levene, 1992; Rock, 1987). Higher frequencies of cluster 1 in the area of Santa Fe (Figure 5a) corresponds well with historical data indicating the Argentinean littoral as one of the most important centers of long-lasting European immigration (Rock, 1987). On the other hand, lower frequencies of cluster 1 in relation to cluster 2 indicate that the central and littoral region is more admixed (Figure 5a). This implicates that besides a widespread European heritage, represented in this sample by cluster 1, other male lineages constitute a considerable fraction of the population in this area, grouped primarily into cluster 4 (Figure 5b). Cluster 4, second in frequency in central and littoral Argentina (Figure 5b), included haplotypes incoming from all over the world (http://www.yhrd.org/). These results support an observed multi-ethnic genetic admixture (Avena *et al.*, 2001) in an area which has been a recursive destination of most recent immigration (Rock, 1987). A differentiation of cluster 3 in the northeast, grouping most probably males of European ancestry (http://www.yhrd.org/), is consistent with historical data as well indicating that this region was populated predominantly by European peasants (Rock, 1987). After the officially promoted immigration decreased, the northeast practically ceased to attract new immigration due to a relative geographical isolation of this region in relation to main industrial and metropolitan centers, located primarily in central and littoral Argentina (Rock, 1987). Further studies might more precisely indicate the differential origins of cluster-1 and cluster-3 haplotypes.

The Argentinean northwest differentiated strongly from the rest of the study region. As mentioned above, the overall highest cluster frequencies (cluster 2) were measured in the region of Jujuy and Salta (Figure 5a). Such difference in frequencies indicates that the northwest is, on an average, less admixed than other regions. Cluster 2 retained the $2^{nd}$ highest frequency in the surrounding area to the south including the provinces of La Rioja, Tucuman, northern Chaco and Formosa. As already mentioned, cluster 2 gathered haplotypes frequently registered in South America (http://www.yhrd.org/), indicating a presumable Amerindian origin (e.g. Alfaro *et al.*, 2005; Marino *et al.*, 2007). These haplotypes belong most probably to the Amerindian populations inhabiting the northwest. According to census data, Jujuy Province counts Argentina's highest percentage of population (10%) identifying him- or herself as an indigenous person or descendant (INDEC, 2005). These are predominantly represented by the Kollas (INDEC, 2005). The Kolla community, one of the last Argentinean Amerindian populations, survivor of the European conquest, resides mainly in the Jujuy Province and extends with lower frequencies to the south (INDEC, 2005). This ethnic group still conserves traditions and habits of the time when it was the most advanced culture in the pre-Columbian Argentinean territory. The spatial distribution of the Kolla community coincides with the geographical regional coverage where cluster 2 showed the maximum and $2^{nd}$ maximum frequency values. Copious studies evaluated the Amerindian contribution to the Argentinean genetic composition (e.g. Alfaro *et al.*, 2005; Avena *et al.*, 2001; Corach *et al.*, 2010; Marino *et al.*, 2007). While Argentina registers a high proportion of Amerindian maternal heritage (Corach *et al.*, 2010), the paternal Amerindian contribution to the whole population is much lower (Corach *et al.*, 2010; Marino *et al.*, 2007). Specifically concerning the northwest, previous studies support a larger Amerindian contribution (Alfaro *et al.*, 2005; Marino *et al.*, 2007). Our findings further reinforce a predominant indigenous paternal heritage in the northwest, much less diluted by either colonial or modern immigration than other Argentinean regions. The spatial coverage of cluster 2, most probably gathering individuals of Amerindian ancestry, strongly represented in the northwest, is in good agreement with prior expectations. All in all, analysis conducted at both single-locus and haplotype level, reinforce the notion of Argentina as an admixed country, with a widespread predominance of male European lineages, a strong component of prevalent Amerindian heritage in the northwest and a strongly admixed fraction in central and littoral Argentina.

## 4. CONCLUSION

An integration of population genetics statistics and geostatistical analysis has allowed the detection of fine-scale spatial, genetic structure of the extant male Argentinean admixture. The complex nature of this genetic structure was revealed through high degrees of resolution by geostatistical methods. Admixture was spatially modeled as the overlapping distribution of several coexistent groups. A systematic, comprehensive search of spatial structures of groups of genetically similar individuals proved a successful approach to identify spatially coherent regions of closely related individuals as well as summarize and display regions of differentiated degrees of admixture.

With this chapter it has been shown that integrating statistical genetics and geostatistics in the framework of GRASS GISS is a successful approach for precisely examining the spatial distribution of groups of genetically similar individuals of a strongly admixed population. The strength of this geostatistical work is the quantification of spatial coverage of groups in relation to others. This task becomes even more challenging when a highly admixed population is being analyzed, which is the case of most studies using samples collected within modern societies. Further advantages of this kind of analysis, as conducted in this chapter, are twofold. First, results presented in the form of maps are intuitive to understand and the most direct way to examine spatial relationships, as it was discussed in Barbujani (2000). Second, precise spatial quantifications of the genetic composition of a population are a suitable basis for a broad scope of related analyses which may include further geostatistical evaluations as well as reporting results in the form of summary statistics.

In the present chapter the genetic admixture of the extant male population in central and northern Argentina was evaluated on the basis of forensic Y-STR loci from a geographical perspective. Admixture was analyzed under two aspects: (a) spatial distribution of most frequent alleles per Y-STR locus, and (b) spatial distribution of most frequent groups of similar Y-STR haplotypes (Y-STR haplotype clusters).

The findings summarized in the composite maps together with the assessed worldwide provenance of most represented haplotypes per cluster further support an expected majority of males with European lineage in the extant Argentinean population (Corach *et al.*, 2010; Marino *et al.*, 2007). This heritage is represented in this sample by two groups of closely related haplotypes, cluster 1 and cluster 3, showing the highest frequencies across the largest extension of the study region. A larger sample or different set of genetic markers would be necessary to more precisely evaluate the difference in origin between these two groups.

Historic, ethnological and census data confirm, explain, and validate the results indicating an exiguous portion of Amerindian component in the largest territories of Argentina and a major component of Amerindian population in the northwest. The largest groups of individuals, who identify themselves as indigenous people or descendants, reside in this region (INDEC, 2005). This expected spatial structure was detected and quantified on the basis of composite maps at two levels: (a) at the single-locus level, by the repeatedly observed pattern of allelic differentiation in the northwest and, (b) at the haplotype level, by the strong representation of cluster 2 in the northwest, which included haplotypes of presumable Amerindian origin. It was through the composite maps presented in this chapter that accurate quantification of spatial coverage, pattern of spatial variation in frequency, and a comparison of the degree of admixture of this group in relation to others could be provided. Specifically, three regions were identified: the northwest, including the provinces of Jujuy and Salta, where this group presents the highest frequency; a surrounding transition zone, where European lineages present similar frequency; and beyond this, the territory where its frequency abruptly declines.

New immigration waves after the 1950's, predominantly affecting central and littoral Argentina (Rock, 1987), might have reintroduced Amerindian lineages from neighboring countries and might have also introduced further lineages arriving from all over the world (Avena et al., 2001). In this chapter such expected strongly admixed group was led back to cluster 4, which gathered haplotypes registered worldwide (http://www.yhrd.org/). A region where cluster 4 is as frequent as other predominant groups was precisely delimited, and it covered central and littoral Argentina. Moreover, on the basis of transects, the pattern of spatial variation in frequency of cluster 4 was compared to others. The broad regional coverage and the substantial contribution of this group to the overall genetic background further support observed changes in the genetic composition of littoral Argentina towards a multi-ethnic population (Avena et al., 2001).

Taking into account that the sampled provinces gathered 75% of the total Argentinean population (INDEC, 2010) and that the study region extended over 80% of the total country, this analysis may be considered representative of the total contemporary male Argentinean population. It is the hope of the authors that the detailed and precise results presented in this chapter in the form of composite maps, and further validated by historical, ethnic, and census data, will provide a basis for future works ranging from investigations in forensic genetics up to studies in closely related areas such as population genetics, genetic epidemiology, as well as ethnology, history, or demographic surveys.

## ACKNOWLEDGMENTS

We sincerely thank Gustavo Penacino for allowing us to use his data. We are greatly thankful to Horacio R. Diaz for his support by reviewing Argentinean history and demographic development. We are also grateful to Thomas F. Wienker for constructive discussions and his help in preparing the manuscript. The authors wish to dearly thank Lodovica Borghese and Markus Leber for their helpful comments and criticisms. We specially thank Birgit Buchholz for her artwork.

## REFERENCES

Alfaro, E.L., Dipierri, J.E., Gutiérrez, N.I., & Vullo, C.M. (2005). Genetic structure and admixture in urban populations of the Argentine North-West. *Ann Hum Biol.*, 32(6), 724-737.

Avena, S., Goycoechea, A., Dugoujon, J., Slepoy, M., Slepoy, A., & Carnese, F.R. (2001). Análisis Antropogenético de los Aportes Indígena y Africano en Muestras Hospitalarias de la Ciudad de Buenos Aires. *Revista Argentina de Antropología Biol.*, 3(1), 79-99.

Barbujani, G. (1985). A two-step test for the heterogeneity of FST values at different loci. *Hum. Hereditas*, 35(5), 292-295.

Barbujani, G. (2000). Geographic patterns: how to identify them and why. *Hum Biol.,* 72, 133-153.

Barbujani, G. & Sokal, R.R. (1990). Zones of sharp genetic change in Europe are also linguistic boundaries. *Proc Natl. Acad. Sci. USA.,* 87(5), 1816-1819.

Bartolome, M.B. (1976). Argentinien. In D. Walter (Ed.), Die Situation der Indios in Südamerika. *Grundlagen der interethnischen Konflikte der nichtandinen Indianer* (pp. 352-398). Wuppertal: Hammer Verlag.

Bosch, E., Calafell, F., Comas, D., Oefner, P.J., Underhill, P.A., & Bertranpetit, J. (2001). High-resolution analysis of human Y-chromosome variation shows a sharp discontinuity and limited gene flow between northwestern Africa and the Iberian Peninsula. *Am J Hum Genet.,* 68(4), 1019-1029.

Brion, M., Quintans, B., Zarrabeitia, M., Gonzalez-Neira, A., Salas, A., Lareu, V., Tyler-Smith, C., & Carracedo, A. (2004). Micro-geographical differentiation in Northern Iberia revealed by Y-chromosomal DNA analysis. *Gene,* 329, 17-25.

Cavalli-Sforza, L.L., Menozzi, P., & Piazza, A. (1994). *The history and geography of human genes.* Princeton, NJ: Princeton University Press.

Corach, D., Lao, O., Bobillo, C., van Der Gaag, K., Zuniga, S., Vermeulen, M., van Duijn, K., Goedbloed, M., Vallone, P.M., Parson, W., de Knijff, P., & Kayser, M. (2010). Inferring continental ancestry of argentineans from Autosomal, Y-chromosomal and mitochondrial DNA. *Ann Hum Genet.,* 74(1), 65-76.

Diaz-Lacava, A., Walier, M., Penacino, G., Wienker, T.F., & Baur, M.P. (2011a). Spatial assessment of Argentinean genetic admixture with geographical information systems. *Forensic Sci Int Genet.* 5, 297-302.

Diaz-Lacava, A., Walier, M., Willuweit, S., Wienker, T.F., Fimmers, R., Baur, M.P., & Roewer, L. (2011b). Geostatistical inference of main Y-STR-haplotype groups in Europe. *Forensic Sci Int Genet.* 5, 91-94.

Dipierri, J.E., Alfaro, E.L., Scapoli, C., Mamolini, E., Rodriguez-Larralde, A., & Barrai, I. (2005). Surnames in Argentina: a population study through isonymy. *Am J Phys Anthropol.,* 128(1), 199-209.

Epperson, B.K. (2003). *Geographical Genetics.* Princeton, NJ: Princeton University Press.

Fechner, A., Quinque, D., Rychkov, S., Morozowa, I., Naumova, O., Schneider, Y., Willuweit, S., Zhukova, O., Roewer, L., Stoneking, M., & Nasidze, I. (2008). Boundaries and clines in the West Eurasian Y-chromosome landscape: insights from the European part of Russia. *Am J Phys Anthropol.,* 137(1), 41-47.

Guillot, G., Estoup A., Mortier, F., & Cosson, J.F. (2005). A spatial statistical model for landscape genetics. Genetics, 170, 1261-1280.

Gusmão, L., Sánchez-Diz, P., Alves, C., Beleza, S., Lopes, A., Carracedo, A., & Amorim, A. (2003). Grouping of Y-STR haplotypes discloses European geographic clines. *Forensic Sci Int.,* 134(2-3), 172-179.

Hardy, O.J. & Vekemans, X. (2002). SPAGeDi: a versatile computer program to analyse spatial genetic structure at the individual or population levels. *Molecular Ecology Notes,* 2, 618-620.

INDEC: National Institute of Statistics and Censuses. (2010). *Censo 2010.* Retrieved from http://www.censo2010.indec.gov.ar/

INDEC: National Institute of Statistics and Censuses. (2005). Encuesta Complementaria de Pueblos Indígenas (ECPI) 2004 - 2005 - Complementaria del Censo Nacional de Población, Hogares y Viviendas 2001. Retrieved from http://www.indec.mecon.ar/

Kayser, M., Krawczak, M., Excoffier, L., Dieltjes, P., Corach, D., Pascali, V., Gehrig, C., Bernini, L.F., Jespersen, J., Bakker, E., Roewer, L., & de Knijff, P. (2001). An extensive analysis of Y-chromosomal microsatellite haplotypes in globally dispersed human populations. *Am J Hum Genet.*, 68(4), 990-1018.

Kayser, M., Lao, O., Anslinger, K., Augustin, C., Bargel, G., Edelmann, J., Elias, S., Heinrich, M., Henke, J., Henke, L., Hohoff, C., Illing, A., Jonkisz, A., Kuzniar, P., Lebioda, A., Lessig, R., Lewicki, S., Maciejewska, A., Monies, D.M., Pawłowski, R., Poetsch, M., Schmid, D., Schmidt, U., Schneider, P.M., Stradmann-Bellinghausen, B., Szibor, R., Wegener, R., Wozniak, M., Zoledziewska, M., Roewer, L., Dobosz, T., & Ploski, R. (2005). Significant genetic differentiation between Poland and Germany follows present-day political borders, as revealed by Y-chromosome analysis. *Hum Genet.*, 117(5), 428-443.

Lao, O., Lu, T.T., Nothnagel, M., Junge, O., Freitag-Wolf, S., Caliebe, A., Balascakova, M., Bertranpetit, J., Bindoff, L.A., Comas, D., Holmlund, G., Kouvatsi, A., Macek, M., Mollet, I., Parson, W., Palo, J., Ploski, R., Sajantila, A., Tagliabracci, A., Gether, U., Werge, T., Rivadeneira, F., Hofman, A., Uitterlinden, A.G., Gieger, C., Wichmann, H.E., Rüther, A., Schreiber, S., Becker, C., Nürnberg, P., Nelson, M.R., Krawczak, M., & Kayser, M. (2008). Correlation between genetic and geographic structure in Europe. *Curr Biol.*, 16, 1241-1248.

Levene, R. (1951). *Las Indias No Eran Colonias.* Buenos Aires: Espasa Calpe.

Levene, R. (1992). *Lecciones de historia argentina,* vol. I. (25th ed.). Buenos Aires: Ediciones Corregidor.

Manel, S., Berthoud, F., Bellemain, E., Gaudeul, M., Luikart, G., Swenson, J.E., Waits, L.P., & Taberlet, P. (2007). A new individual-based spatial approach for identifying genetic discontinuities in natural populations. *Mol Ecol.*, 16, 2031-2043.

Manel, S., Schwartz, M.K., Luikart, G., & Taberlet, P. (2003). Landscape genetics: combining landscape ecology and population genetics. *Trends in Ecology & Evolution,* 18, 189-197.

Marino, M., Sala, A., Bobillo, C., & Corach, D. (2008). Inferring genetic sub-structure in the population of Argentina using fifteen microsatellite loci. *Forensic Sci. Int.: Genetics Supplement Series,* 1(1), 350-352.

Marino, M., Sala, A., & Corach, D. (2007). Genetic attributes of the YHRD minimal haplotype in 10 provinces of Argentina. *Forensic Sci Int Genet.*, 1(2), 129-133.

Mitasova, H. & Mitas, L. (1993). Interpolation by regularized spline with tension: I. Theory and implementation. *Math. Geol.*, 25, 641-655.

Neteler, M. & Mitasova, H. (2004). *Open Source GIS: A GRASS GIS Approach* (second edition). Boston: Kluwer Academic Publishers/Springer.

Novembre, J., Johnson, T., Bryc, K., Kutalik, Z., Boyko, A.R., Auton, A., Indap, A., King, K.S., Bergmann, S., Nelson, M.R., Stephens, M., & Bustamante, C.D. (2008). Genes mirror geography within Europe. *Nature,* 456(7218), 98-101.

Rock, D. (1987). *Argentina, 1516-1987: from Spanish colonization to Alfonsín.* Los Angeles: University of California Press.

Roewer, L., Croucher, P.J., Willuweit, S., Lu, T.T., Kayser, M., Lessig, R., de Knijff, P., Jobling, M.A., Tyler-Smith, C., & Krawczak, M. (2005). Signature of recent historical events in the European Y-chromosomal STR haplotype distribution. *Hum Genet.*, 116(4), 279-291.

Rosser, Z.H., Zerjal, T., Hurles, M.E., Adojaan, M., Alavantic, D., Amorim, A., Amos, W., Armenteros, M., Arroyo, E., Barbujani, G., Beckman, G., Beckman, L., Bertranpetit, J., Bosch, E., Bradley, D.G., Brede, G., Cooper, G., Côrte-Real, H.B., de Knijff, P., Decorte, R., Dubrova, Y.E., Evgrafov, O., Gilissen, A., Glisic, S., Gölge, M., Hill, E.W., Jeziorowska, A., Kalaydjieva, L., Kayser, M., Kivisild, T., Kravchenko, S.A., Krumina, A., Kucinskas, V., Lavinha, J., Livshits, L.A., Malaspina, P., Maria, S., McElreavey, K., Meitinger, T.A., Mikelsaar, A.V., Mitchell, R.J., Nafa, K., Nicholson, J., Nørby, S., Pandya, A., Parik, J., Patsalis, P.C., Pereira, L., Peterlin, B., Pielberg, G., Prata, M.J., Previderé, C., Roewer, L., Rootsi, S., Rubinsztein, D.C., Saillard, J., Santos, F.R., Stefanescu, G., Sykes, B.C., Tolun, A., Villems, R., Tyler-Smith, C., & Jobling, M.A. (2000). Y-chromosomal diversity in Europe is clinal and influenced primarily by geography, rather than by language. *Am J Hum Genet.*, 67(6), 1526-1543.

Sala, A., Penacino, G., & Corach, D. (1998). Comparison of allele frequencies of eight STR loci from Argentinian Amerindian and European populations. *Hum Biol.*, 70(5), 937-947.

Sanchez-Albornoz, N. (1994). *La Poblacion de America latina: desde los tiempos precolombinos al año 2005.* Madrid: Editorial Alianza.

Storfer, A., Murphy, M.A., Evans, J.S., Goldberg, C.S., Robinson, S., Spear, S.F., Dezzani, R., Delmelle, E., Vierling, L., & Waits, L.P. (2007). Putting the "landscape" in landscape genetics. *Heredity*, 98(3), 128-142.

Toscanini, U., Gusmão, L., Berardi, G., Amorim, A., Carracedo, A., Salas, A., & Raimondi, E. (2007). Testing for genetic structure in different urban Argentinian populations. *Forensic Sci Int.*, 165(1), 35-40.

Zerjal, T., Beckman, L., Beckman, G., Mikelsaar, A.V., Krumina, A., Kucinskas, V., Hurles, M.E., & Tyler-Smith, C. (2001). Geographical, linguistic, and cultural influences on genetic diversity: Y-chromosomal distribution in Northern European populations. *Mol Biol Evol.*, 18(6), 1077-1087.

In: Forensic Science
Editors: N. Yacine and R. Fellag

ISBN 978-1-61324-999-4
© 2012 Nova Science Publishers, Inc.

*Chapter 3*

# HUMAN PIGMENTATION GENES: FORENSIC PERSPECTIVES, GENERAL ASPECTS AND EVOLUTION

*Caio Cesar Silva de Cerqueira[a], Carlos Eduardo Guerra Amorim[a], Francisco Mauro Salzano[a], Maria Cátira Bortolini[a,*]*

[a]Genetics Department, Biosciences Institute, Federal University of Rio Grande do Sul, Porto Alegre, RS, Brazil

## ABSTRACT

Despite the growing number of registered DNA forensic profiles, the rate of profile hits is far below the expected. When a given profile is not found with the standard kits, any available information is important. Ancestry Informative Markers (AIM) have been employed for the identification of the person's ethnicity. However, this is not an adequate approach in certain cases, as, for instance, individuals living in ethnically admixed populations, in which the physical appearance is not necessarily associated with ethnicity. Hence, the use of AIMs in such populations has few or no advantage. The interest in the search for alleles directly linked to physical characteristics is therefore rapidly increasing, resulting in the commercialization of kits for the identification of skin, hair and eye pigmentation phenotypes based on genetic variation of candidate genes such as *ASIP, HERC2, MC1R, OCA2,* and *TYR*. This genetic variation may affect different stages of the pigmentation process, including melanogenesis, the stabilization and transport of enzymes during melanin synthesis, melanosome production and maintenance, and the balance between the synthesis of different types of melanin. In this chapter we examine the most important genes associated to human hair, skin and eye pigmentation, discussing the evolutionary background for the observed variation and their functional relevance for the physiological mechanisms involved with pigmentation, highlighting the forensic application of this knowledge. We will also discuss better ways of collecting pigmentation phenotypic data in human populations for forensic and general studies. It is expected that in the near future we may be able to predict with high reliability the externally visible human characteristics based on DNA analyses.

---

[*] Correspondence: Dr. Maria Cátira Bortolini, Programa de Pós-Graduação em Genética e Biologia Molecular, Departamento de Genética, Instituto de Biociências, Universidade Federal do Rio Grande do Sul, Caixa Postal 15053, 91501-970 Porto Alegre, RS, Brazil. Email: maria.bortolini@ufrgs.br; Telephone: +55 (51) 3308-9844.

# 1. INTRODUCTION

## 1.1. General Considerations

With the advent of forensic genetics and attempts to include information of phenotypic characteristics of possible suspects in police databases, it is desirable to generate data about these traits and additionally to explore and integrate the information generated by the scientific community (see recent discussion in Enserink, 2011). However, it is necessary to uncover the relationship of each gene in particular with its phenotype, something nontrivial due to the enormous complexity of the genotype → phenotype connections. Specific morphological characteristics of plants, animals or humans are products of processes that involve the spatial and temporal expression of several genes that interact during development, despite the existence of variants in genes of major effect, which may lead to great morphological changes (Major gene effect hypothesis; Nei, 2007). The indicated major gene effect hypothesis suggests that morphological evolution can occur by the action of a small number of mutations of large effect on structural and/ or regulatory genes. Thus, when dealing with human pigmentation, it is expected that several genes may be involved in this trait, as well as environmental and epigenetic factors.

Many hypotheses predict how we can find pigmentation variation over human populations. For many authors, skin color is one of the most illustrative examples of the action of natural selection. This factor would be responsible for the elimination of genetic variants associated with light skin in areas with high levels of ultraviolet radiation, as a form of protection to sun damage (i.e. burns, malignant melanoma, basal and squamous cell carcinoma) (Blum, 1961; Kollias et al., 1991). The photoprotective properties of a highly melanized skin and the recent African origin of modern humans suggest that the ancestral phenotype would be dark skin (Jablonski & Chaplin, 2000; Rogers et al., 2004). Thus, the appearance of white skin would have occurred after the departure of modern humans from Africa, and two possibilities exist for its increase in frequency: (a) relaxation of functional constraints, and drift of the derived alleles (Brace, 1963); or (b) in regions of low UV radiation, positive selection favoring the fixation of mutations that resulted in a clear skin as a way to maximize cutaneous vitamin D synthesis (Rana et al., 1999; Jablonski & Chaplin, 2000).

# 2. PIGMENTATION AND GENETIC VARIATION

## 2.1. Mechanisms of Development

Human hair, eye, and skin pigmentation are the most visible examples of the human phenotypic diversity (Sulem et al., 2007). Since Darwin's first studies, it was believed that human pigmentation variation could be a consequence of natural selection (Darwin, 1871). Skin color is associated to latitude, with people having increasingly fairer skin as far as they live away from the equator (Relethford, 1997). On the other hand, the most diverse eye and hair pigmentation is found in the European and Euro-derived populations. The others present mainly brown eyes and dark hair. In contrast to skin color, the adaptive significance of a loss of eye pigmentation is less evident. The high degree of exposure to light of the white region of the eyeball around the iris is unique to humans and has been proposed as a factor to enhance signals stare, for example (Kobayashi & Kohshima, 2001).

One suggestion that seems to have little support is that the iris pigmentation could influence visual acuity in low-light environments. Although albinism is an exception, with obvious eye problems due to loss in the ability of melanin synthesis, there are reports of the effects of eye color on reaction time and involvement in specific sports (Rowe & Evans, 1994), associations with shyness in childhood (Coplan et al., 1998), links with hearing loss (Da Costa et al., 2008), and sexual selection (Frost, 2006). The latter may have been a cofactor for the loss of pigmentation in humans. Haplotype analyses suggest that the blue eye color has originated about 10,000 years ago, independently of albinism, as a founder mutation shared by several European populations (Eiberg et al., 2008). There are also reports that the ability to recover from the seasonal affective disorder (SAD), a major depressive illness, is linked to blue eyes (Goel et al., 2002; Terman & Terman, 1999). Extrapolating these results, perhaps individuals with blue eyes might have been able to better adapt to darkness in Neolithic Europe gloomy winter's day better than those with brown eyes.

The organic pigment melanin is synthesized and stored inside melanosomes in the melanocytes – dendritic cells located between dermis and epidermis in skin, in the hair bulb and in the iris (Hida et al., 2009). During ontogenesis primary melanocytes – the melanoblats – migrate from the neural crest to the skin, to hair follicles and to eyes, and are directly responsible for the pigmentation of such regions (Sturm et al., 2001). The variation in human pigmentation is associated to melanin type, number, size, and density of melanosomes, and also their pH. There are two main types of melanin: feomelanin (red – yellow) and eumelanin (black – brown), which are synthesized according to the chemical and hormonal environment present inside the melanosomes (Barsh, 2006). Tanning, for instance, is associated to eumelanin production, which is synthesized in response to ultraviolet radiation (Nan et al., 2009a), to protect the skin from damage. The melanosome's pH works as a regulatory factor for melanin synthesis (Cheli et al., 2009; Lamason et al., 2005).

The number of melanocytes does not appear to differ between different eye colors (Imesch et al., 1997). However, it has been reported that the total number of melanocytes in the iris may be lower in Asians as compared to Africans and Europeans, due to the smaller area of the iris or low density of melanocytes in that group (Albert et al., 2003). Unlike skin and hair, where melanin is continuously produced and secreted, in the iris melanosomes are retained and accumulated in the melanocytes cytoplasm within the iris stroma. Melanin type has also been studied chemically between eye colors, and blue iris is associated with minimal pigment content, while the eumelanic and pheomelanic forms were detected in other eye colors (Prota et al., 1998; Wielgus & Sarna, 2005). Thus, change in packaging, the quality and quantity of melanin pigment is what causes the observed spectrum of the eyes, hair and skin hues.

The pigmentation candidate genes that were identified up to the present act during many different stages of the process, including melanogenesis, stabilization and transport of enzymes during melanin synthesis, melanosome production and maintenance, and balance between the synthesis of different melanin types (Norton et al., 2007). The basic mechanisms of human pigmentation regulation involve a series of processes. Melanocites respond to the peptide alfa-MSH hormones (alfa-melanocite stimulant hormone) and to ACTH (adenocorticotropic hormone) through a protein-G-coupled receptor (Mc1r) to drive melanin production, which is derived from the enzymatic oxidation of tyrosine (Sturm et al., 2001). Alfa-MSH binds to the product of the *MC1R* gene, increasing the intracellular cyclic adenosine monophosphate (cAMP, Buscà & Ballotti, 2000) and activating the microphthalmia transcription factor (Mitf; Goding, 2000). It activates many enzymes in the melanosomes, the first being tyrosinase (Tyr; Marks & Seabra, 2001), which acts on tyrosine to produce dopaquinone; the latter links to cysteine molecules, if they are available in the cellular environment. After these interactions, the product of this reaction (cysteinylDOPA) is then oxidized to produce feomelanin (Ito, 2003). The *MITF* gene product also stimulates the tyrosine-related protein (*Tyrp1*) and the dopachrome tautomerasis (*Dct*; Marks & Seabra, 2001). Without cysteine, the dopainones found at the melanocites are transformed in other compound to produce eumelanin through the action of *Tyrp1* and *Dct* (Ito, 2003). The *Pmel17, Matp, Oca2,* and *Nckx5* proteins are all required for optimal melanin synthesis. *Pmel17* forms the fibrilar matrix where eumelanin is formed (reviewed by Theos et al., 2005). The *SLC45A2, OCA2,* and *SLC24A5* gene products are involved in inter-membrane transportation (Lee et al., 1995; Newton et al., 2001, Lamason et al., 2005), driving eumelanin production and eumelanosome maturation. The *ASIP* gene product binds to the *MC1R* gene product, blocking its association to alfa-MSH and modifying melanin production. Many genome-wide association studies (GWAS) indicated the importance of the above-mentioned genes through the identification of single-nucleotide polymorphisms (SNPs) and other types of genetic variation (Pho & Leachman, 2010).

A study of *SLC24A5, SLC45A2* and *TYR* polymorphisms found highly significant associations between their variation and skin reflectance measurements, an indirect measure of melanin content (Stokowski et al., 2007). The additive association found in these three genes accounts for a large fraction of the natural variation in skin pigmentation found in South Asian populations. This was the first study analyzing polymorphisms across the genome to find possible genetic determinants of natural variation in pigmentation within a human population. Norton et al. (2007), on the other hand, showed evidence that at least two other genes (*ASIP* and *OCA2*) work in shaping light and dark pigmentation around the globe, and also identified several other candidate loci that have a significant effect on regional pigmentation phenotypes worldwide. The data of Norton et al. (2007) are important because they showed independent genetic effects for light skin in Europeans and East Asians, which probably arose after their divergence. Details of the aforementioned genes, and other possibly involved in pigmentation, as well as some of their variants, will be discussed in greater detail in the following items.

## 2.1. *MC1R*

One of the most important systems regulating human pigmentation is the melanocortin 1 receptor (*MC1R*), G-protein coupled (Sturm, 2009). The genetic mechanisms of normal variation in skin color were only better understood after the discovery of mutations in this gene, encoding the Mc1r receptor (Makova & Norton, 2005, Valverde et al., 1995). The *MC1R* gene is located on chromosome 16q24.3 (Gantz et al., 1994), has 5 exons in humans, and its product is a cell surface receptor of melanocytes, working towards the production of melanin. It also participates in the regulation of eumelanin and pheomelanin production. The gene produces a 317 aminoacids protein (Sturm, 2009) and is polymorphic (Box et al., 1997;

Rana et al., 1999). Many of its variants are related to red hair and fair skin, increased risk for skin cancer and poor tanning ability, and it shows interactions with the *OCA2* gene (King et al., 2003).

Nine common *MC1R* alleles have been analyzed through the expression of the variant protein in studies in vitro (Beaumont et al., 2007). The Arg151Cys and Arg160Trp polymorphisms (rs1805007, rs1805008) produce changes in the cellular localization of the receptor encoded by the *MC1R* gene (Schioth et al., 1999; Beaumont et al., 2005). Another polymorphism, Asp294His (rs1805009), interferes with the coupling ability of the G protein in the cell membrane surface (Schioth et al., 1999; Duffy et al., 2004). In a GWAS study conducted by Nan et al. (2009a), a highly significant association between some SNPs outside the *MC1R* gene on chromosome 16 and the hair color phenotype, disappear after adjustment for functional variants (Arg151Cys, Arg160Trp, Asp294His) of the *MC1R* gene.

## *2.2. OCA2*

The *OCA2* gene has 24 exons and is located on chromosome 15q11.2-15q12 (Sturm & Frudakis, 2004), produces a protein with 838 aminoacids (Sturm, 2009) and its function is not well established (Rebbeck et al., 2002): it was suggested to be a channel (antiporter) of $Na^+/H^+$ (Ancans et al., 2001; Puri et al., 2000) or a glutamate transporter (Lamoreux et al., 1995). Both functions indicate that *OCA2* is involved in supplying substrates for tyrosinase in melanin biosynthesis (Ancans *et al.*, 2001). Alternatively, *OCA2* may be involved in the intracellular pathway of tyrosinase during melanosome maturation (Toyofuku et al., 2002). Duffy et al. (2007) proposed that variations within the regulatory 5' control region are responsible for 90% of the variation in eye color pigmentation. Puri et al. (2000) also suggested that the *OCA2* gene product, a membrane melanosomal protein, can serve as an anion transporter, thereby helping to regulate the melanosomal pH.

Recent studies have revealed that the interaction between *OCA2* and *HERC2* may be responsible for determining the blue eye color in humans. In an association study with *OCA2* and *HERC2,* Branicki et al. (2009) verified possible interaction effects with other genes (*MC1R*, *ASIP*, and *SLC45A2*) also associated with variation in eye, hair and skin color in some populations. They concluded that the rs1800407 (Arg419Gln) polymorphism in the *OCA2* gene is associated with eye color and that there are significant interactions between *MC1R* and *HERC2* in determining skin and hair color in their Polish sample. Sturm (2009), on the other hand, found that variants in *OCA2* increase by 2.4 times the amount of melanin in melanocytes culture. In another study on a sample of individuals of Asian ancestry, Edwards et al. (2010) verified that the non-synonymous polymorphism His615Arg (rs1800414) of the *OCA2* gene is associated with skin pigmentation. Individuals with the G derived allele, which codes for the aminoacid arginine, showed less melanin index than those with the ancestral allele A, which encodes the aminoacid histidine. The methodology and analysis performed by Edwards et al. (2010) are consistent with other findings, also indicating that the evolution of light skin occurred at least in part independently in Europeans and Asians.

## 2.3. *SLC45A2 (MATP)*

The Membrane Associated Transporter Protein (*MATP*), known as *SLC45A2* (solute carrier family 45, member 2), has 7 exons and is located on chromosome 5p. The matp protein has 530 aminoacids (Sturm, 2009) and is considered a regulator of tyrosinase activity in human melanocytes (Smith et al., 2004). In the GWAS conducted by Nan et al. (2009a), they suggested that the rs16891982 in the *SLC45A2* gene is the most likely causal variant or is in strong linkage disequilibrium with the causal variant related to tanning ability.

Polymorphisms in the gene encoding the *Matp* protein proved to be related to variation in normal and abnormal skin color in Europeans. Lucotte et al. (2010) showed that the frequency of the Phe374Leu (rs16891982) polymorphism in Western Europe and North Africa may reflect the level of ultraviolet radiation received and the associated variation in skin color of individuals in these regions. This same polymorphism would also be associated with protection against the development of malignant melanoma (Guedj et al., 2008, Fernandez et al., 2008). Yuasa et al. (2006), in turn, suggested that the 374Phe allele may be an important causative factor in hypopigmentation in Caucasian populations. Cook et al. (2009) also analyzed the same polymorphism and found that the 374Leu allele was associated with high levels of tyrosinase and the homozygotes for it had lower levels of Matp transcripts in the European sample analyzed. Sturm (2009) observed that the these 100 homozygotes showed 2.6 times the amount of melanin in cultured melanocytes, as compared to the 374Phe homozygotes. The heterozygous genotype possessed an intermediate melanin index, suggesting an additive effect. Finally, in the genome-wide study conducted by Sabeti et al. (2007) it was found that the *SLC45A2* gene is probably under positive selection in Europeans, since the 374Phe allele is nearly fixed in this population, but absent in Asian and African samples.

## 2.4. *TYR*

Melanin synthesis also occurs with the participation of tyrosinase-related proteins (Huang et al., 2008). Tyrosinase has a critical role in cellular melanogenesis and therefore has been a target for skin pigmentation studies, including pharmacological tests involved in the care and esthetic maintenance of this pigmentation (An et al., 2009). The *TYR* gene, coding for tyrosinase, has five exons, is located on chromosome 11q, and produces a molecule of 529 aminoacids (Sturm, 2009).

*TYR* is one of the classic genes related to oculocutaneous albinism (Hutton & Spritz, 2008), and Meyler & Guldberg (2009) suggested that its product has a major effect on the hair and skin pigmentation. Bishop et al. (2009), on the other hand, related them to sun-sensitive skin, freckles, and a specific melanoma. An et al. (2009) used *TYR* small interfering RNA to test the effect of silencing this gene in some cell types. *TYR* silencing resulted in the suppression of melanin synthesis and decreased the viability of cells exposed to ultraviolet radiation.

In the GWAS conducted by Nan et al. (2009a), several SNPs were found significantly associated with tanning ability in a USA population of European ancestry, among them SNPs in the *TYR* gene. One of them (rs1393350) was the only which remained significant after adjusting for the analysis conducted. The SNP is also in strong linkage disequilibrium with rs1126809 (Arg402Gln), a common and widely studied tyrosinase polymorphism. Tyrosinase is critical for melanosomal maturation, leading also to eumelanosome formation (Jimbow et al., 2000).

Fukai et al. (1995) and Morell et al., (1997) reported that one allele of the Arg402Gln polymorphism was correlated with reduced iris and retina pigmentation, due to low tyrosinase activity. In another study Nan et al. (2009b) also showed that this same allele was significantly related to tanning ability and skin color. Sturm (2009), in turn, showed that polymorphisms in other genes (*SLC45A2, SLC24A5* and *OCA2*) also cause variations in the tyrosinase activity. For example, in the *SLC24A5,* Ala111Thr polymorphism 111Ala/111Ala homozygotes showed 1.7x increased tyrosinase activity, compared to 111Thr/111Thr homozygotes. *SLC45A2* (Leu374Phe) and *OCA2* (rs12913832 T> C) polymorphisms were also correlated with tyrosinase activity. Homozygotes for *SLC45A2* 374Leu and *OCA2* TT independently presented a higher tyrosinase activity (2.8x and 2.1x, respectively), compared to 374PhePhe (*SLC45A2*) and CC (*OCA2*) genotypes.

## 2.5. *ASIP*

The gene encoding the agouti signaling protein (*ASIP*) has 3 exons and is located on chromosome 20q. Its product, together with other ligands, regulates the exchange between the synthesis of eumelanin and pheomelanin in melanocytes (Hida et al., 2009). It is known that *ASIP* regulates the pigmentation in mice, but its functional role in other animals and humans has not been well elucidated (Norris & Whan, 2008). The *ASIP* gene encodes a molecule with 132 aminoacids (Sturm, 2009), which coordinates melanocytes in the hair follicle to produce yellow or black pigment. The unregulated expression of agouti in mice carrying the dominant (yellow) allele is associated with pleiotropic effects including increased yellow fur pigmentation, obesity, diabetes and increased susceptibility to tumors (Perry et al., 1995).

Anno et al. (2008) attempted to identify alleles at multiple loci associated with differences in skin color in peoples of various origins using SNP genotyping and linkage disequilibrium. They analyzed 20 SNPs of several (*ASIP, TYR, OCA2, MC1R,* and others) genes in Canadians and Japanese and found significant differences between the two groups. Although the Asip protein was presented as a competitive antagonist of the *MC1R* gene product, the possibility of having other independent activity could not be ruled out, according to Hunt & Thody (1995). These authors showed that the rodent agouti protein causes suppression of melanin production in cultured melanoma cells. Moreover, this same protein decreased melanogenesis in human epidermal melanocytes in culture. Recent studies also suggest that the *ASIP* gene product regulates the expression of the *SLC24A5* gene (Nadeau et al., 2008).

Bonilla et al. (2005) showed that the 8818A allele acts as a strong antagonist to alpha-MSH, binding to Mc1r and then blocking the signaling mediated by cAMP in the melanocyte. The production of pheomelanin is thus favored, leading to the maturation of feomelanosomes and lighter coloring.

## 2.6. SLC24A5 (NCKX5)

One of the genes of the family of solute carriers (*SLC24A5*) encodes the *Nckx5* protein with 500 aminoacids, has 9 exons and is located on chromosome 15q (Sturm, 2009). Giardina et al., (2008) showed that the G (rs1426654 - Thr111Ala) allele together with two other intragenic markers (rs2555364 and rs16960620) vary in frequency among populations with different skin pigmentation.

Ginger et al. (2008) were the first to demonstrate that expression of the *SLC24A5* gene product is required for the production of melanin in differentiating human epidermal melanoblasts. It is believed that the *SLC24A5* gene encodes a calcium/sodium potassium dependent transporter present in the melanosomal membrane, and calcium may be required for the activation of a gene to produce Pmel17, required to form mature eumelanosome involved in eye color variation (Frudakis et al., 2003); melanosome pH regulation may also be a function of the SLC24A5 protein (Lamason et al., 2005). The role of pH in melanogenesis has been studied in detail, and there is evidence that pH changes affect tyrosinase maturation and its catalytic activity (Smith et al., 2004; Watabe et al., 2004).

*SLC24A5*, which is orthologous to the golden gene in zebrafish, has been widely cited in studies of human pigmentation. For example, in a study by Dimisianos et al. (2009) in Greece the rs1426654 (Thr111Ala) SNP was analyzed and the results were correlated with pigmentation traits and with *MC1R* genotypes. It was shown that the 111Thr allele was more prevalent among Greeks of darker skin, although this study shows a bias, since the majority of subjects (99%) were homozygous for this allele. *TYR*, *SLC45A2* and *SLC24A5* polymorphisms were studied in South Asian populations and their alleles may account for differences in skin reflectance (darker or lighter skin) through a simple additive model (Sturm, 2009). On the other hand, *SLC45A2/MATP*, *SLC24A5/NCKX5* and *OCA2/P* SNPs have been associated with natural variation of pigmentation traits in several human populations (Cook et al., 2009).

In a genome-scan for the detection and characterization of positive selection in human populations Sabeti et al. (2007) verified that *SLC24A5* and *SLC45A2* are subjected to this type of selection, while *EDAR* and *EDAR2R* were involved in the development of the hair follicle. It was also found that the *SLC24A5* gene Thr111Ala polymorphism showed the strongest signal of positive selection. Its ancestral allele (111Ala) predominates in Amerindians, Africans and East Asians. Conversely, 111Thr is almost fixed in Europeans and is also correlated with skin lighter pigmentation in admixed populations (Lamason et al., 2005). In a functional study conducted by Sturm (2009) it was found that the AlaAla genotype increases 2.2 times the amount of melanin in cultured melanocytes, compared to ThrThr. Heterozygous subjects possessed an intermediate level of melanin, suggesting an additive effect.

## 2.7. ADAM17

The gene encoding the Adam17 protein (*ADAM17* - a disintegrin and metalloprotease) has 19 exons and is located on chromosome 2p. Its product encodes 824 aminoacids and it is part of the Adam family of proteolytic enzymes, acting in the cleavage of other enzymes (Corrias et al., 2010; Yamamoto et al., 2010). It is also called *TACE* (Tumor necrosis factor-Alpha Converting Enzyme), and codifies a metalloprotease associated with the cell membrane that is expressed in endothelial cells (Weskamp et al., 2010), adipocytes (Junyent et al., 2010) and is the primary enzyme responsible for catalyzing the release of membrane proteins anchored in the cell surface of Metazoan organisms (Caescu et al., 2009).

These metalloproteinases can rapidly modulate signaling events in the cell surface through proteolytic release of soluble forms of pro-ligands for cell receptors, and many regulatory pathways are affected by the *Adam17* activity; the detailed mechanisms of its activity, however, are not well understood (Willems et al., 2010). *Adam17* has pleiotropic effects and is therefore also associated with various diseases such as those leading to neurodegeneration, cancer and inflammation (Hoettecke et al., 2010, Long et al., 2010). Norton et al. (2007) have detected significant evidence of natural selection in *ADAM17* and *ATRN*. They found evidence of positive selection in these genes in Asians comparable to the *MATP* and *SLC24A5* signals found in Europeans.

## 2.8. HERC2

*HERC2* is located upstream of *OCA2* (Eiberg et al., 2008). In three independent GWAS analyses the 15q13.1 region, which covers 38cM in the genome and includes genes *OCA2* and *HERC2*, was found to be the predominant region involved in human iris color (Kayser et al., 2008). Estimates indicated that 74% of the variance in human eye color could be explained by this region. The *HERC2* gene contains 93 exons, and the detailed function of its product is still unknown, but the gene encodes domains of conserved functional proteins involved in spermatogenesis, ubiquitin-mediated proteolysis and intracellular transport (Ji et al., 2000). Interactions between *OCA2* and *HERC2* through epistatic effects were observed (Kayser et al., 2008).

The melanin pigment within the iris is responsible for the human eye color (Sturm & Larsson, 2009). Fine mapping of this region identified a single base variation (rs12913832 - T/C) in *HERC2* intron 86, which explains much of the association with blue-brown eye color. Eiberg et al. (2008) had already identified two SNPs (rs12913832 and rs1129038) within the 15q13.1 region that were strongly associated with blue and brown eye colors. Kayser et al. (2008) also claimed that no other region on genes showed so consistent evidence of association with iris color. They also suggested that the testing of *OCA2-HERC2* markers could be used in forensic applications to predict eye color phenotypes of unknown persons of European origin. Partial *OCA2-HERC2* deletions are known in the Prader-Willi and Angelman syndromes, which are associated with oculocutaneous albinism or reduced pigmentation (Spritz et al., 1997).

So far the most consistent reports concerning eye color have been the association of three SNPs of *OCA2* intron 1 and two *HERC2* (rs129113832 and rs1129038) SNPs (Iida et al., 2009). Humbert (2008) suggested that blue eye color could be due to the change of an element located in *HERC2* suppressing *OCA2* expression.

## 2.9. TPCN2

The *TPCN2* (Two-Pore Channel segment 2) gene has 25 exons and is located on chromosome 11q. Its encoded protein has 752 aminoacids (Sturm, 2009). This protein influences calcium transport, similarly to those of the *SLC24A4* (Sulem et al., 2007) and *SLC24A5* (Lamason et al., 2005) genes. Sulem et al. (2008) found that two coding polymorphisms (rs35264875 - Met484Leu and rs3829241 - Gly734Glu) could explain the difference between blond and brown hair individuals in Iceland.

## 2.10. Other Pigmentation Genes

The loci involved in pigmentation are related to a variety of physiological processes, including DNA damage responses, immunity and hypo/hyperpigmentation (Stinchcombe et al., 2004), melanocyte migration, melanogenesis control, hormone responses (MSH-like and sex hormones or vitamin D), or prostaglandin synthesis. The latter may mediate changes in post-inflammatory pigmentation by modulating melanocyte dendricity and melanin synthesis (Scott et al., 2004). These loci include *ADAMTS20, AP3D1, AP3M2, AR, ASMT, ATRN, BLOC1S3, BRCA1, CHS1* (*LYST*), *CNO, CYP24A1, CYP27B1, DC6, DCT, DDC, EDA, EDN3, EDNRB, ERCC2, ESR1, ESR2, GGT1, GPR143, HPS1, HPS2* (*AP3B1*), *HPS3, HPS5, HPS6, HPS7* (*DTNBP1*), *IKBKG, IRF4, KIT, KITLG, MAGMAS, MAMAL1, MDM2, MGRN1, MITF, MLANA, MLPH, MTNR1A, MTNR1B, MUTED, MYO5A, MYO7A, OSTM1, PAR2, PAX3, PER1, PGR, PKCb, PLDN, POMC, PTGER1, PTGER2, PTGER3, PTGFR, PTGIR, RAB27A, RABGGTA, RAD50, RXRA, SILV* (*PM17*), *SOX10, TBX2, TH, TP53, TP53BP1, TYRP1, TYRP2* (*DCT*), *VDR, VDRIP, VPS18, VPS33A, YARS*, and *ZNFN1A1*, besides those already mentioned above.

Many of these genes show no robust evidence for positive selection (Izagirre et al., 2006; Myles et al., 2007; Norton et al., 2007), differently from those previously mentioned. But this is expected due to the complex nature of the phenotypes considered.

## 3. FORENSIC APPLICATION AND PERSPECTIVES

The initial attempt to apply human DNA analysis to forensic investigations was based in DNA "fingerprints", individual-specific genetic profiles defined by a set of hypervariable markers' genotypes (Jeffreys et al., 1985). These "fingerprints" could be analyzed with southern-blot hybridization and used for human identification and parenthood testing. Since then, however, the repertoire of genetic markers used in forensic routine has grown substantially and several advances in molecular biology had brought much progress to the forensic sciences.

One of such advances is the possibility to infer the person's ethnicity and/or physical appearance by using genetic markers. Ancestry Informative Markers (AIMs), genetic loci showing alleles with large frequency differences between continental populations (Shriver et al., 2003), have been employed for this purpose. These markers enhance the power of an already effective system of DNA analysis based on microsatellite variation for the identification of unmatched samples in, for instance, cases such as mass-disasters due to terrorist attacks. It is believed that these markers could also provide information about the general appearance of a person (Budowle and Van Daal, 2008). But although they could provide some lead in certain populations, AIMs may not be completely associated to human physical appearance in admixed populations (Parra et al., 2003).

In cases where police investigations fail to identify the attackers, and especially when the biological evidence found at crime scenes do not match those existing in the DNA police database, it is expected the development in the near future of predictions of externally visible features (Externally Visible Characteristics - EVCs) based on DNA (Kayser & Schneider, 2009). Physical features that are explained by a small number of loci and few alleles, easy to detect using standard methods of linkage analysis and genetic association, are the most promising.

Usually the first step in analyzing a crime-scene sample is to produce a profile of short tandem repeats (STRs) using multiplex amplification kits. When this profile do not match those of a police database, any additional information is extremely valuable (Werrett, 2005), including tests for predicting specific phenotypes (Tully, 2007). SNPs on the Y chromosome (Y-SNPs) are usually investigated for their potential to predict the geographic origin of a given male suspect. Unfortunately, due to the presence of admixed individuals, it is occasionally difficult to predict the geographic ancestry of an individual using Y-SNPs only. In a study conducted by Sims & Ballantyne (2008), using the *SLC24A5* gene variants in combination with Y-SNPs and other lineage markers, the authors were able to blindly differentiate Africans, Europeans and Asians. The eye color prediction could also be of great value in certain crime investigations. Mengel-From et al., (2010), for instance, developed predictive values for various SNP combinations in *HERC2*, *OCA2*, and *SLC45A2* (*MATP*) genes for blue/brown eye color.

Grimes et al., (2001) described a multiplex minisequencing protocol to quick scan DNA samples for the presence of 12 variants of the *MC1R* gene. In another study Frudakis et al. (2003) tested 754 SNPs in 851 individuals, and identified 61 SNPs associated with iris color. Nearly half of these SNPs were independently associated with this characteristic, while the remainder was associated only if considered as part of a haplotype or diplotype. Some companies already provide multiplex PCR-based tests for predicting iris color, and based on the literature, it is estimated that the inferences are correct in 92% of the cases.

With regard to ethical issues, the forensic scientific community recommends to avoid typing markers that are predictive of disease susceptibility, to protect the privacy of the persons involved (Tully, 2007).

## 4. EVOLUTIONARY BACKGROUND

The genetic basis underlying the normal variation in skin, hair and eye pigmentation has been the subject of intense research to verify the presence of any adaptive component. A combination of approaches has been used, including comparative genomics of candidate genes, identification of regions of the human genome under positive selection, allele-specific association studies, and genome-wide scans (Sturm, 2009).

Although the combination of fair skin and intense sun exposure results in a significant individual health risk, it is unclear whether this risk has evolutionary significance at the population level. Therefore, several adaptive hypotheses have been proposed to explain the evolution of human skin pigmentation, such as photo-protection against sun-induced cancer, sexual selection, vitamin D synthesis or photo-protection from photo-unstable compounds. It is expected that if skin pigmentation is adaptive, we could detect signs of the action of positive selection in some of the genes involved (Izagirre et al., 2006).

Several regions of the human genome have recently been identified as subjected to the action of positive selection. The combination of new methods, including large SNP banks at the population level, as well as new and robust analytic methodologies show clear evidence for selection acting on several pigmentation genes in different populations (Voight et al., 2006; Norton et al., 2007; Sabeti et al., 2007; Williamson et al., 2007; Johansson & Gyllensten, 2008). These studies also showed that the process probably occurred many times in multiple geographic locations around the globe, in ancient and recent human populations.

Jablonski & Chaplin (2000) and Chaplin (2004), for example, have confirmed a strong positive correlation between skin pigmentation and intensity of ultraviolet radiation. However, although there is strong evidence that the variation in pigmentation have been influenced by natural selection, little is known about how selection has affected the genetic architecture of pigmentation loci in different populations, even when these populations have experienced similar levels of ultraviolet radiation in their evolutionary trajectory. The dark skin that characterizes many African populations south of the Sahara and Melanesians may be due to shared ancestral variants or new genetic adaptations. Similarly, the light skin of Europeans and East Asians may have a common genetic origin or can be the result of independent adaptations to environments of low ultraviolet radiation.

Norton et al. (2007) described the allele frequencies of polymorphisms in the *ASIP* (A8818G), *OCA2* (A355G), *TYR* (Ser192Tyr), *MATP* (Phe374Leu), and *SLC24A5* (Thr111Ala) in various populations. They wanted to verify the presence of positive selection for these polymorphisms in Africans, Asians, Europeans and a small group of Native Americans. An evolutionary model for the independent selection of variants of pigmentation genes in East Asian, European and West African populations was proposed, leading to the conclusion of convergent evolution in the case of lighter colored skin (McEvoy et al., 2006; Norton et al., 2007). In Europeans and Asians, signs of positive selection were confirmed for *SLC24A5* (Lamason et al., 2005; Norton et al., 2007) and *SLC45A2* (Soejima et al., 2006; Norton et al., 2007) gene variants, which result in lighter skin. Norton et al. (2007) also concluded that light pigmentation in Europeans is due, at least in part, to the effects of sexual selection and/or positive directional selection, and not simply by relaxation of functional constraints, as previously suggested.

Izagirre et al., (2006) and Myles et al., (2007) used public data banks (HapMap and Pelergen), with African, African-American, European and East Asian genotypic information and performed an $F_{st}$ analysis. Under a neutral model, $F_{st}$ is determined by the demographic history (basically gene flow and drift) of the groups considered and would affect all loci in a similar way. In contrast, under the action of selection, specific loci would show different patterns. Balancing or purifying selection tend to reduce $F_{st}$ values while positive selection would lead to increased values when compared to those of other genomic regions. The two studies identified signs of selection in *SLC24A5* and *SLC45A2* (*MATP*) in European and East Asian individuals. In contrast, no signs of selection were found for *MC1R*.

## 5. IMPROVING PIGMENTATION PHENOTYPIC DATA FOR FORENSIC AND GENERAL STUDIES

In studies that seek to relate genotype-phenotype in pigmentation characteristics, it is recommended that these characteristics should be examined as objectively as possible, avoiding qualitative ratings for skin pigmentation such as 'black', 'dark brown', 'light brown' or 'white', since classification criteria may be diverse in different countries and ethnicities.

It is suggested that frontal photographs should be made of the study participants, to make a data log archive of eyes and face pigmentation. Photographs of the back of the head can also be made to obtain data from hair color. Quantitative measurements of pigmentation through the contents of melanin in exposed/non-exposed regions, as described by Stokowski et al. (2007), are recommended. These measures could be made by reflectance spectrophotometry, for instance, DermaSpectrometer, Cortex Technology, Hadsund, Denmark. This instrument emits light at the green (568nm) and red (655nm) regions of the visible spectrum and the photo-detector measures the amount of light reflected by the skin. These measures are used to estimate the melanin content of skin, which is expressed as a Melanin Index (M). In human populations M ranges from about 20 (people with lighter skin) to near 100 (individuals with darker skin). For more accurate readings, these measures should be carried out preferably indoors and in a well-lighted room. More information about the DermaSpectrometer can be found in Shriver & Parra (2000).

A traditional method for hair classification involves its observation under a microscope considering such characteristics as color, length, diameter, pigment granules and other morphological traits (Saferstein, 2001; Bednarek, 2004; SWGMAT, 2005). Reflectance spectrophotometry is also used to determine hair color, which is more consistent than digital image analysis (Vaughn et al., 2008, 2009b). The CIE L*a*b* apparatus is used both for digital image analysis by microscopy, or for measuring macroscopic color (Vaughn et al., 2009a). The CIE L*a*b* model was developed by the *Commission Internationale de l'Eclairage* and measures the color in three axes, that correspond to the trichromatic human perception and reflects the degree of change in color that humans can perceive (Ford & Roberts, 1998). In this system, the brightness or intensity of a color is measured in the L* axis on a scale from 0 (black) to 100 (white). Color, in turn, is measured first along the a* axis, varying from -100 (green) to +100 (red); and then in the *b*\* axis, varying from -100 (blue) to +100 (yellow). The L*a*b* unit is regarded as the minimum difference that the human eye can observe (TASI, 2004).

Iris color categorization has been carried out using a variety of descriptive terms for self-assessment, as well as the use of a trained observer to describe, or qualitatively classify it using photographic standards (Seddon et al., 1990; Franssen et al., 2008). None of these methods is completely reliable and thus automated photographic methods have been developed to improve the accuracy in classification (Takamoto et al., 2001; Niggemann et al., 2003). A method which uses a digital camera and a computer software to analyze the light reflected from the iris was described in detail, with the sum of a range of color and brightness values used to derive an expression called the Iris Melanin Index (IMI), suitable for categorizing a population survey, but possibly still missing details of the iris pattern (Frudakis, 2008).

The most important point to emphasize is that objective, not subjective classifications should be used. Qualitative subdivision of continuous traits also oversimplify their nature (Liu et al., 2010). If indeed it is not possible to quantitatively measure hair and eye colors, care must be taken that the classification is made in accordance with previous studies, with the help of color standards. The most common hair characterizations involve 'black', 'brown' (without subdivisions, to avoid a subjective qualification), 'red', 'blond' or 'white'; while eye pigmentation may be characterized as 'black', 'brown', 'blue', 'green ' or 'grey'; whenever possible, the presence of brown spots around the pupil or any other eye brown spot should also be recorded (Eiberg et al., 2008).

## 6. REFERENCES

Albert, DM; Green, WR; Zimbric, ML; Lo, C; Gangnon, RE; Hope, KL; Gleiser, J. Iris melanocyte numbers in Asian, African American, and Caucasian irides. *Trans. Am. Ophthalmol. Soc.* 101: 217–222. 2003.

An, SM; Koh, JS; Boo, YC. Inhibition of melanogenesis by tyrosinase siRNA in human melanocytes. *BMB Rep.* 42(3):178-183. 2009.

Ancans, J; Tobin, DJ; Hoogduijn, MJ; Smit, NP; Wakamatsu, K; Thody, AJ. Melanosomal pH controls rate of melanogenesis, eumelanin/ phaeomelanin ratio and melanosome maturation in melanocytes and melanoma cells. *Exp Cell Res.* 268: 26–35. 2001.

Anno, S; Abe, T; Yamamoto, T. Interactions between SNP alleles at multiple loci contribute to skin color differences between caucasoid and mongoloid subjects. *Int J Biol Sci.* 4(2):81-86. 2008.

Barsh, GS. Regulation of pigment type switching by agouti, melanocortin signaling, attractin and mahoganoid. In *The Pigmentary System,* 2nd edn J.J. Nordlund, R.E. Boissy, V.J. Hearing, R.A. King, W.S. Oetting, and J.P. Ortonne, eds (Massachusetts: Blackwell Publishing), pp. 395–409. 2006.

Beaumont, KA; Newton, RA; Smit, DJ; Leonard, JH; Stow, JL; Sturm, RA. Altered cell surface expression of human MC1R variant receptor alleles associated with red hair and skin cancer risk. *Hum Mol Genet.* 14: 2145–2154. 2005.

Beaumont, KA; Shekar, SN; Newton, RA; James, MR; Stow, JL; Duffy, DL; Sturm, RA. Receptor function, dominant negative activity and phenotype correlations for MC1R variant alleles. *Hum Mol Genet.* 16: 2249–2260. 2007.

Bednarek, J. An attempt to establish objective criteria for morphological examinations of hairs using the image analysis system. *Probl Forensic Sci* 56: 65–77. 2004.

Blum, H. Does the melanin pigment of human skin have adaptive value? *Q Rev Biol.* 36:50–63. 1961.

Bonilla, C; Boxill, LA; Donald, SA; Williams, T; Sylvester, N; Parra, EJ; Dios, S; Norton, HL; Shriver, MD; Kittles, RA. The 8818G allele of the agouti signaling protein (ASIP ) gene is ancestral and is associated with darker skin color in African Americans. *Hum Genet.* 116 (5): 402–406. 2005.

Box, N; Wyeth, J; O'Gorman, L; Martin, NG; Sturm, RA. Characterization of melanocyte stimulating hormone receptor variant alleles in twins with red hair. *Hum Mol Genet.* 6 (11): 1891–1897. 1997.

Brace, C. Structural reduction in evolution. *Am Nat.* 97:39–49. 1963.

Branicki, W; Brudnik, U; Wojas-Pelc, A. Interactions between HERC2, OCA2 and MC1R may influence human pigmentation phenotype. *Ann Hum Genet.* 73(2):160-170. 2009.

Budowle, B & Van Daal, A. Forensically relevant SNP classes. *BioTechniques.* 44 (5): 603-610 (25th Anniversary Issue, April 2008). 2008.

Buscà, R & Ballotti, R. Cyclic AMP a key messenger in the regulation of skin pigmentation. *Pigment Cell Res.* 13(2): 60–69. 2000.

Caescu, CI; Jeschke, GR; Turk, BE. Active-site determinants of substrate recognition by the metalloproteinases TACE and ADAM10. *Biochem J.* 424(1):79-88. 2009.

Chaplin, G. Geographic distribution of environmental factors influencing human skin coloration. *Am J Phys Anthropol.* 125:292–302. 2004.

Cheli, Y; Luciani, F; Khaled, M; Beuret, L; Bille, K; Gounon, P; Ortonne, JP; Bertolotto, C; Ballotti, R. {alpha}MSH and Cyclic AMP elevating agents control melanosome pH through a protein kinase A-independent mechanism. *J Biol Chem.* 284(28):18699-18706. 2009.

Cook, AL; Chen, W; Thurber, AE; Smit, DJ; Smith, AG; Bladen, TG; Brown, DL; Duffy, DL; Pastorino, L; Bianchi-Scarra, G; Leonard, JH; Stow, JL; Sturm, RA. Analysis of cultured human melanocytes based on polymorphisms within the SLC45A2/MATP, SLC24A5/NCKX5, and OCA2/P loci. *J Invest Dermatol.* 129(2):392-405. 2009.

Coplan, RJ; Coleman, B; Rubin, KH. Shyness and little boy blue: iris pigmentation, gender, and social wariness in preschoolers. *Dev. Psychobiol.* 32: 37–44. 1998.

Corrias, MV; Gambini, C; Gregorio, A; Croce, M; Barisione, G; Cossu, C; Rossello, A; Ferrini, S; Fabbi, M. Different subcellular localization of ALCAM molecules in neuroblastoma: association with relapse. *Cell Oncol.* 32(1-2):77-86. 2010.

Darwin, C. The descent of man. Princeton University Press, Princeton. 1871.

Da Costa, EA; Castro, JC; Macedo, ME. Iris pigmentation and susceptibility to noise-induced hearing loss. *Int. J. Audiol.* 47: 115–118. 2008.

Dimisianos, G; Stefanaki, I; Nicolaou, V; Sypsa, V; Antoniou, C; Poulou, M; Papadopoulos, O; Gogas, H; Kanavakis, E; Nicolaidou, E; Katsambas, AD; Stratigos, AJ. A study of a single variant allele (rs1426654) of the pigmentation-related gene SLC24A5 in Greek subjects. *Exp Dermatol.* 18(2):175-177. 2009.

Duffy, DL; Box, NF; Chen, W; Palmer, JS; Montgomery, GW; James, MR; Hayward, NK; Martin, NG; Sturm, RA. Interactive effects of MC1R and OCA2 on melanoma risk phenotypes. *Hum Mol Genet.* 13: 447–461. 2004.

Duffy, DL; Montgomery, GW; Chen, W; Zhao, ZZ; Le, L; James, MR; Hayward, NK; Martin, NG; Sturm, RA. A three single-nucleotide polymorphism haplotype in intron 1 of OCA2 explains most human eye-color variation. *Am J Hum Genet.* 80: 241–252. 2007.

Edwards, M; Bigham, A; Tan, J; Li, S; Gozdzik, A; Gozdzik, A; Ross, K; Jin, L; Parra, EJ. Association of the OCA2 Polymorphism His615Arg with melanin content in East Asian populations: further evidence of convergent evolution of skin pigmentation. *PLoS Genet.* 6(3): e1000867. 2010.

Eiberg, H; Troelsen, J; Nielsen, M; Mikkelsen, A; Mengel-From, J; Kjaer, KW; Hansen, L. Blue eye color in humans may be caused by a perfectly associated founder mutation in a regulatory element located within the HERC2 gene inhibiting OCA2 expression. *Hum Genet.* 123(2):177-187. 2008.

Enserink, M. Can this DNA sleuth help catch criminals? *Science.* 331: 838-840. 2011.

Fernandez, LP; Milne, RL; Pita, G; Avilés, JA; Lázaro, P; Benítez, J; Ribas, G. SLC45A2: a novel malignant melanoma-associated gene. *Hum Mutat.* 29(9):1161-1167. 2008.

Ford, A & Roberts, A. *Colour space conversions.* Available at www.poynton.com/PDFs/coloureq.pdf, accessed February 1, 2007. 1998.

Franssen, J; Coppens, JE; Van Den Berg, TJTP. Grading of iris color with an extended photographic reference set. *J Optom.* 1: 36–40. 2008.

Frost, P. European hair and eye color: a case of frequency dependent sexual selection? *Evol Hum Behav.* 27: 85–103. 2006.

Frudakis, TN. *Molecular Photofitting – Predicting Ancestry and Phenotype Using DNA* (Burlington, MA, USA: Academic Press). 2008.

Frudakis, T; Thomas, M; Gaskin, Z; Venkateswarlu, K; Chandra, KS; Ginjupalli, S; Gunturi, S; Natrajan, S; Ponnuswamy, VK; Ponnuswamy, KN. Sequences associated with human iris pigmentation. *Genetics.* 165(4): 2071–2083. 2003.

Fukai, K; Holmes, SA; Lucchese, NJ; Siu, VM; Weleber, RG; Schnur, RE; Spritz, RA. Autosomal recessive ocular albinism associated with a functionally significant tyrosinase gene polymorphism. *Nat Genet.* 9:92–95. 1995.

Gantz, I; Yamada, T; Tashiro, T; Konda, Y; Shimoto, Y; Miwa, H; Trent, JM. Mapping of the gene encoding the melanocortin-1 (alpha-melanocyte stimulating hormone) receptor (MC1R) to human chromosome 16q24.3 by fluorescence in situ hybridization. *Genomics.* 19 (2): 394–395. 1994.

Giardina, E; Pietrangeli, I; Martínez-Labarga, C; Martone, C; de Angelis, F; Spinella, A; De Stefano, G; Rickards, O; Novelli, G. Haplotypes in SLC24A5 gene as ancestry informative markers in different populations. *Curr Genomics.* 9(2):110-114. 2008.

Ginger, RS; Askew, SE; Ogborne, RM; Wilson, S; Ferdinando, D; Dadd, T; Smith, AM; Kazi, S; Szerencsei, RT; Winkfein, RJ; Schnetkamp, PPM; Green, MR. SLC24A5 encodes a trans-Golgi network protein with potassium-dependent sodium-calcium exchange activity that regulates human epidermal melanogenesis. *J Biol Chem.* 283 (9): 5486–5495. 2008.

Goding, CR. Mitf from neural crest to melanoma: signal transduction and transcription in the melanocyte lineage. *Genes Dev.* 14(14): 1712–1728. 2000.

Goel, N; Terman, M; Terman, JS. Depressive symptomatology differentiates subgroups of patients with seasonal affective disorder. *Depress Anxiety* 15, 34–41. 2002.

Grimes, EA; Noake, PJ; Dixon, L; Urquhart, A. Sequence polymorphism in the human melanocortin 1 receptor gene as an indicator of the red hair phenotype. *Forensic Sci Int.* 122(2-3): 124–129. 2001.

Guedj, M; Bourillon, A; Combadières, C; Rodero, M; Dieudé, P; Descamps, V; Dupin, N; Wolkenstein, P; Aegerter, P; Lebbe, C; Basset-Seguin,N; Prum, B; Saiag, P; Grandchamp, B; Soufir, N; MelanCohort Investigators. Variants of the MATP/SLC45A2 gene are protective for melanoma in the French population. *Hum Mutat.* 29(9):1154-1160. 2008.

Hida, T; Wakamatsu, K; Sviderskaya, EV; Donkin, AJ; Montoliu, L; Lynn Lamoreux, M; Yu, B; Millhauser, GL; Ito, S; Barsh, GS; Jimbow, K; Bennett, DC. Agouti protein, mahogunin, and attractin in pheomelanogenesis and melanoblast-like alteration of melanocytes: a cAMP-independent pathway. *Pigment Cell Melanoma Res.* 22(5): 623-634. 2009.

Hoettecke, N; Ludwig, A; Foro, S; Schmidt, B. Improved synthesis of ADAM10 inhibitor GI254023X. *Neurodegener Dis.* 7(4):232-238. 2010.

Huang, YH; Lee, TH; Chan, KJ; Hsu, FL; Wu, YC; Lee, MH. Anemonin is a natural bioactive compound that can regulate tyrosinase-related proteins and mRNA in human melanocytes. *J Dermatol Sci.* 49(2):115-123. 2008.

Humbert, P. Quoi de neuf en recherche dermatologique? *Ann Dermatol Venereol.* 135 Suppl 7:S326-334. 2008.

Hunt, G & Thody, AJ. Agouti protein can act independently of melanocyte-stimulating hormone to inhibit melanogenesis. *J Endocrinol.* 147(2):R1-R4. 1995.

Hutton, SM & Spritz, RA. A comprehensive genetic study of autosomal recessive ocular albinism in Caucasian patients. *Invest Ophthalmol Vis Sci.* 49(3):868-872. 2008.

Iida, R; Ueki, M; Takeshita, H; Fujihara, J; Nakajima, T; Kominato, Y; Nagao, M; Yasuda, T. Genotyping of five single nucleotide polymorphisms in the OCA2 and HERC2 genes associated with blue-brown eye color in the Japanese population. *Cell Biochem Funct.* 27(5):323-327. 2009.

Imesch, PD; Wallow, IH; Albert, DM. The color of the human eye: a review of morphologic correlates and of some conditions that affect iridial pigmentation. *Surv Ophthalmol.* 41(Suppl 2): S117–S123. 1997.

Ito, S. The IFPCS presidential lecture: a chemist's view of melanogenesis. *Pigment Cell Res.* 16(3): 230–236. 2003.

Izagirre, N; García, I; Junquera, C; de la Rúa, C; Alonso, S. A scan for signatures of positive selection in candidate loci for skin pigmentation in humans. *Mol Biol Evol.* 23(9):1697-1706. 2006.

Jablonski, NG & Chaplin, G. The evolution of human skin coloration. *J Hum Evol.* 39:57–106. 2000.

Jeffreys, AJ; Wilson, V; Thein, SL. Hypervariable minisatellite regions in human DNA. *Nature.* 314:67-73. 1985.

Ji, Y; Rebert, NA; Joslin, JM; Higgins, MJ; Schultz, RA; Nicholls, RD. Structure of the highly conserved HERC2 gene and of multiple partially duplicated paralogs in human. *Genome Res.* 10(3): 319–329. 2000.

Jimbow, K; Hua, C; Gomez, PF; Hirosaki, K; Shinoda, K; Salopek, TG; Matsusaka, H; Jin, HY; Yamashita, T. Intracellular vesicular trafficking of tyrosinase gene family protein in eu- and pheomelanosome biogenesis. *Pigment Cell Res.* 13(Suppl 8):110–117. 2000.

Johansson, A & Gyllensten, U. Identification of local selective sweeps in human populations since the exodus from Africa. *Hereditas.* 145: 126–137. 2008.

Junyent, M; Parnell, LD; Lai, CQ; Arnett, DK; Tsai, MY; Kabagambe, EK; Straka, RJ; Province, M; An, P; Smith, CE; Lee, YC; Borecki, I; Ordovás, JM. ADAM17_i33708A>G polymorphism interacts with dietary n-6 polyunsaturated fatty acids to modulate obesity risk in the Genetics of Lipid Lowering Drugs and Diet Network study. *Nutr Metab Cardiovasc Dis.* 20(10): 698-705. 2010.

Kayser, M & Schneider, PM. DNA-based prediction of human externally visible characteristics in forensics: motivations, scientific challenges, and ethical considerations. *FSI Genetics.* 3: 154–161. 2009.

Kayser, M; Liu, F; Janssens, AC; Rivadeneira, F; Lao, O; Van Duijn, K; Vermeulen, M; Arp, P; Jhamai, MM; Van Ijcken, WF; Den Dunnen, JT; Heath, S; Zelenika, D; Despriet, DD; Klaver, CC; Vingerling, JR; De Jong, PT; Hofman, A; Aulchenko, YS; Uitterlinden, AG;

Oostra, BA; Van Duijn, CM. Three genome-wide association studies and a linkage analysis identify HERC2 as a human iris color gene. *Am J Hum Genet.* 82(2):411-423. 2008.

King, R; Willaert, R; Schmidt, R; Pietsch, J; Savage, S; Brott, MJ; Fryer, JP; Summers, CG; Oetting, WS. MC1R mutations modify the classic phenotype of oculocutaneous albinism type 2 (OCA2). *Am J Hum Genet.* 73 (3): 638–645. 2003.

Kobayashi, H & Kohshima, S. Unique morphology of the human eye and its adaptive meaning: comparative studies on external morphology of the primate eye. *J Hum Evol.* 40: 419–435. 2001.

Kollias, N; Sayer, R; Zeise, L; Chedekel, M. Photoprotection by melanin. *J Photochem Photobiol* B. 9:135–160. 1991.

Lamason, RL; Mohideen, MA; Mest, JR; Wong, AC; Norton, HL; Aros, MC; Jurynec, MJ; Mao, X; Humphreville, VR; Humbert, JE; Sinha, S; Moore, JL; Jagadeeswaran, P; Zhao, W; Ning, G; Makalowska, I; McKeigue, PM; O'donnell, D; Kittles, R; Parra, EJ; Mangini, NJ; Grunwald, DJ; Shriver, MD; Canfield, VA; Cheng, KC. SLC24A5, a putative cation exchanger, affects pigmentation in zebrafish and humans. *Science.* 310(5755):1782-1786. 2005.

Lamoreux, ML; Zhou, BK; Rosemblat, S; Orlow, SJ. The pinkeyed-dilution protein and the eumelanin/pheomelanin switch: in support of a unifying hypothesis. *Pigment Cell Res.* 8: 263–270. 1995.

Lee, ST; Nicholls, RD; Jong, MT; Fukai, K; Spritz, RA. Organization and sequence of the human P gene and identification of a new family of transport proteins. *Genomics.* 26(2): 354–363. 1995.

Liu, F; Wollstein, A; Hysi, PG; Ankra-Badu, GA; Spector, TD; Park, D; Zhu, G; Larsson, M; Duffy, DL; Montgomery, GW; Mackey, DA; Walsh, S; Lao, O; Hofman, A; Rivadeneira, F; Vingerling, JR; Uitterlinden, AG; Martin, NG; Hammond, CJ; Kayser, M. Digital quantification of human eye color highlights genetic association of three new loci. *PLoS Genet.* 6(5):e1000934. 2010.

Long, C; Wang, Y; Herrera, AH; Horiuchi Dagger, K; Walcheck, B. In vivo role of leukocyte ADAM17 in the inflammatory and host responses during E. coli-mediated peritonitis. *J Leukoc Biol.* 87(6):1097-1101. 2010.

Lucotte, G; Mercier, G; Diéterlen, F; Yuasa, I. A decreasing gradient of *374F* allele frequencies in the skin pigmentation gene SLC45A2, from the north of West Europe to North Africa. *Biochem Genet.* 48(1-2):26-33. 2010.

Makova, K & Norton, H. Worldwide polymorphism at the MC1R locus and normal pigmentation variation in humans. *Peptides.* 26: 1901–1908. 2005.

Marks, MS & Seabra, MC. The melanosome: membrane dynamics in black and white. *Nat Rev Mol Cell Biol.* 2(10): 738–748. 2001.

McEvoy, B; Beleza, S; Shriver, MD. The genetic architecture of normal variation in human pigmentation: an evolutionary perspective and model. *Hum Mol Genet.* 15 (Spec no. 2): R176–R181. 2006.

Mengel-From, J; Børsting, C; Sanchez, JJ; Eiberg, H; Morling, N. Human eye colour and HERC2, OCA2 and MATP. *Forensic Sci Int Genet.* 4(5): 323-328. 2010.

Morell, R; Spritz, RA; Ho, L; Pierpont, J; Guo, W; Friedman, TB; Asher, JH Jr. Apparent digenic inheritance of Waardenburg syndrome type 2 (WS2) and autosomal recessive ocular albinism (AROA). *Hum Mol Genet.* 6(5):659-664. 1997.

Myles, S; Somel, M; Tang, K; Kelso, J; Stoneking, M. Identifying genes underlying skin pigmentation differences among human populations. *Hum Genet.* 120: 613–621. 2007.

Nadeau, NJ; Minvielle, F; Ito, S; Inoue-Murayama, M; Gourichon, D; Follett, SA; Burke, T; Mundy, NI. Characterization of Japanese quail yellow as a genomic deletion upstream of the avian homolog of the mammalian ASIP (agouti) gene. *Genetics.* 178(2):777-786. 2008.

Nan, H; Kraft, P; Qureshi, AA; Guo, Q; Chen, C; Hankinson, SE; Hu, FB; Thomas, G; Hoover, RN; Chanock, S; Hunter, DJ; Han, J. Genome-wide association study of tanning phenotype in a population of European ancestry. *J Invest Dermatol.* 129: 2250–2257. 2009a.

Nan, H; Kraft, P; Hunter, DJ; Han, J. Genetic variants in pigmentation genes, pigmentary phenotypes, and risk of skin cancer in Caucasians. *Int J Cancer.* 125(4):909-917. 2009b.

Nei, M. The new mutation theory of phenotypic evolution. *Proc Natl Acad Sci USA.* 104 (30): 12235-12242. 2007.

Newton, JM; Cohen-Barak, O; Hagiwara, N; Gardner, JM; Davisson, MT; King, RA; Brilliant, MH. Mutations in the human orthologue of the mouse underwhite gene (uw) underlie a new form of oculocutaneous albinism, OCA4. *Am J Hum Genet.* 69(5): 981–988. 2001.

Niggemann, B; Weinbauer, G; Vogel, F; Korte, R. A standardized approach for iris color determination. *Int J Toxicol.* 22, 49–51. 2003.

Norris, BJ & Whan, VA. A gene duplication affecting expression of the ovine ASIP gene is responsible for white and black sheep. *Genome Res.* 18(8):1282-1293. 2008.

Norton, HL; Kittles, RA; Parra, E; McKeigue, P; Mao, X; Cheng, K; Canfield, VA; Bradley, DG; McEvoy, B; Shriver, MD. Genetic evidence for the convergent evolution of light skin in Europeans and East Asians. *Mol Biol Evol.* 24(3):710-722. 2007.

Parra, FC; Amado, RC; Lambertucci, JR; Rocha, J; Antunes, CM; Pena, SDJ. Color and genomic ancestry in Brazilians. *Proc Natl Acad Sci USA.* 100:177–182. 2003.

Perry, WL; Hustad, CM; Swing, DA; Jenkins, NA; Copeland, NG. A transgenic mouse assay for agouti protein activity. *Genetics.* 140(1):267-274. 1995.

Pho, LN & Leachman, SA. Genetics of pigmentation and melanoma predisposition. *G Ital Dermatol Venereol.* 145(1):37-45. 2010.

Prota, G; Hu, DN; Vincensi, MR; Mccormick, SA; Napolitano, A. Characterization of melanins in human irides and cultured uveal melanocytes from eyes of different colors. *Exp Eye Res.* 67, 293–299. 1998.

Puri, N; Gardner, JM; Brilliant, MH. Aberrant pH of melanosomes in pink-eyed dilution (P) mutant melanocytes. *J Invest Dermatol.* 115: 607–613. 2000.

Rana, B; Hewett-Emmett, D; Jin, L; Chang, BH; Sambuughin, N; Lin, M; Watkins, S; Bamshad, M; Jorde, LB; Ramsay, M; Jenkins, T; Li, WH. High polymorphism at the human Melanocortin 1 Receptor locus. *Genetics.* 151 (4): 1547–1557. 1999.

Rebbeck, TR; Kanetsky, PA; Walker, AH; Holmes, R; Halpern, AC; Schuchter, LM; Elder, DE; Guerry, D. P gene as an inherited biomarker of human eye color. *Cancer Epidemiol Biomarkers Prev.* 11: 782–784. 2002.

Relethford, JH. Hemispheric difference in human skin color. *Am J Phys Anthropol.* 104: 449–457. 1997.

Rogers, A; Iltis, D; Wooding, S. Genetic variation at the MC1R locus and time since loss of human body hair. *Curr Anthropol.* 45:105–108. 2004.

Rowe, PJ & Evans, P. Ball color, eye color, and a reactive motor skill. *Percept Mot Skills.* 79: 671–674. 1994.

Sabeti, PC; Varilly, P; Fry, B; Lohmueller, J; Hostetter, E; Cotsapas, C; Xie, X; Byrne, EH; McCarroll, SA; Gaudet, R; Schaffner, SF; Lander, ES; International HapMap Consortium. Genome-wide detection and characterization of positive selection in human populations. *Nature.* 449(7164):913-918. 2007.

Saferstein, R. *Criminalistics.* Upper Saddle River, NJ: Prentice Hall. 2001.

Schioth, HB; Ohillips, SR; Rudzish, R; Birch-Mahin, MA; Wikberg, JE; Rees, JL. Loss of function mutations of the human melanocortin 1 receptor are common and associated with red hair. *Biochem Biophys Res Commun.* 260: 488–491. 1999.

Scott, G; Leopardi, S; Printup, S; Malhi, N; Seiberg, M; Lapoint, R. Proteinase-activated receptor-2 stimulates prostaglandin production in keratinocytes: analysis of prostaglandin receptors on human melanocytes and effects of PGE2 and PGF2alpha on melanocyte dendricity. *J Investig Dermatol.* 122: 1214–1224. 2004.

Seddon, JM; Sahagian, CR; Glynn, RJ; Sperduto, RD; Gragoudas, ES. Evaluation of an iris color classification system. The Eye Disorders Case-control Study Group. *Invest Ophthalmol Vis Sci.* 31: 1592–1598. 1990.

Shriver, MD & Parra, EJ. Comparison of narrow-band reflectance spectroscopy and tristimulus colorimetry for measurements of skin and hair color in persons of different biological ancestry. *Am J Phys Anthropol.* 112: 17–27. 2000.

Shriver, MD; Parra, EJ; Dios, S; Bonilla, C; Norton, H; Jovel, C; Pfaff, C; Jones, C; Massac, A; Cameron, N; Baron, A; Jackson, T; Argyropoulos, G; Jin, L; Hoggart, CJ; McKeigue, PM; Kittles RA. Skin pigmentation, biogeographical ancestry and admixture mapping. *Hum Genet.* 112 (4): 387–399. 2003.

Sims, LM & Ballantyne J. The golden gene (SLC24A5) differentiates US sub-populations within the ethnically admixed Y-SNP haplogroups. *Leg Med (Tokyo).* 10(2):72-77. 2008.

Smith, DR; Spaulding, DT; Glenn, HM; Fuller, BB. The relationship between $Na(+)/H(+)$ exchanger expression and tyrosinase activity in human melanocytes. *Exp Cell Res.* 298:521–534. 2004.

Soejima, M; Tachida, H; Ishida, T; Sano, A; Koda, Y. Evidence for recent positive selection at the human AIM1 locus in a European population. *Mol Biol Evol.* 23: 179–188. 2006.

Spritz, RA; Bailin, T; Nicholls, RD; Lee, ST; Park, SK; Mascari, MJ; Butler, MG. Hypopigmentation in the Prader-Willi syndrome correlates with P gene deletion but not with haplotype of the hemizygous P allele. *Am J Med Genet.* 71: 57–62. 1997.

Stinchcombe, J; Bossi, G; Griffiths, CM. Linking albinism and immunity: the secrets of secretory lysosomes. *Science.* 305: 55–59. 2004.

Stokowski, RP; Pant, PV; Dadd, T; Fereday, A; Hinds, DA; Jarman, C; Filsell, W; Ginger, RS; Green, MR; Van der Ouderaa, FJ; Cox, DR. A genomewide association study of skin pigmentation in a South Asian population. *Am J Hum Genet.* 81(6):1119-1132. 2007.

Sturm, RA. Molecular genetics of human pigmentation diversity. *Hum Mol Genet.* 18(R1):R9-R17. 2009.

Sturm, RA & Frudakis, TN. Eye colour: portals into pigmentation genes and ancestry. *Trends in Genetics.* 20 (8): 327-332. 2004.

Sturm, RA & Larsson, M. Genetics of human iris colour and patterns. *Pigment Cell Melanoma Res.* 22(5):544-562. 2009.

Sturm, RA; Teasdale, RD; Box, NF. Human pigmentation genes: identification, structure and consequences of polymorphic variation. *Gene.* 277: 49–62. 2001.

Sulem, P; Gudbjartsson, DF; Stacey, SN; Helgason, A; Rafnar, T; Magnusson, KP; Manolescu, A; Karason, A; Palsson, A; Thorleifsson, G; Jakobsdottir, M; Steinberg, S; Pálsson, S; Jonasson, F; Sigurgeirsson, B; Thorisdottir, K; Ragnarsson, R; Benediktsdottir, KR; Aben, KK; Kiemeney, LA; Olafsson, JH; Gulcher, J; Kong, A; Thorsteinsdottir, U; Stefansson, K. Genetic determinants of hair, eye and skin pigmentation in Europeans. *Nat Genet.* 39 (12): 1443-1452. 2007.

Sulem, P; Gudbjartsson, DF; Stacey, SN; Helgason, A; Rafnar, T; Jakobsdottir, M; Steinberg, S; Gudjonsson, SA; Palsson, A; Thorleifsson, G; Pálsson, S; Sigurgeirsson, B; Thorisdottir, K; Ragnarsson, R; Benediktsdottir, KR; Aben, KK; Vermeulen, SH; Goldstein, AM; Tucker, MA; Kiemeney, LA; Olafsson, JH; Gulcher, J; Kong, A; Thorsteinsdottir U, Stefansson K. Two newly identified genetic determinants of pigmentation in Europeans. *Nat Genet.* 40(7):835-837. 2008.

SWGMAT (ScientificWorking Group on Materials Analysis). Forensic human hair examination guidelines. *Forens Sci Communicat.* 7(2). Available at http://www.fbi.gov/hq/lab/fsc/backissu/april2005/standards/2005_04_standards02.htm. 2005.

Takamoto, T; Schwartz, B; Cantor, LB; Hoop, JS; Steffens, T. Measurement of iris color using computerized image analysis. *Curr Eye Res.* 22, 412–419. 2001.

TASI. Technical Advisory Service for Images. *Colour theory: Understanding and modelling colour.* University of Bristol. Available at http://www.tasi.ac.uk/advice/creating/pdf/colour. pdf, accessed December 5, 2007. 2004.

Terman, JS & Terman, M. Photopic and scotopic light detection in patients with seasonal affective disorder and control subjects. Biol Psychiatry. 46: 1642–1648. 1999.

Theos, AC; Truschel, ST; Raposo, G; Marks, MS. The Silver locus product Pmel17/gp100/Silv/ME20: controversial in name and in function. *Pigment Cell Res.* 18(5): 322–336. 2005.

Toyofuku, K; Valencia, JC; Kushimoto, T; Costin, GE; Virador, VM; Vieira, WD; Ferrans, VJ; Hearing, VJ. The etiology of oculocutaneous albinism (OCA) type II: the pink protein modulates the processing and transport of tyrosinase. *Pigment Cell Res.* 5: 217–224. 2002.

Tully, G. Genotype versus phenotype: human pigmentation. *Forensic Sci Int: Genetics.* 1 (2): 105–110. 2007.

Valverde, P; Healy, E; Jackson, I; Rees, JL; Thody, AJ. Variants of the melanocyte stimulating hormone receptor gene are associated with red hair and fair skin. *Nat Genet.* 11 (3): 328–330. 1995.

Vaughn, MR; Brooks, E; van Oorschot, RA; Baindur-Hudson, S. A comparison of macroscopic and microscopic hair color measurements and a quantification of the relationship between hair color and thickness. *Microsc Microanal.* 15(3):189-193. 2009a.

Vaughn, M; van Oorschot, R; Baindur-Hudson, S. A comparison of hair colour measurement by digital image analysis with reflective spectrophotometry. *Forensic Sci Int* 183, 97–101. 2009b.

Vaughn, M; van Oorschot, R; Baindur-Hudson, S. Hair color measurement and variation. *Am J Phys Anthropol.* 137(1): 91–96. 2008.

Voight, BF; Kudaravalli, S; Wen, X; Pritchard, JK. A map of recent positive selection in the human genome. *PLoS Biol.* 4: e72. 2006.

Watabe, H; Valencia, JC; Yasumoto, K; Kushimoto, T; Ando, H; Muller, J; Vieira, WD; Mizoguchi, M; Appella, E; Hearing, VJ. Regulation of tyrosinase processing and trafficking by organellar pH and by proteasome activity. *J Biol Chem.* 279(9):7971-7981. 2004.

Werrett, DJ. The new frontiers of forensics. *Policy Today.* 11: 29–31. 2005.

Weskamp, G; Mendelson, K; Swendeman, S; Le Gall, S; Ma, Y; Lyman, S; Hinoki, A; Eguchi, S; Guaiquil, V; Horiuchi, K; Blobel, CP. Pathological neovascularization is reduced by inactivation of ADAM17 in endothelial cells but not in pericytes. *Circ Res.* 106(5):932-940. 2010.

Wielgus, AR & Sarna, T. Melanin in human irides of different color and age of donors. *Pigment Cell Res.* 18, 454–464. 2005.

Willems, SH; Tape, CJ; Stanley, PL; Taylor, NA; Mills, IG; Neal, DE; McCafferty, J; Murphy, G. Thiol isomerases negatively regulate the cellular shedding activity of ADAM17. *Biochem J.* 428(3):439-450. 2010.

Williamson, SH; Hubisz, MJ; Clark, AG; Payseur, BA; Bustamante, CD; Nielsen, R. Localizing recent adaptive evolution in the human genome. *PLoS Genet.* 3:e90. 2007.

Yamamoto, T; Suganami, T; Kiso-Narita, M; Scherle, PA; Kamei, Y; Isobe, M; Higashiyama, S; Ogawa, Y. Insulin-induced ectodomain shedding of heparin-binding epidermal growth factor-like growth factor in adipocytes in vitro. *Obesity.* 18(10): 1888-1894. 2010.

Yuasa, I; Umetsu, K; Harihara, S; Kido, A; Miyoshi, A; Saitou, N; Dashnyam, B; Jin, F; Lucotte, G; Chattopadhyay, PK; Henke, L; Henke, J. Distribution of the F374 allele of the SLC45A2 (MATP) gene and founder-haplotype analysis. *Ann Hum Genet.* 70 (Pt 6):802-811. 2006.

In: Forensic Science
Editors: N. Yacine and R. Fellag

ISBN 978-1-61324-999-4
© 2012 Nova Science Publishers, Inc.

Chapter 4

# BLOODSTAIN INVESTIGATION: A REVIEW

*Ana Castelló[1*], Francesc Francés[2†]*

[1]University of Valencia EG, Facultad de Medicina, U. D. Medicina Legal, Av/
Blasco Ibañez, n°15,
46010 Valencia, Spain

[2]University of Valencia EG, Facultad de Medicina, U. D. Medicina Legal, Av/
Blasco Ibañez, n°15, 46010 Valencia, Spain

## ABSTRACT

In criminal investigations, there are three successive stages involved in studying bloodstains: search and orientation, confirmation and individualisation

The first of these tests, called presumptive tests, are responsible for locating latent remains and providing some preliminary information on the possible blood content of the sample.

The second stage consists of establishing the origin of the stain. The question to be answered is: Is this really a human stain?

Confirmatory tests have to be undertaken for two reasons:

- To show that the stain contains a human biological fluid. By undertaking this test, a genetic analysis – longer and more costly- on stains that may appear to be blood, but which are not, can sometimes be avoided.
- To confirm the type of biological fluid that has been found. Clearly, biological samples are destined for genetic analysis, but to discover the type of fluid under consideration it is also essential to reconstruct and understand the events.

The need to determine the nature of the evidence is reflected in the latest bibliography that includes interesting studies where all these methods have been thoroughly studied. It is necessary to know the possible causes of false positives and negatives as well as the ways of trying to prevent them.

---

[*] Biochemist Ph D.Sci, Professor of Legal Medicine, Telephone: +34 963983774; E-mail: Ana.Castello@uv.es.
[†] MD, PhD., Professor of Legal Medicine; Telephone: +34 963864655;   E-mail: Francesc.Frances@uv.es.

In this chapter, we propose to review the methods for search, presumptive and confirmation test of bloodstains, including the most recent works published.

## INTRODUCTION

"If it were possible to spray the house with chemical products, it may be possible to literally resurrect the scene. Blood forms clots, it oozes, drips, splashes and screams in brilliant red. It gets into cracks and crannies and hides under floors and upholstery, Although it may disappear with washing and fade over the years, it never entirely goes away".

"The stains, smudges, splashes and latent prints that we had been examining provided us with the most accurate picture ever seen in crime reconstruction"

Cornwell, Patricia D. Cruel and Unusual (1993) [1]

This fragment of Patricia Cornwell's novel describes and illustrates, what can be expected of a bloodstain study at the scene of a crime. It is true that the study of physical, chemical and serological aspects of stains can lead to the following:

- The participation of individuals or objects in a criminal action
- A clearer idea of how a certain event took place
- Identification of an unknown body
- Through toxicologycal analysis, the cause of death
- Finally, by bringing these and other data together, knowledge of whether we are dealing with death by homicide, suicide, accident or natural causes.

Consequently, the search for and later study of bloodstains should always be undertaken when an act of violence act is suspected.

Before going into a detailed description of investigation systematics, it may be of interest to provide a brief history on how different evidence from bloodstain analysis has developed [2,3,4,5,6,7].

## A BRIEF HISTORY

The first method to be found in the bibliography was proposed in 1828 by Barruel.

Some years later, in 1853, Ludwig Teichmann-Stawlarsky described a more rigorous procedure, known as the Teichmann test. This was based on obtaining the characteristic crystals derived from hemoglobin.

In 1861, Van Deen proposed another that consisted of demonstrating the existence of peroxidases in the sample to be analysed by causing the oxidation of the guaiac tincture by oxygen and, in 1863, Schönbein described yet another one in which the sample was checked to see whether it contained catalase or not by adding hydrogen peroxide.

At around the same time, the year 1859 marked the beginning of the development of another important group of techniques based on the analysis of the absorption spectra of blood.

It was not until 1901 that Paul Uhlenhuth published a study entitled "*A method for differentiating different types of blood and, in particular, to prove, by means of a differential diagnosis, the existence of human blood*". This came to be considered as the most important innovation in Forensic Medicine in the 19th century.

In that same year, Landsteiner discovered the presence of different blood groups in human beings. This he called the ABO system. In 1902, Richter tried to apply this system to the identification of dry blood, but this was not possible until 1916, using a technique developed by Leone Lattes.

Kastle and Scheede in 1903 and, later, Meyer, proposed a method based on the oxidation of phenolphthalein.

In 1904, Adler described a blood identifying technique using benzidine and, later, in 1911, Von Furth, replaced benzidine with leucomalachite green. In 1912 Ruttan and Hardisty proposed using o-tolidine as it was a less dangerous compound.

Another method for identifying blood, this time based on blood luminescence, was described in 1937 by Walter Specht [8].

However, from 1927 there were a series of important discoveries took place that led to the development of methods providing a diagnosis of blood stain type.

Outstanding among these was the possibility of detecting antigens of the blood in other body fluids such as saliva and semen, described by Landsteiner, and Levine, and, simultaneously, by Yamakami.

Also noteworthy was the discovery in 1940 by Landsteiner and Weiner of the existence of the RH factor in blood and, in 1945, the description of the Coombs Test, proposed by Coombs, Mourant and Race, for detecting antiRh anti-bodies.

In 1949, Ouchterlony described a technique based on the antigen-antibody reaction and, in 1960, Stuart Kind used a new procedure that applied the absorption-dilution technique and which could be used on dry blood.

From 1962, techniques based on luminescence were introduced and electroscopic techniques rapidly developed during the 1970s and 80s.

A decisive step, which at the moment is in full development, was taken in 1985 when Jeffreys proposed a process based on obtaining what is now called "*genetic fingerprinting*".

In 1987, Kary Mullis described the technique called the Polymerase Chain Reaction that has proved to be a great leap forward in the application of DNA studies to Forensics.

## INVESTIGATION PROCEDURE

### I. Visual Examination and Search

The location, distribution and appearance of bloodstains that are found at the scene of a crime can be of great help when it comes to reconstructing and interpreting the facts [9].

The bibliography contains several very interesting studies, such as the use of a bloodstain distribution study on hands and the weapons used in supposed suicides [10]. This analysis was undertaken in five cases of suicide and in all of them information was obtained to clarify the etiology of death. The authors point out that these studies should be undertaken before reagents are used to detect shot remains.

In any case, the study of the position and the pattern of blood traces is extremely complex and, in order to correctly interpret the results from the observations made, it will be necessary to compare them with laboratory models, obtained using materials equal to those found at the real scene of the crime [11,12].

Stains that are found at the scene of a crime may have been produced in various ways:

1. *By projection:* These are formed by the spraying of blood to a certain distance and in various directions or also when blood drips from a certain height. In the study of stains produced by projection the following must be borne in mind:
   - The angle of impact of the blood. Drops of blood move in accordance with the laws of physics. As it is a viscous liquid it produces drops of a perfectly defined shape. When a drop of blood falls upon a flat surface forming a right angle with the surface, stains of a circular shape are formed. The diameter as well as the contour will vary depending on the height. On increasing the height, the diameter is greater and the contour more irregular as it bursts and small drops are formed around it. When the projection is oblique, the stain acquires an ellipse form. Depending on the angle of incidence, speed and quantity of blood, the axis of the ellipse will be more or less elongated, satellite drops perhaps being formed at the point. The study of the shape and axis of the ellipse will help to calculate the trajectory of the drop of blood that caused the stain.

     The trajectories of drops of blood are studied on Cartesian axes (X, Y and Z) and knowing them may help to determine the place where the aggression took place. To do this, the variation from the axis of the elliptical stains that have been formed are measured. The angle of impact on the surface is also studied by measuring the ratio between the two axes of the ellipse and then calculating the ratio between the shorter and longer axis that will correspond, as trigonometry teaches us, to the value of the core of the impact angle.

     If the trajectories of each drop are represented by a string that joins the different points of reference, it will be seen that that all the different strings pass through a coinciding point. This point of convergence corresponds to the origin of the blood.

     There are now information technology applications that analyse all the data and, by making comparisons with patterns, provide information on the trajectories and points of origin of blood. This is what is known as directional analysis of bloodstains.
   - The texture of the surface (hardness and porosity): On smooth and hard surfaces, the contour of stains will be regular. On rough surfaces they are expected to be irregular and that they may even form small surrounding drops as a consequence of exploding. On absorbent surfaces, the drop impregnates the substratum and spreads to a greater or lesser degree depending on the absorption capacity of that surface.
2. *By dripping:* Blood drips and flows to form trickles and pools. Studying those trickles will provide information on the possible changes in the position of the victim.

   Similarly, the situation of the pools provides important information on the position of the victim and possible changes of the same.

3. *By contact or impregnation:* This occurs when a bloody object comes into contact with a substratum. If this is an absorbent material, the blood will spread and soak into it resulting in uniform stains with clean edges. The study of the dimensions of the stains on clothing, for example, will provide some idea of when contact took place and, should coagulation have taken place, can also indicate how long the victim survived.

The prints made by hands and feet that have been in contact with blood are very important. Studying them can, if they are clear enough, help to identify the person to whom they belong, as well as provide useful information when it comes to reconstructing the events. Analysing the prints left by the soles of shoes or slippers can also prove to be very interesting.

When they have been located and their distribution studied and photographed, the stains are then gathered and taken to the laboratory. The correct gathering, conservation and transportation, strictly fulfilling the custody conditions, will be essential when it comes to considering the clue valid as valid evidence.

## II. And when they Cannot be Seen?: The Search for Latent Stains

Sometimes stains are not seen by the naked eye or those that are seen pose doubts on the nature of the blood. It should be borne in mind that the look of bloodstains will vary greatly depending on various factors:

- The age of the stain,
- Atmospheric conditions,
- The backing,
- Washing, etc.

They may remain hidden either by accident or by a deliberate attempt to remove any clues. However, with the help of chemical reagents, they can be revealed.

One of the best-known and most-used products for this purpose is luminol [13]. This is how it works:

### *Basis of the Method*
Some proteins have a non-protein component called the prosthetic group, which is responsible for developing the biological function of the protein. In hemoglobin, it is the haemo that is involved in the transportation of oxygen. This group contains iron in oxidation state II. This means that the Hemoglobin, in the development of its biological function, contains $Fe(II)$. However, in the stain, $Fe(II)$ gradually oxidises to $Fe(III)$, so forming metahemoglobin.

Luminol (3-aminophtalhydrazide) is a chemiluminescent compound, i.e., it is capable of emitting light during a chemical reaction. When it is made to react with blood in basic pH and in the presence of an oxidant, the formation of a brilliant luminescence can be observed that indicates the possible presence of blood.

Although different authors have studied the mechanism of the luminol-blood reaction, it is not yet fully understood.

Latest research points to the fact that probably the haemin group acts as a catalyst in the luminol oxidation reaction in basic media. This reaction would not be produced or would be very slow in the absence of a catalyst.

The positive reaction of luminol would indicate the possibility that blood exists in the area that has been treated with the reagent.

## *Method*

Notes on reagent preparation:

The reagent can be prepared to different formulae which, according to what has been published, yield very similar results. In the second edition of the manual *Interpretation of bloodstain evidence at crime scenes*[1], quoted earlier as a reference, many preparation possibilities are described. Basically, it must have:

- Luminol (3-aminophtalhydrazide)
- A base to achieve a basic pH: sodium hydroxide Na(OH) and sodium carbonate have been used.
- An oxygen provider: Normally sodium perborate or hydrogen peroxide.
- Distilled water as a solvent.

Logically proportions vary depending on the components chosen. The preparation is very simple. It consists in obtaining either a solid or a solution mixture (depending on the type of basic compound chosen) of luminol and base. At the moment of undertaking the test, the oxidant will be added. All the reagents must be fully dissolved. The resulting solution will be stored in a plastic bottle with a spraying device. What remains following the search must not be stored, not even in the fridge.

Carrying out the test:

Luminol is applied by spraying onto the areas in which the possible presence of blood is being investigated. Obviously, it is obligatory to work in the dark. If deemed necessary, the test can be repeated on the same area provided that it is left to dry first.

When stains are located, they have to be taken for analysis. If the object on which they are found can be easily transported, it is best that they be taken to the laboratory for analysis. If not, traces are collected using sterile cotton swabs. The sample must always be left to dry before being transported, adequately protected, to the laboratory.

The area to be studied must be photographed in order to have graphic evidence of the test results.

## *Sensitivity*

Some researchers have stated that sensitivity reaches 1/1000000 (ml blood/ml total of sample). This means that luminol can detect blood on samples containing 1 cubic centimeter of blood for each thousand litres of sample. However, other studies have stated that they only identified traces of blood up to a concentration of 1/300000 (one cubic centimeter per three hundred litres), on stains prepared in the laboratory [14].

---

[1] James SH., Eckert WG. Interpretation of bloodstain evidence at crime scenes 2ª Ed. New York: CRC Press, 1999.

Whatever the case, the reagent is sufficiently effective to reveal stains valid for DNA studies and it has also been shown that samples containing amounts not detectable by luminol have not been useful for extracting DNA [15]. Nevertheless, it is clear that the extraordinary advances in research techniques suggest that we will be able to obtain DNA from ever smaller quantities of blood, even under the most adverse circumstances – a fire scene for example [16] - so making it necessary to improve the reactions that allow the clues to be located.

This reagent, luminol, is capable of detecting both recent and old stains, although it is less effective with very fresh blood. Despite some studies proposing the prior treatment of the sample using hydrochloric acid in order to facilitate the degradation of the haemo group [17], it has been shown that this prior process can interfere in later analyses.

## *Interpretation of Results*

*Positive:* This would indicate the possible existence of traces of blood. Different studies have shown that vegetables, pulp and fruit juice, as well as commercial and domestic oils, cleaning products and glues, paints and varnishes can interfere with this [18,19]. In a recent work, the possible interference of 205 substances was investigated. In the conclusions there is a list of 9 substances that are capable of producing a luminescence comparable to that of hemoglobin. They are: vegetables such as parsnip, turnip and horseradish, commercial bleach, several furniture polishes, some enamel paints and several fabrics used in the interior of vehicles.

Other studies propose methods for detecting and hindering false positives that bleach or products containing hypochlorites produce. The presence of bleach (and similar products) is easily detected because the luminescence that it produces is different from that observed in the reaction with blood. In the former, luminescence is brilliant and of short duration. In the second, it is more difficult to see but remains for a fairly long time.

It has been shown that the spectrum that is obtained on treating a bloodstain with luminol has an absorption peak at a different wavelength from when the emission is produced by the effect of products containing bleach. This difference allows us to confirm the presence of a contaminant and, therefore, a false positive [20].

Another possible way of eliminating interference is that proposed by E. J. Kent et al. [21]. These researchers added an amine (the 1,2-diaminoethane) to the luminol formula. This is a compound that reacts very quickly with the hypochlorite of bleach so eliminating its interference in the reaction.

In a later study [22] glycine was used: Although its addition hindered the false positive result, it complicated the preparation of the reagent and also reduced its sensitivity.

The recommended method, therefore, is to begin the search with a traditional solution and distribute it on a small area of the place or object to be examined. If the reaction makes one suspect the presence of bleach, the modified formula should then be used.

Another alternative is to take advantage of the fact that hypochlorites are not stable in contact with air. By letting sufficient time pass by, they will self-destruct. It has been shown that when working on non-absorbent surfaces, the waiting period is minimal.

In the laboratory of Forensic Sciences at the Faculty of Medicine, Valencia, we studied the effect of drying on porous surfaces [23]. Our conclusion is that by waiting the necessary time, the effect of the contaminant is eliminated. When there is no hurry, this, perhaps, is the best option.

*Negative:* It has been shown that the presence of reducing compounds as sample contaminants (e.g. ascorbic acid) can cause a false negative result. In the case of luminol, the concentration of contaminant must necessarily be high in relation to the blood for the false negative to be produced.

Another cause of error is due to the use of new cleaning products that contain active oxygen. It has been shown that stains washed with these detergents give a negative result to luminol, as well as to all other presumptive tests (to which we will refer later) [24].

### *Effects on Later Analyses*

It has been shown that luminol does not interfere in the development of other presumptive or confirmatory tests, nor in the amplification of DNA by PCR [25].

It is a useful reagent for detecting the presence of blood and also for the study of its distribution. By using it, traces of blood can be found corresponding to footprints, fingerprints, signs of pulling, etc. The use of photography provides a material that may prove fundamental for the possible reconstruction of the events at the scene of a crime. However, the interpretation of the traces observed following the test demand great experience from the investigator, which is only acquired with practice in the laboratory together with the study of real cases, always under the guidance of an expert.

The effectiveness of the luminol test is continually put to the test in laboratories as is its ability to detect blood on new materials and also surfaces treated with the new cleaning products that regularly appear on the market. For example, in 2004, an interesting study was published that analysed the capacity of luminol to detect blood on different vehicle accessories such as seats, foot mats and plastic components [26]. The possibility of obtaining false positives in determining whether there was any blood or not due to a reaction to the surface and also the effect of washing and heat was studied.

Another compound with luminescent properties that has also been used for detecting latent bloodstains is fluorescein. This reagent is applied in the same way as luminol, i.e. by spraying onto the areas where one is trying to locate traces of blood. After, it has to be illuminated with a forensic light and if luminescence is observed, the possibility arises that blood has been detected. It has been shown that its sensitivity is similar to that of luminol and that DNA can be extracted from stains found using this reagent [27].

From luminol and fluorescein, other products have been formulated that, with the same chemical basis, are easier to use and prepare. The first of these is called Bluestar Forensic®[2] This is a derivative of luminol that, according to the product manufacturers, is much more effective. The advantages over the original solution lie mainly in the fact that a more brilliant luminescence is produced and that it is less affected by the interferences of hypochlorites. Furthermore, preparing it is very simple; one only has to dissolve a tablet in distilled water.

Works published by independent groups show that, although it is true that its reaction with peroxidases is very intense, Bluestar forensic® gives rise to more false positives than its predecessor, or what amounts to the same, it is less specific [28].

Using fluorescein as the main reagent, HemaScein®[3] has been produced. At the moment of writing, there is no more information available than that provided by the product

---

[2] www.bluestar-forensic.com/
[3] http://www.abacusdiagnostics.com/hemasceinmoreinfo.htm

manufacturer. The results of studies undertaken by independent laboratories remain to be seen.

Whatever the case, the crime scene investigator will be the person who must assess which is the best choice.

Another procedure for locating non-visible stains consists of using a forensic light.

Well diluted bloodstains, when illuminated with a forensic light at an appropriate wavelength (400-430 nm for blood), appear as dark shadows that contrast with the light, thus revealing them to the naked eye. Indeed, it has been claimed that forensic light is the only means of locating bloodstains when these have been covered in paint [29].

Another possibility is that of working with the infrared range. It has been shown that blood absorbs the nearby infrared area and that this is a good method for locating it on different types of fabrics [30].

To end this section devoted to the search for bloodstains, we would like to mention several luminol applications that, although not related with the analysis of bloodstains, are curious and illustrate how a single reagent may have very different applications:

The first example is its use in determining the age of skeletal remains from the reaction they cause with the traces of blood remaining in the bone tissue. The intensity of the reaction, which can be measured, is related to the age of the bones [31].

In the second example the reagent is used to analyse the anti-oxidant characteristics of Martinis and to check whether it is better to "shake rather than stir" (as recommended by James Bond) [32] in order to maintain these antioxidant properties.

A third example is its use in determining the antioxidant content of wastewater in the olive oil making process with the aim of preventing environmental damage [33].

As a fourth and final example, its use in checking the degree of cleanliness in operating theatres [34].

Clearly, its only limits are an individual's imagination.

## III. Presumptive Tests

### Basis of the Method

Regardless of the reagent used, all are based on the same type of chemical reaction. It should be remembered that:

Hemoglobin is an enzyme that has a peroxidase activity, i.e. capable of catalysing (i.e. facilitating, accelerating) the decomposition of hydroperoxide and liberating oxygen.

A reagent is chosen which, on changing from the reduced form to the oxidated form, changes colour.

If the reagent, followed by hydrogen peroxide, is added to a sample containing peroxidases, the decomposition of the peroxide will take place and the corresponding liberation of oxygen. This gas will cause the oxidation of the reagent and the colour change corresponding to the oxidated form will be observed.

Perhaps the best-known reagent is benzidine. At first, it was used in the clinic to detect blood in faeces until Adler proposed its use in criminology for studying bloodstains [35].

Other components that perform in the same way are reduced phenolphthalein and leucomalachite green. Later, and because the carcinogenic nature of benzidine has been shown, the use of methylated derivatives of that product were introduced such as O-tolidine and tetramethylbenzidine. O-toluidine is another of the compounds that has been used, although it is less known.

Reagents must be prepared at the moment of use and conserved in the refrigerator. It is essential to carry out control tests that ensure their perfect state (with stains prepared in the laboratory), and the negative reaction from the backing bearing the sample.

## *Method*

Notes on preparing the reagent:

Preparation is very simple and basically consists of dissolving the corresponding reagent, using the appropriate solvent (e.g. glacial acetic acid).

In the case of reduced phenolphthalein, the process is a little more complicated, because it requires prior treatment of the compound. Fortunately, laboratories specialising in criminal investigation provide prepared reagents delivered in single-use ampoules.

Undertaking the test:

It can be undertaken directly on the sample. Another possibility (more recommendable) consists of dampening a cotton swab with distilled water and passing it over the surface where the presence of blood is suspected.

The test is then undertaken on the cotton swab. For all reagents the method is similar:

- Apply a few drops of reagent onto the sample or cotton swab.
- Check that no colour change takes place. If it does take place, the test will be invalid.
- Add a few drops of hydrogen peroxide.

A change in the reagent will indicate if the test is positive. The colour change must be observed at once (10 seconds).

## *Sensitivity and Specificity*

Reagents are highly sensitive although some differences of opinion exist among researchers about the concentration of blood that they are capable of detecting. Data varies for benzidine and tolidine between 1/300000 and 1/500000, 1/100000 for leucomalachite green and 1/1000000 in the case of reduced phenolphthalein, although these values must be considered only as a guide and will always depend on the experimental conditions in which they have been determined.

## *Interpreting Results*

**Positive**

Indicates the existence of enzymes with peroxidase properties in the sample. They may, therefore, be of a bloody nature.

It should be borne in mind at this point that vegetable compounds also contain peroxidases and, therefore, they are equally capable of being positive in the test.

Nevertheless, there are several factors that allow us to deduce the presence of plant peroxidases and in some cases eliminate them.

Firstly, plant peroxidases are not found in the sap, but in plant fibres, so observation through the microscope of the sample could allow us to detect the presence of foreign fibres and to suspect their nature. On the other hand, plant peroxidases are less stable than animal ones and besides are easily destroyed by the effects of heat. It is possible, taking advantage of these differences to eliminate them as interference, provided that care is taken not to damage the sample [36].

**Negative**

There are several contaminants that can cause a false negative result of the test.

These are reducing agents that interfere in the reaction and hinder the observation of the change in colour that indicates positive [37]. The presumptive reagents which are commonly used are much more sensitive to this type of contamination than luminol.

In our laboratory we have undertaken an investigation with the aim of determining the effectiveness of reagents on bloodstains contaminated by other products such as different types of drinks, washing-up liquids, iodine, etc. The results show that in some cases the mixture with other products may give rise to false positives as well as to false negatives [38].

In addition, it should be borne in mind that – as has been stated earlier on- washing with detergents containing active oxygen can annul presumptive reactions.

This problem is especially serious because it has also been shown that, from samples treated with these cleaning products and which proved negative in the presumptive test, it was possible to extract DNA [39].

Continuing along this line of research, another study was designed to determine the sensitivity of tests on samples subjected to real degradation conditions. In short the experiment consisted of forming blood stains on fabric and wood and leaving them in different environments for different periods of time. More specifically these were:

- One part of the samples was left in the open air without any form of protection.
- Another was buried in a field,
- And a third was preserved in the laboratory also without protection.

Tests took place at two, four, eight and twelve months after depositing them. The results show that there are presumptive reagents -benzidine and luminol- that bear the bad conditions of the sample better than others (phenolphthalein, tolidine) [40].

*Effects on Later Analyses*

The bibliography suggests that reagents do not cause adverse effects in later DNA analyses. However, the latest studies indicate that degradation of DNA is detected in samples treated with benzidine 48 hours after applying the reagent. This, however, only underlines the need to undertake the analysis as soon as possible [41].

In any case, normal practice recommends the test application only on part of the sample, or on a cotton swab, as mentioned above.

In this section of presumptive tests we have not included luminol because traditionally it has been used in the search for blood at the scene of a crime, and especially when one needs to comb large surfaces. However, even in the case of small objects, it is useful for determining, with considerable accuracy, whether there is blood in the sample.

## IV. Confirmatory Tests

Currently, these tests are increasingly less common as they have been replaced by kits that detect human hemoglobin. These are similar to those normally applied in the clinic for detecting blood in faeces.

Traditional confirmatory tests are very specific but not very sensitive. They are based on proving the presence in the sample of any of the components of blood. Using them, one does not determine if the blood analysed is human or not. The best-known are [42]:

*Microscopic Tests*

These consist of observing the stain through a microscope. This can be done by:

- Direct examination-
    The sample is observed through a special microscope with which opaque bodies can be viewed (Leitz Ultropack). Red blood cells form structures that look like a stack of coins. If the blood is well conserved one can determine whether the cells have a nucleus or not and also their shape, which helps one to identify the animal species to which they belong.
- By examining the sample previously subjected to a process of isolation and tincture of the red and white blood cells
- Microchemical or crystallographic techniques -
    In these tests the sample is subjected to the action of various reagents in order to obtain certain derivatives of hemoglobin. These derivates form colour crystals and characteristic shapes that are identified by observation through a microscope and allow us to confirm whether there is blood on the sample under analysis:

**Basis of the Method**

Treating blood with the appropriate reagents allows one to separate the hemo group from the rest of the protein and to obtain derivatives obtained that form characteristic crystals that can be detected and recognised by observation through a microscope.

**Method**

Notes on preparing the reagents:

*Teichmann test:* Glacial acetic acid is used. The presence of sodium chloride in the blood is taken advantage of to obtain haematin from the halogenated derivative.

*Takayama test:* The reagent has a haematinizing agent (sodium hydroxide), a reducing agent (glucose, sucrose, ascorbic acid) and a nitrogenous base (pyridine).

Undertaking the test:

The test is undertaken on a blood scab formed on a slide. Having covered the slide, several drops of the reagent are added by capillary action. It is important to check that contact takes place with the scab. To facilitate the reaction, it is heated gently using a flame. Finally, the possible formation of crystals is observed through a microscope. In the event of having used the Teichmann reagent, the crystals obtained (hematin chloride) are of a dark grey colour and elongated prisms in shape. If the Takayama reagent has been applied, the crystals (hemochromogen) are orangey and form arborescent structures. The process may be repeated if at the first attempt, no crystals are observed.

**Sensitivity**

Although the bibliography does not provide information on this point, it is generally agreed that these are methods of little sensitivity. In tests undertaken in the Criminology Laboratory at the Legal Medicine Teaching Unit., no crystals in dilutions greater than 1/1000 were observed.

**Interpreting Results**

*Positive:*
Confirms that the sample contains blood.
*Negative:*
A negative result may be due to the absence of blood in the sample, but also to the fact that either its concentration is low, or it is deteriorated or even to a bad application of the method. That it is to say, the negative result does not allow us to discard the bloody nature of the sample.

We will now go on to give a brief explanation of others traditional methods used in diagnosing and confirming bloodstains.

- *Luminescent examination:* In this technique, the stain that one wishes to identify is studied using Wood's lamp.

The first step is to illuminate the sample directly. Then several drops of concentrated sulphuric acid are added and it is again examined by Wood's lamp. The stain under study may be said to contain blood provided that in direct observation no luminescence was observed, and then, on repeating the examination using Wood's lamp, after further treatment with sulphuric acid, a red luminescence is observed.

This test renders the sample useless for any further analysis, so its undertaking must be duly calibrated.

- *Spectroscopic techniques:* These consist of confirming the presence of blood in a stain by obtaining the absorbance spectrum of the hemoglobin and its derivatives, obtained by adding different reagents.
- *Chromatographic techniques:* The blood sample is identified by chromography on Whatmann n° 1 paper, or on a fine layer of silica gel, using methanol, acetic acid and

water in a proportion of 90:3:7 as a solvent. Benzidine or its derivatives are used as the revealing agent.

## V. Specific Diagnosis

These are tests undertaken to establish whether the blood is human or not. This diagnosis can be obtained, as was said above in the previous section, with the human Hemoglobin Kit. And it is this method that is increasingly being used as it is quick and simple. However, traditionally other methods have been used which we now list below:

### *Study of Elements Forming the Blood*
The microscopic study, either directly on the sample or following its prior preparation, points one in the direction of the type of blood to which the sample belongs, as a result of the differences that are observed in the red and white blood cells, with regard to the shape of the cell and its nucleus. Obviously, the sample must be well preserved and contain a sufficient concentration of blood.

### *Hemoglobin Study*
By various methods:
   a. Crystallographic: these consist of analysing the difference in the crystals that the hemoglobin produces for different species.
   b. Spectographic .
   c. Structural differences: Obtaining aminoacid sequences.
   d. Differences in physical-chemical parameters: This includes studies on solubility, denaturalisation, chromographic and electrophoretic mobility and antigenic differences.

### *Techniques Based on, the Antigen-Anti-body Reaction [43]*
These are based on the fact that when a protein (antigen) of the same species is introduced into the organism of a different one, a defensive reaction takes place with the appearance of anti-bodies.

As the antigen reacts exclusively with its complementary antibody, one can discover if there is a certain antigen in a sample by adding the complementary antibody to it and observing whether a reaction takes place or not.

## VI. Human Hemoglobin Diagnosis Using Kits

These Kits were designed to detect blood in faeces. Therefore, so that they may be used with forensic samples, they have to be validated given that the conditions of the sample are, obviously, different. At first, the sensitivity and specificity of the kit that the manufacturer stated referred to its use in clinical samples and was not for use on forensic samples.

There are now several kits are on offer for forensic tests, although in principle, they are designed to detect hidden blood in faeces[4].

The basis of all of them is identical. Generally speaking, the sample is mixed with a liquid that acts as transport and several drops of this mixture pass through the kit. Hemoglobin reacts with a conjugated compound formed by coloured particles, together with a monoclonal human anti-hemoglobin anti-body and forms an immunocomplex. The latter migrates until finding a second human anti-hemoglobin anti-body, which catches the hemoglobin so forming a coloured line indicating a positive result.

The conjugated compound continues moving until arriving at a second zone in which there is a line of anticonjugated anti-bodies that immobilise it, so forming a second coloured line that indicates that the kit has worked correctly. This is the line of control.

There are several studies that support the use of these kits in forensic analysis. As far back as 1991, Hochmeister et al. published a work which evaluated its effectiveness (specifically the OneStep ABAcard® HemaTrace®) in forensic identification of human blood. They studied the sensitivity and specificity of the kit with this type of sample and concluded that, in principal, they were valid for analysing forensic samples, although in samples that had been dried with driers or had been in contact with dirt and were, therefore, fairly contaminated, good results were not obtained [44].

Several researchers have detected problems of false positives in semen and saliva. Nevertheless, it is arguable that the positive may not be due to the presence of traces of blood in the sample. For HemaTrace®, it has been shown that it provides positive results for saliva and semen up to a concentration of 1/100. With more diluted samples this result is not observed. As always happens in forensic investigation, the effectiveness of the test will depend on the state of the sample, its age and degree of contamination, etc. However, in any case, the use of kits is a simple and considerably effective alternative for determining the presence of human hemoglobin. Although a negative result cannot be exclusive, given that it may be due to the conditions in which the clue was found.

In our laboratory, the effectiveness of a standard hemoglobin kit was tested on blood samples subjected to real conditions of degradation. The results show that a negative result can never be interpreted as the absence of human blood in the sample, given that it may be due to those bad conditions.

Furthermore, we found that stains washed with detergents containing active oxygen do not give a positive result to the test. The results of this study can be found in an article published in Naturwissenschaften -*Active oxygen doctors the evidence*- which is referred to in the bibliography.

As an alternative to human hemoglobin, the use of human Glycophorin A has been proposed. This is a protein found in the membranes of red blood cells and for which a kit has been prepared which functions in a similar way to that of the Hemoglobin Kit [45].

Furthermore, more recent research has been evaluating the application of the study of specific markers located in the RNA messenger for semen. Also RAMAN spectroscopy has been proposed as a technique to be used in the future [46,47].

---

[4] For example: Hexagon OBTI® test http://www.bluestar-forensic.com/gb/hexagon.php or Hematrace® http://www.abacusdiagnostics.com/hematrace.htm

## VII. Individual Diagnosis

Recent spectacular advances in Molecular Biology have led, as a consequence, to individual diagnosis centring on the analysis of DNA profiles and other techniques. Serological methods and those that use polymorphic enzymes are increasingly less used.

The application of DNA analysis techniques in criminal investigation is subject that must be dealt with in depth, requiring an entire chapter to itself. Here, we will limit ourselves to making only a few commentaries on DNA studies when dealing with a sample of a bloody nature.

In this case, DNA is extracted from the white blood cells, which have to be separated from the other components of the blood using a process of controlled rupture and separation by centrifugation. The sample is treated with certain reagents which, selectively, "break down" the components of blood that are of no interest. After centrifuging, the whole white blood cells are found in the bottom of the tube and a floating mass consisting of the rest of the cellular components. By eliminating (decanting) the liquid, we are left with the white blood cells.

Once the white blood cells have been isolated, they will have to be broken (lyse) in order to release the DNA. They are treated with an appropriate lysis buffer and the DNA is obtained mixed with proteins and other cellular remains, now ready for extraction and purification.

The samples with which we work in Criminology present additional problems in analysis. Generally speaking, if the stain has not been dried and adequately preserved, it is difficult to achieve good results in amplification.

Also the backing can pose a serious impediment to developing the test. In the case of non-absorbent backings or natural fabrics (provided they are quite clean), the extraction method that seems to give the best results is that of extraction by Chelex. In absorbent backings (e.g. carpets, upholstery, etc.) organic extraction, applied after purification of the sample, should be tried.

Alternatively there are extraction kits and robots, which will be referred to in chapter five.

Another factor to be taken into account is the inhibitor effect that hemoglobin has on the Taq-Polymerase (which is the enzyme that is used in amplification). Although well preserved samples do not present problems, difficulties may arise in degraded samples containing derivatives of hemoglobin capable of blocking the enzyme, so hindering amplification. This is the case with liquid blood taken from cadavers or also from badly preserved stains) for example those found outdoors or buried that have been subject to rain, wind, damp, etc).

## VIII. Other Problems of Medical-legal Importance

Other problems of medical-legal importance, with regard to bloodstains are as follows:

### *Diagnosis of the Sex of the Individual to whom the Sample Belongs*

In 1969 Zech described a technique that is based on quinacrine staining of the distal portion of the Y chromosome, with which a characteristic fluorescence can be obtained. Phillips and Gaten, in 1971, used this procedure for forensic purposes. However, later on it was shown that there were cases of the Y chromosome not presenting luminescence, so the technique does not allow us to definitely determine the sex of the individual, as a false negative result may be obtained if the blood is old or, as mentioned above, when it belongs to an individual with negative Y fluorescence.

Currently sex is determined through DNA analysis. Various methods have been described. Some are based on the study of the amelogenin gene, which is found in the sex chromosomes. The fact that it is a different size in chromosome X and Y is very useful for distinguishing between the masculine and feminine sex. The amelogenin test is now included in the DBNA Kits for PCR [48].

Another possibility is to try amplifying the STRs corresponding to the Y chromosomes. If amplification is achieved and the alleles studied, it will be clear whether the sample is of masculine origin.

Analysis of the SRY gene has also be used in the identification of sex. This gene, which is found in chromosome Y, has proved its usefulness in determining sex in forensic samples in various investigations.

Comparisons of the effectiveness of the various methods have been made by various authors [49].

## *Determining the Anatomic Region from where the Blood Comes*

This is done through a cytological study of the cells that the stain may contain. For example, if buccal epithelial cells can be detected in the sample, the origin of the blood that formed the stain can be determined.

## *Studying the Age of the Blood Shed*

Discovering the age of a bloodstain found at a scene of a crime is an important item of information. If it is known when the event took place, it can be deduced whether the blood is related with that crime or not. If it is not known, the age of the stain will provide a good indication of when.

It should be borne in mind that, when calculating age, there will always be considerable error due to the fact that many factors intervene in the process of aging that could lead to confusing a recent stain with an old one.

Some of the methods traditionally employed for determining this parameter are:

- The appraisal of the elution speed of the stain in an appropriate solvent,
- The chloride diffusion test, proposed by Professors Gisbert and Iborra in 1957,
- And the study of protein fraction degradation.

Other authors have put forward alternatives:

In 1992 high performance liquid chromatography (HPLC) was used on bloodstains and fresh blood. In the chromatogram, the presence of a peak called "X" was noted that only appeared in the samples corresponding to stains. Moreover, the first data indicated that the peak area could be related with the age of the stain [50].

Some years later, in 1997, this study was widened and the effect of temperature on the results of the HPLC was determined. It was shown that this factor did not produce any variation in the peak "X" area [51].

In other experiments the relationship between oxyhemoglobin and total hemoglobin was studied and related to age. The authors, however, state that it is essential to know the temperature to which the stain has been subjected, which is a clear drawback in the case of forensic samples [52].

Years later another research group used the PCR technique for calculating age from the relationship between the mRNA and the rRNA. Their work showed that the relationship between both types of RNA varies in a linear way with age. The advantage of this method lies in the fact that it can be applied on very small samples and that it can also include DNA analysis [53,54].

Lastly, in 2010, several works have been published with new proposals:

For example the use of UV-VIS spectrometry to study the changes that take place in the hemoglobin and then to relate them to the age of the sample [55] or to study circadian biomarkers (melatonin and cortisol) and their variation over time [56].

We have now come to the end of this text. We hope we have been able to show that the investigation of bloodstains is not limited to a few laboratory techniques aimed at discovering one or two pieces of information. On the contrary, it is a wide open field of study for experts in highly diverse branches of knowledge: Photography, Mathematics, Statistics, Biology, Law among others, are disciplines that can find fascinating topics of research into different aspects of blood stain analysis. This is what makes blood stains so interesting.

## REFERENCES

[298] Cornwell, Patricia D. *Cruel and Unusual,* 1993.
[299] Balthazard V. *Manual de Medicina Legal.* Barcelona: Salvat, 1933.
[300] Thorwald J. *el siglo de la investigación criminal.* Barcelona: Labor S.A., 1966.
[301] Eckert W G, James S H. *Interpretation of bloodstains evidence at crime scenes.* New York: Elsevier, 1989.
[302] Ferreira A. A pericia técnica em Criminología e Medicina Legal. Sao Paulo: Imprenta E. G. *Revista des Tribunais Lda (sin referencia editorial),* 1948.
[303] Thoinot L. *Tratado de Medicina Legal vol 2.* Barcelona: Salvat S.A., 1928.
[304] Pérez Argilés V. *Prácticas de Medicina Legal y Toxicología.* Zaragoza: Librería General, 1940.
[305] Specht W. Die chemiluminiscenz des hämins, ein hilfsmittel zur auffindung und erkennung forensisch wichtiger blutspuren. Deustsche Ztschr. *f. d. ges. gerichtl. Med,* 1937; 28:225.
[306] Karger B, Rand S, Fracasso T, Pfeiffer H. Bloodstain pattern analysis—Casework experience. *Forensic Sci. Int.* 2008; 181:15–20.
[307] Yen K, Thali MJ, Kneubuehl BP, Peschel O, Zollinger U, Dirnhofer R. Blood-spatter patterns: hands hold clues for the forensic reconstruction of the sequence of events. *Am J Forensic Med Pathol.* 2003 Jun;24(2):132-140.
[308] James SH., Eckert WG. *Interpretation of bloodstain evidence at crime scenes* 2ª Ed. New York: CRC Press, 1999.
[309] http://home.iprimus.com.au/ararapaj/craigslea_testbed/Forensic%20Web%20Test%20Site/blood_spatter_analysis.htm

[310] Barni F, Lewis S W, Berti A, Miskelly G M, Lagoa G. Forensic application of the luminol reaction as a presumptive test for latent blood detection. *Talanta* 2007;72:896–913.

[311] Castelló A, Alvarez M, Verdú F. Accuracy, Reliability and safety of Luminol in bloodstain investigation. *Journal of Canadian Society of Forensic Science,* 2002; vol 35(3):113-121.

[312] Castelló A, Alvarez M, Miquel M, Verdú F. "Revelado de manchas latentes: efectividad del luninol y evaluación de su efecto sobre el estudio del DNA" Cuadernos de Medicina Forense, *abril* 2002; 28:33-36.

[313] Tontarski K L, Hoskins K A, Watkins T G, Brun-Conti L, Michaud A L. Chemical Enhancement Techniques of Bloodstain Patterns and DNA Recovery After Fire Exposure. *J Forensic Sci, January* 2009; 54(1):37-48.

[314] Proescher F, Moody A M. Detection of blood by means of chemiluminiscence. *The Journal of Laboratory and Clinical Medicine* 1939; 24:1183-1189.

[315] Quickenden TI, Creamer JI. A study of common interferences with the forensic luminol test for blood. *Luminescence* 2001 Jul-Aug;16(4):295-298.

[316] Creamer JI, Quickenden TI, Apanah MV, Kerr KA, Robertson P. A comprehensive experimental study of industrial, domestic and environmental interferences with the forensic luminol test for blood. *Luminescence,*2003 Jul-Aug;18(4):193-198.

[317] Quickenden TI, Cooper PD. Increasing the specificity of the forensic luminol test for blood. *Luminescence* 2001 May-Jun;16(3):251-253.

[318] Kent EJ, Elliot DA, Miskelly GM. Inhibition of bleach-induced luminol chemiluminescence. *J Forensic Sci* 2003 Jan; 48(1):64-67.

[319] King R, Miskelly G M. The inhibition by amines and amino acids of bleach-induced luminol chemiluminescence during forensic screening for blood. *Talanta* 2005; 67: 345–353.

[320] Castelló A, Francès F, Verdú F. Bleach interference in forensic luminol tests on porous surfaces: More about the drying time effect. *Talanta* 2009; 77:1555–1557.

[321] Castelló A, Francès F, Corella D, Verdú F. Active oxygen doctors the evidence. *Naturwissenschaften* 2009; 96:303–307.

[322] Gross A M et al. The effect of Luminol on presumptive tests and DNA analysis using the polymerase chain reaction. *J. Forensic Science* 1999; 44(4):837-840.

[323] Quickenden TI, Ennis CP, Creamer JI. The forensic use of luminol chemiluminescence to detect traces of blood inside motor vehicles. *Luminescence* 2004 Sep-Oct; 19(5):271-277.

[324] Budowle B, Leggitt JL, Defenbaugh DA, Keys KM, Malkiewicz SF. The presumptive reagent fluorescein for detection of dilute bloodstains and subsequent STR typing of recovered DNA.*J Forensic Sci.* 2000 Sep; 45(5):1090-1092.

[325] Tobe SS, Watson N, Daeíd NN. Evaluation of Six Presumptive Tests for Blood, Their Specificity, Sensitivity, and Effect on High Molecular-Weight DNA. *J Forensic Sci.* 2007 January; 52(1):102-109.

[326] Vandenberg N, van Oorschot R A H. The Use of Polilights in the Detection of Seminal Fluid, Saliva, and Bloodstains and Comparison with Conventional Chemical-Based Screening Tests. *J Forensic Sci. March* 2006; 51(2): 361-370.

[327] Chun-Yen Lin A, Hsing-Mei Hsieh, Li-Chin Tsai, Linacre A, Chun-I Lee J. Forensic Applications of Infrared Imaging for the Detection and Recording of Latent Evidence. *J Forensic Sci,* September 2007; 52(5): 1148-1150.

[328] Ramsthaler F, Kreutz K, Zipp K,Verhoff MA. Dating skeletal remains with luminol-chemiluminescence. Validity, intra- and interobserver error. *Forensic Sci Int* 2009; 187:47–50.

[329] Trevithick C C, Chartrand M M, Wahlman J, Rahman F, Hirst M, Trevithick J R. Shaken, not stirred: bioanalytical study of the antioxidant activities of Martinis. *BMJ* 1999; 319:1600-1602.

[330] Atanassova D, Kefalas P, Psillakis E.Environ. Measuring the antioxidant activity of olive oil mill wastewater using chemiluminescence.*Int.* 2005 Feb; 31(2):275-280.

[331] Bergervoet PWM et al. Application of the forensic Luminol for blood in infection control. *Journal of Hospital Infection* 2008; 68:329-333.

[332] Adler O, Adler R. Über das Verhalten gewisser organischer Verbindungen gegenüber Blut mit besonderer Berücksichtigung das Nachweises von Blut. *Hoppe-Seyler's Zeitschrift fur Physiologiste Chemie* 1904; 41:59-67. (artículo en alemán)

[333] Culliford BJ, Nickols LC. The Benzidine test. A critical review. *Journal of Forensic Sciences,* 1964 January; 9(1):175-191.

[334] Culliford BJ, Nickols LC. The Benzidine test. A critical review. *Journal of Forensic Sci* 1964 January; 9(1):175-191.

[335] Negre C, Castelló A, Gil P, Verdú F. ¿Manchas de sangre?: Seguridad en pruebas de orientación. *Cuadernos de Medicina Forense* 2003; 34:29-34.

[336] Castelló A, Francés F, Verdú F. DNA Evidence Uncompromised by Active Oxygen. *The Scientific World Journal* 2010; 10:387–392.

[337] Castelló A, Negre M C, Verdú F. Influencia del ambiente en el estudio criminalístico de muestras biológicas: el caso de las manchas de sangre. *Revista Brasileira de Medicina Legal* 2004; II(1)

[338] PivadeAlmeida J, Glesse N, Bonorino C. *Effect of presumptive tests reagents on human blood confirmatory tests and DNA análisis using real time polimerase chain reaction.* Forensic Sci Int 2010 doi:10.1016/j.forsciint.2010.06.017 (artículo en prensa)

[339] Gisbert Calabuig J A. Medicina Legal y Toxicología 5ª Ed. Salvat, Barcelona, 1998.

[340] Saferstein R. *Criminalistics. An introduction to Forensic Science* 5ª Ed. Prentice Hall, USA, 1995.

[341] Hochmeister MN, Budowle B, Sparkes R, Rudin O, Gehrig C, Thali M, Schmidt L, Cordier A, Dirnhofer R. Validation studies of an immunochromatographic 1-step test for the forensic identification of human blood. *J Forensic Sci.* 1999 May; 44(3):597-602.

[342] Schweers BA, Old J, Boonlayangoor PW, Reich KA. Developmental validation of a novel lateral flow strip test for rapid identification of human blood (Rapid Stain Identification--Blood). *Forensic Sci Int Genet.* 2008 Jun;2(3): 243-247.

[343] Zubakov D, Kokshoorn M, Kloosterman A, Kayser M. New markers for old stains: stable mRNA markers for blood and saliva identification from up to 16-year-old stains. *Int J Legal Med.* 2009; 123:71–74.

[344] Virkler K, Lednev IK. Raman spectroscopic signature of blood and its potential application to forensic body fluid identification. *Anal Bioanal Chem.* 2010; 396:525–534.

[345] Francès F, Castelló A, Verdú F. El diagnóstico genético del sexo mediante el test de la amelogenina: Métodos y posibles fuentes de error. *Cuad Med Forense* 2008; 14(52):119-125.

[346] Steinlechner M, Berger B, Niederstter H, Parson W. Rare failures in the amelogenin sex test. *Int J of Leg Medicine* 2002; 116(2):117-120.

[347] Inoue H, Takabe F, Iwasa M, Maeno Y, Seko Y. A new marker for estimation of bloodstain age by high performance liquid chromatography. *Forensic Sci Int.* 1992 Nov; 57(1):17-27.

[348] Andrasko J. The estimation of age of bloodstains by HPLC análisis. *J Forensic Sci.* 1997 Jul; 42(4):601-607.

[349] Matsuoka T, Taguchi T, Okuda J. Estimation of bloodstain age by rapid determinations of oxyhemoglobin by use of oxygen electrode and total hemoglobin. *Biol Pharm Bull.* 1995 Aug;18(8):1031-1035.

[350] Anderson S, Howard B, Hobbs GR, Bishop CP. A method for determining the age of a bloodstain. *Forensic Sci Int.* 2005 Feb 10; 148(1):37-45.

[351] Zubakov D, Hanekamp E, Kokshoorn M, van Ijcken W, Kayser M. Stable RNA markers for identification of blood and saliva stains revealed from whole genome expression analysis of time-wise degraded samples. *Int J Legal Med.* 2008 Mar; 122(2):135-142.

[352] Hanson E K, Ballantyne J. A Blue Spectral Shift of the Hemoglobin Soret Band Correlates with the Age (Time Since Deposition) of Dried Bloodstains. *PLoS ONE* 2010; 5(9). doi: 10.1371/journal.pone.0012830

[353] Ackermann K, Ballantyne K N, Kayser M. Estimating trace deposition time with circadian biomarkers: a prospective and versatile tool for crime scene reconstruction. *Int J Legal Med.* 2010; 124:387–395.

In: Forensic Science
Editors: N. Yacine and R. Fellag

ISBN 978-1-61324-999-4
© 2012 Nova Science Publishers, Inc.

*Chapter 5*

# DNA BASED KINSHIP ANALYSIS AND MISSING PERSON IDENTIFICATION

## *Jianye Ge**

Institute of Investigative Genetics, University of North Texas Health Science Center
Ft Worth, TX 76107, U. S.

## 1. INTRODUCTION

Over the past two decades, forensic DNA typing has become widely accepted as a powerful tool in criminal and civil investigations. This technology has become invaluable in many missing-person identifications. There are a number of scenarios in which person identification is required: war victims in mass graves, missing soldiers or military personnel from past wars, murdered peoples, remains from mass disasters due to natural catastrophes or terrorism attacks. In attempts to identify these individuals, DNA profiles from unidentified people may be compared with direct reference samples of the missing person, such as buccal swabs collected before their disappearance, or items they have used, such as toothbrushes, hairbrushes or preserved dental casts. In some cases, direct comparisons are not possible because no direct reference is available or the chain of custody may not be established reliably. Alternatively, a missing person may be identified by kinship analysis using family reference samples (e.g., parents, offspring, siblings or cousins) of the person to be identified.

In this chapter, first, the general principle of likelihood ratio (LR) method is explained [1,2]. Second, the pedigree likelihood ratio (PLR) method based on autosomal STR markers is introduced [2], in which jointly considers the DNA profile data of all available family reference samples with both population substructure and mutation model incorporated. Third, a more sophisticated algorithm for calculating the pedigree likelihood ratio of the lineage markers (i.e., Y chromosome STRs and mitochondrial DNA) is described [3]. Fourth, guidelines are given on which and how many relatives should be selected and typed for missing person identification so that efficiency can be optimized under the constraints of limited resources [4].

---

* Email: Jianye.Ge@unthsc.edu.

## 2. GENERAL PRINCIPLES

To evaluate whether a missing person (*MP*) belongs to a family pedigree (*P*), one or more reference family members from the putative pedigree are typed. Identification is assessed by comparing two alternative hypotheses: (i) $H_p$: *MP* is the specific member of the putative pedigree and (ii) $H_d$: *MP* is unrelated to the known reference members of the putative pedigree.

The LR is calculated based on probability of the DNA evidence under each hypothesis, represented by the general expression (Equation 1):

$$LR = \frac{\Pr(G_{MP}, G_P \mid H_p)}{\Pr(G_{MP}, G_P \mid H_d)} \tag{1}$$

where $G_{MP}$ refers to the DNA profile of the missing-person and $G_P$ is the joint DNA profile of all typed family members in the pedigree, computed conditions imposed by the hypotheses $H_p$ and $H_d$, respectively. $H_p$ is favored if the LR is > 1; when the LR is < 1, $H_d$ is better supported. For $H_p$, the position of *MP* in *P* is usually fixed. However, several scenarios could apply to $H_d$; for example, the biological mother but not biological father of *MP* is already in *P*, *MP* is a half sibling but not a full sibling of someone in *P*, or *MP* is not related to anyone in *P*. Multiple LRs can be compared in terms of different $H_d$. If no prior information of *MP* is provided to specify $H_d$, *MP* may be regarded as not related to anyone in *P*.

## 3. PEDIGREE LIKELIHOOD RATIO WITH MUTATIONS AND POPULATION SUBSTRUCTURE

In this section, the method to calculate the pedigree likelihood based on the classic Elston–Stewart (ES) algorithm [5] was improved by incorporating both population substructure and mutations. Population substructure was incorporated to comply with recommendation 4.1 in the NRCII Report [6]. A realistic mutation model is also embedded to address potential mismatches between true biological relatives. The details of genotype inference for the untyped family members in the reference pedigree were also disclosed. The computational complexity of the pedigree LR was presented.

### 3.1. Pedigree Likelihood Algorithm

The ES algorithm [5] calculates the probability by 'peeling' the pedigree into multiple nested nuclear families. In brief, the ES algorithm can be adapted to the likelihood of a pedigree as:

$$L = \sum_{G_1} \cdots \sum_{G_n} \Pr(G_{founder}) \prod_{founder} \prod_{\{o, f, m\}} \Pr(G_o \mid G_f, G_m), \tag{2}$$

in which $G_i$ represents the genotype (at a specific locus) of the *i*-th person of a pedigree, and each member is classified as either a founder (that is, a person without antecedent relatives in the pedigree, with their genotype represented as $G_{founder}$), or an offspring ($G_o$) from a given mother ($G_m$) and father ($G_f$). The locus-specific likelihood ($L$) of a pedigree is the summation over all possible genotype combinations, $G_i$, for each member (of course, for the typed members in the pedigree, the observed genotypes are considered as the only possibility). Within the summation, the probability of each possible genotype combination of a pedigree is computed as the product of two factors: (i) joint probability of all founder genotypes, $Pr(\prod G_{founder})$ and the product of each of the probabilities of offspring genotypes conditional on parental genotypes for trios, $Pr(G_o|G_f, G_m)$ or (ii) the probability of allele transmission in the pedigree. Computed in this fashion, values for $L$ across all loci are multiplied to get a combined $L$ value, denoted by $Pr(G_{MP}, G_P)$, which is in turn used in the final LR calculation (see equation 1). The computational complexity of the ES algorithm increases linearly with the number of trios in a complete pedigree (i.e., a pedigree with all family members typed).

## 3.2. Genotype Inference of Untyped Persons

In some situations, not all family members of a reference pedigree may be typed. Genotypes of these untyped individuals can only be inferred from those of the typed relatives, such as parents, offspring and spouse. If mutation is considered, the genotype of untyped individuals theoretically can be all possible genotypes at that locus. However, not all genotypes need to be inferred for each untyped individual in the pedigree. The computational complexity can be reduced by reducing the number of individuals with inferred genotypes. For nuclear families with a single offspring and a single typed parent, the genotypes of the untyped parent are not needed. For nuclear families with several offspring, the genotypes of both parents should be inferred, because the probabilities of allele transmissions from the untyped parent to multiple offspring are not independent. To reduce computational complexity, an untyped individual, defined as one whose genotypes has to be inferred, is termed an *untyped connector* (*UC*), which includes (1) untyped founders with > 1 offspring, (ii) untyped founders with a single offspring but an untyped spouse, (iii) untyped non-founders who are not leaf or bottom nodes in the pedigree tree.

For nuclear families with single offspring, one untyped parent, and one typed or *UC* parent, the single offspring is defined as an 'offspring with single typed parent' (*OSTP*). *OSTP*s are important in population substructure adjustment because the transmitted allele from the typed or UC parent is undecided. Figure 1 gives an example to illustrate both definitions. *A*, *B*, *E* and *F* in this example are *UC*s, and *G* is an OSTP. The genotype of *C* does not need to be inferred because there is only one offspring *G* in the nuclear family {*C*, *D*, *G*}.

## 3.3. Population Substructure Correction

Population substructure induces a degree of correlation of uniting gametes in randomly chosen individuals from the population. Hence, population substructure corrections for the probability calculations were recommended by previous publications [6-8]. This correlation is measured by the co-ancestry coefficient ($\theta$), that is, the probability that random sampled alleles from two individuals are identical by descent. The probability that an allele $A$ will be observed, given that $x$ alleles of type $A$ have been observed in all observed $n$ alleles, is

$$\Pr(A \mid \text{Observed Alleles}) = \frac{x\theta + (1-\theta)p(A)}{1+(n-1)\theta} \qquad (3)$$

where $p(A)$ is the allele frequency of allele $A$ [7, 8]. According to the NRCII recommendation, $\theta$ is set at 0.01 for large populations and 0.03 for small, isolated populations, but can be set to population- and even locus-specific $\theta$ values.

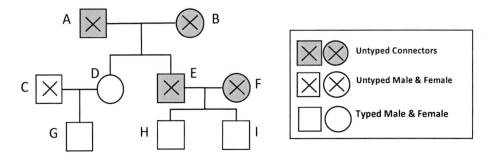

Figure 1. A, B, C, E and F are untyped family members; D, G, H and I are typed members. *Untyped Connectors (UC)* include A, B, E and F. G is an *Offspring with Single Typed Parent (OSTP)*.

The likelihood of founder alleles can be calculated by selecting all founder alleles one by one based on formula (3). For example, the likelihood of two typed founders, {A, B} and {C, D}, is

$$L = \Pr(A)\Pr(B \mid A)\Pr(C \mid AB)\Pr(D \mid ABC) \qquad (4)$$

The probability of transmission from parents to offspring {E, F} is calculated as shown in equation 5, if both parents are typed.

$$\begin{aligned} P(EF \mid AB, CD) = &\ 1/2 \times [\Pr(A \to E) + \Pr(B \to E)] \\ &\times 1/2 \times [\Pr(C \to F) + \Pr(D \to F)] \\ &+ 1/2 \times [\Pr(A \to F) + \Pr(B \to F)] \\ &\times 1/2 \times [\Pr(C \to E) + \Pr(D \to E)] \end{aligned} \qquad (5)$$

For cases with a single typed parent {A, B} and a typed offspring {E, F}, transmission likelihoods need to be calculated with caution, because the allele transmitted from the parent is undetermined, that is, either E or F could be the transmitted allele or founder allele. If there is only one *OSTP* in the pedigree, two possible scenarios are considered: E is transmitted from the typed parent and F is the founder allele, and *vice versa*. The transmission probability within the trio is based on the summation of transmission probabilities for both scenarios.

$$L = 1/2 * [\Pr(A \to E) + \Pr(B \to E)]\Pr(F \mid AB)$$
$$+ 1/2 * [\Pr(A \to F) + \Pr(B \to F)]\Pr(E \mid AB) \quad (6)$$

If there is > 1 OSTP in the pedigree, all possible transmission patterns are considered, and the transmission likelihood of the pedigree is calculated by summarizing likelihoods of all transmission patterns. For a pedigree with all genotypes of *UCs* assigned, *n* (number of *OSTPs* in the pedigree) generates $2^n$ possible patterns, and pedigree likelihoods can be calculated by

$$L = \sum_{O_1} ... \sum_{O_n} \Pr(Pedigree \mid O_1,...O_n) \quad (7)$$

where $O_i$ is the *i*-th OSTP. Each $O_i$ has two possibilities: the first or the second allele is a founder allele. In this situation, the likelihood of founders and the likelihood of transmission cannot be clearly separated, because they are not independent.

## 3.4. Mutation Correction

The most applicable mutation model for most human STR or microsatellite markers is the Two Phase Model [9], which is a symmetrical mutation model allowing alleles to change by adding or subtracting an absolute number of *x* repeat units. The transmission probability of two identical allele is $1-\mu$. The probability of a mutation event with *x* step (*x* > 0) is

$$\Pr(X = x) = \mu\alpha(1-\alpha)^{x-1} \quad (8)$$

where $\alpha$ is the probability of being a one step mutation and $\mu$ is the mutation rate of the locus. Equal probabilities for gaining or losing repeats are assumed.

According to the AABB annual report [10], > 95% of mutations result in one-step differences, hence $\alpha$ was set at 0.95; mutations of > 2 steps are unlikely, but several mutation steps are allowed in this model. The mutation rates of the forensically used STR loci are on the order of $10^{-3}$ to $10^{-4}$ per locus per generation [10, 11]. Because males have higher mutation rates than females [10], different locus-specific mutation rates must be used for the father and mother within a pedigree. The mechanism of mutations between integer (e.g., 10) and fractional (e.g., 10.2) STR alleles is different from slippage-based mutation. The probability of a partial repeat mutation should be lower than the average STR mutation rates and higher than the SNP mutation rates (for example, $10^{-8}$). Because there are no data on partial repeat mutations, we arbitrarily set the probability at $10^{-5}$, but further investigations are needed to establish a more meaningful probability.

## 3.5. Computational Complexity Analysis

The computational complexity of a pedigree LR calculation generally depends on the number of markers (*NM*), the number of UCs (*NUC*), the number of possible genotypes of each UC (*NGUC*) and the number of *OSTP*s (*NO*). The complexity or the number of pedigrees with genotypes of *UC*s assigned, can be presented as

$$NM * \prod_{i=1...NUC} NGUC_i * 2^{NO} \tag{9}$$

The genotypes are not inferred for all untyped individuals but *OSTP* is defined because *NGUC* is always > 2 with the possibility of mutation. By *OSTP*, the computation could be several orders of magnitudes faster for large pedigrees with several untyped individuals. Thus, *NUC* and *NGUC* make up the major contribution for complexity. Without mutation, *NGUC* is small compared with the number of all possible genotypes. However, with the presence of mutation, *NGUC* is close to its maximum possible number. One approach to reduce *NGUC* is to summarize all alleles that were not observed in the pedigree as a new allele '*X*'. The frequency of '*X*' is the complement of the sum of frequencies of all possible present alleles, including possible mutated alleles.

## 3.6. Software

A software MPKin was developed based on the methods and models described above. The results were compared with two other kinship analysis software. LRs of each locus of three pedigrees calculated by DNAView, Familias and MPKin were identical. Familias and MPKin can further calculate LRs accommodating population substructure and mutation. Familias may also give LR with mutations, but with different mutation models. Details can be found at http://www.investigativegenetics.com/content/1/1/8/additional.

## 4. PEDIGREE LIKELIHOOD RATIO FOR LINEAGE MARKERS

In kinship analysis cases, lineage markers often are used as an adjunct tool to the autosomal STR markers. The general principle of kinship analysis of lineage markers is the same as that of autosomal markers. However, the prosecution or kinship hypothesis usually considers the haplotypes in the same lineage instead of a fixed relationship of the questioned person in the reference family. In most cases, this probability is simply set at 1 if the number of mismatched loci or nucleotides between the questioned person and the references is less than a predefined threshold (e.g., less than 2 mismatched nucleotides infers that mtDNA sequence cannot be excluded as possibly being from the same lineage [12]). Mutations and inconsistent haplotypes among the questioned person and the reference(s) were taken into account in the likelihood calculation. Rolf *et al.* [13] suggested a method for calculating the probability of segregating the haplotypes in multiple generations. Unfortunately, no mutation model to deal with multiple step mutations and complex mutation events was incorporated. In addtion, the details of the pedigree structure were not considered in [13]. Instead, only the number of transmission events or generations between individuals was considered.

In this study, we provide a sophisticated method to formalize the likelihood calculations of both Y-STR and mtDNA haplotypes, in which the likelihood is calculated in a pedigree fashion, same as the way for autosomal markers, and the kinship hypothesis is based on a fixed relationship rather than solely on lineage. The computational complexity is analyzed and methods to reduce the complexity are discussed. Preliminary mutation models for the mtDNA are introduced to calculate the transmission probability between mtDNA haplotypes.

## 4.1. Pedigree Likelihood for Y-STR

The pedigree likelihood based on the Y-STR haplotypes is the product of the haplotype frequency of the founder (i.e., the person without antecedent relatives in the pedigree) and the transmission probability from the founder to all descendants, which is dependant on the mutation steps between each father-son transmission event. The whole pedigree is regarded as a directed acycling graph [14], in which vertices are the family members and the directed edges represent the genetic transmission from fathers to sons (see Figure 2 as an example).

Suppose there are $N$ father-son pairs (i.e., $FS_1$, $FS_2$, ..., $FS_N$) in the pedigree and the genotype of each individual in the pedigree is known, the cumulative transmission probability of the pedigree, $TP$, is the cumulative product of the transmission probability of each father-son pair at each locus (Equation 10), assuming the mutation events at each locus are independent:

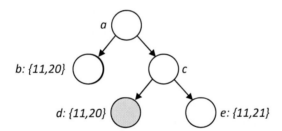

Figure 2. A two-locus Y-STR pedigree including individuals from $a$ to e. The vertices represent individuals and the directed edges are father-son transmissions. $b$, $d$, and $e$ have Y-STR genotypes available; $a$ and $c$ are untyped. Individual $d$ is the questioned person with genotype {11,20}, and the true person d has a brother $e$ and an uncle $b$ as the family references.

$$TP = \prod_{i=1}^{N}\prod_{k=0}^{K} TP(FS_{ik}) \qquad (10)$$

where $TP(FS_{ik})$ is the transmission probability of $i$-th father-son pair at $k$-th locus and it can be calculated using the same mutation model, Two Phase model, as used for autosomal STRs.

The pedigree likelihood is the product of the haplotype frequency of the founder, Pr(*founder*), and the transmission probability within the pedigree (Equation 11). The computational complexity is on the order of $N \times K$ for a pedigree with all individuals having unambiguous genotypes.

$$L = \Pr(founder) \times TP \tag{11}$$

In situations where genotypes are not available at some loci for some individuals in the pedigree, the genotypes are inferred. The likelihood of the pedigree with untyped individuals is the sum of the likelihood of all possible subpedigrees with all individual's genotypes typed or inferred. Note that different subpedigrees may have different founder profiles.

The genotype assignment with minimum mutation steps to explain the pedigree is preferred. It is assumed that the genotypes of the untyped individuals can only be composed of one or more of the observed alleles in the pedigree or the alleles between these observed alleles. The number of alleles should be the same as those of the majority of the observed genotypes in the pedigree. Suppose all individuals have the same number of observed alleles ($m$), there are $X$ number of observed alleles in the whole pedigree and $Y$ number of untyped individuals at a specific locus, the number of possible subpedigrees ($NP$) at this locus is

$$NP = \begin{cases} \binom{X}{m} * Y & X > 1 \\ 1 & X = 1 \end{cases} \tag{12}$$

When the numbers of observed alleles are different among the individuals, in the worst case, the complexity is on the order of the product of $Y$ and the permutation of $X$, which is not polynomial. Fortunately, in most real cases, $X$ is less than 3 or 4, which is acceptable and the computation can be completed in a reasonable time (i.e., less than 1 second with the current computation ability). For any pedigrees or subpedigrees with all the genotypes determined, the computational complexity is linear to the number of transmission with the pedigrees (i.e., the number of edges in the acycling graph).

### 4.2. Pedigree Likelihood for mtDNA

The algorithm for pedigree likelihood calculation based on mtDNA haplotypes is the same as that for Y-STR haplotypes, except that the mtDNA and Y-STR loci have different mechanisms and rates of mutation. mtDNA mutations are due to base substitution (i.e., transition and transversion), deletion or insertion. The independence of mutation events between bases is assumed.

The mutation rates for the mtDNA genome are known to be higher than those of nuclear DNA [15,16]. Many nucleotide substitution models [17] have been proposed, such as Kimura model, Tamura model, HKY model, and unrestricted model, etc. Unfortunately, there has been no systematic study for which model is the best fit for human mtDNA sequences. The Kimura model [18] was used (simply as a starting point), which assigns different substitution rates to transitions and transversions, but the substitution rates of two different transitions, as well as two different transversions, are assumed equal. The mutation rates are assumed to be even for all nucleotides, although relatively high mutation rates were observed at some hotspots [19,20]. More sophisticated models can be implemented with further data. According to the summarized data in Howell et al [21], 15 mutations in 1,246 transmission events were observed in HVI and HVII, which leads to an average mutation rate $2.0 \times 10^{-5}$ across HVI and HVII (i.e., 15/(1,246*610)). Table 1 summarizes the mutation rates of HVI and HVII for the Kimura model [22, 23].

**Table 1. Human Mitochondrial DNA nucleotides mutation rates ($\times 10^{-6}$) assuming Kimura model**

| Nucleotides | Mutations | | | | | |
|---|---|---|---|---|---|---|
| | A | T | C | G | insertion | deletion |
| A | | 0.2 | 0.2 | 3.6 | 0.5 | 0.5 |
| T | 0.2 | | 3.8 | 0.2 | 0.5 | 0.5 |
| C | 0.2 | 3.6 | | 0.2 | 0.5 | 0.5 |
| G | 3.6 | 0.2 | 0.2 | | 0.5 | 0.5 |

To accommodate heteroplasmy, the mtDNA pedigree likelihood of a base position is the sum of likelihood of subpedigrees with a nucleotide fixed for each individual. For untyped individuals at a base position, the genotype can be all four possible nucleotides (although transitions tend to be favoured over transversions at many sites). Suppose there are $m$ mtDNA typed individuals in a pedigree with $T_1, T_2, ..., T_m$ number of nucleotides, respectively, the number of possible subpedigrees with fixed nucleotides for all typed individuals is the product of the number of nucleotides of individuals (i.e., $\prod_{k=1}^{m} T_k$). To save the computational time, the transmission probability may be directly set at 1 for bases at which all individuals share at least one nucleotide. Subpedigrees with transversion mutation may be ignored if there are other subpedigrees which only contain transition mutations or no mutation.

### 4.3. Haplotype Frequency

There are many reasonable suggestions to estimate haplotype frequency of the lineage markers. Let $n$ be the database size and $x$ be the number of observations of the lineage profile. The suggested haplotype frequency estimates mainly include the followings.

4. $p = \dfrac{x}{n}$;
5. $p = \dfrac{x+2}{n+2}$ [8, 24];
6. $p = 1 - \alpha^{1/n}$, where α is (1 – confidence interval), usually 0.05 [24,25];
7. The "surveying" methods [26,27];
8. $p = \dfrac{x}{n} + \theta\left(1 - \dfrac{x}{n}\right)$ [28, 29], where θ is the measure of population substructure;

9. Upper bound of 95% binomial confidence interval [29]; the Clopper and Pearson's binomial confidence interval is suggested.

## 5. Choosing Relatives for Missing Persons Identifications

Increasing the likelihood ratio to obtain reliable identification is the primary goal of the missing person identifications. There are two ways to increase the likelihood ratio: 1) type more markers; and 2) type more relatives. The number of markers that can be typed will be limited by the quality and quantity of DNA derived from a remains. In many cases, the quality and quantity of DNA is poor. Increasing the number of reference relatives can increase the chances of identifying remains and particularly for challenged samples. Typing all relatives of a large pedigree can be costly and may not be necessary to reach a certain threshold for identification. Since there are information and cost factors regarding the selection and number of relatives, respectively, some selection criteria should be considered to guide identity testers. The probabilities of identity with certain combinations of relatives are more powerful than are other combinations.

In this section, the 37 most common relative combination scenarios in missing person identifications were selected and using the 13 CODIS STRs as genetic profile data large numbers of pedigrees (e.g., 1,000,000) were simulated for each scenario. The distribution of LRs for each scenario was evaluated to first confirm the well-known single relative reference scenarios and second to determine the most informative combinations of relatives for identifying an unknown person. Thus guidance is given on which and how many relatives should be selected and typed for kinship analyses for identification so that efficiency can be optimized under the constraints of limited resources.

### 5.1. Method

Thirty-seven common reference scenarios (ranging from a single relative as a reference sample to combinations of relatives for kinship analysis) were selected. The pedigrees consisting of DNA profiles for each scenario were simulated using the Caucasian population data on the 13 CODIS STR loci [30] assuming no population substructure and mutation (Table 2). To generate simulated data the alleles of founders (i.e., individuals without parents in the pedigree) were randomly assigned according to the allele frequencies of each locus [30] and each locus was treated independently. Founders transmitted with equal probability a single allele at each locus to his/her offspring. One million pedigrees were simulated for most scenarios. Due to the computational complexity of the LR calculation, only thousands or tens of thousands of pedigrees were simulated for some complex scenarios. Logarithm base 10 of the likelihood ratios, $Log_{10}(LR)$, were calculated by comparing the probabilities of observing a DNA profile under two hypotheses: the missing person belongs to the pedigree under a specified relationship or the missing person is unrelated to the pedigree.

## 5.2. Results

Table 2 shows the mean and variance of the $\text{Log}_{10}(\text{LR})$ distributions of reference scenarios, as well as the 5th, 1[th], 0.1[th] percentiles of the distributions (i.e., 95%, 99%, 99.9% confidence level, respectively) and number of simulations in each scenario. As already well known, for pedigrees containing a single reference relative (Figure 3), informativeness of relationships can be ranked as follows:

- Parent/child
- Fullsib
- Grandparent/grandchild, uncle/nephew, halfsib
- First Cousin

This part of the study was performed to establish that the simulations were providing reliable data on relationship and information content for kinship analysis. The parent or child is the most preferred reference among singe relative scenarios with all LRs greater than one. The fullsib scenario has the highest variance of LRs among all single reference relative scenarios, due to the wide distribution of Identity by Descent (IBD) alleles with fullsibs (i.e., 1/4, 1/2 and 1/4 for IBD = 0, 1, 2, respectively). Grandchild, uncle and halfsib essentially have the same distributions. The majority of LRs (i.e. 99.5%) with a first cousin scenario (cousin in short) were less than 100, which is consistent with the known relationship of that of a cousin and that such genetic data (i.e., STRs) typically do not provide much information for missing person identification.

**Table 2. Means, variances, 5th, 1[th] and 0.1[th] percentiles of $\text{Log}_{10}(\text{LR})$ of relative scenarios**

| Relative scenarios | Mean | Variance | 5% | 1% | 0.1% | simulations |
|---|---|---|---|---|---|---|
| 3 children + spouse | 12.4199 | 3.72 | 9.31 | 8.054 | 6.646 | 1,000,000 |
| 4 children | 10.4023 | 3.2167 | 7.481 | 6.216 | 4.725 | 1,000,000 |
| **Both parents** | 10.2561 | 2.0865 | 8.071 | 7.337 | 6.5855 | 1,000,000 |
| 2 spouses + 2 children (1 each) | 10.1768 | 3.3654 | 7.303 | 6.258 | 5.141 | 1,000,000 |
| 2 children + spouse | 10.1122 | 3.4419 | 7.197 | 6.133 | 4.9875 | 1,000,000 |
| 3 children | 9.057 | 3.2728 | 6.14 | 4.958 | 3.6355 | 1,000,000 |
| 1 parent + 3 fullsibs | 8.8683 | 2.9959 | 6.07 | 4.878 | 3.504 | 1,000,000 |
| 1 child + 1 parent + spouse | 8.8089 | 2.6358 | 6.285 | 5.356 | 4.369 | 1,000,000 |
| Spouse + 1 child + 1 child with 2nd spouse | 8.8088 | 2.6381 | 6.288 | 5.35 | 4.36 | 1,000,000 |
| 4 fullsibs | 8.5438 | 3.419 | 5.493 | 4.147 | 2.593 | 1,000,000 |
| 1 fullsib + 1 child + spouse | 8.1415 | 3.1616 | 5.314 | 4.231 | 3.046 | 1,000,000 |
| 1 parent + 2 fullsibs | 7.9474 | 3.2484 | 5.03 | 3.839 | 2.5135 | 1,000,000 |
| 3 fullsibs | 7.5199 | 3.74 | 4.346 | 2.985 | 1.4155 | 1,000,000 |
| 1 child + 1 parent | 7.2595 | 2.2328 | 4.925 | 4.03 | 3.0285 | 1,000,000 |
| 2 children | 6.9823 | 2.8332 | 4.334 | 3.346 | 2.304 | 1,000,000 |
| 1 fullsib + 1 child | 6.5897 | 3.4195 | 3.628 | 2.457 | 1.15 | 1,000,000 |
| 1 fullsib + 1 parent | 6.3159 | 3.3385 | 3.39 | 2.248 | 1.01 | 1,000,000 |

| Relationship | | | | | | |
|---|---|---|---|---|---|---|
| **1 child + spouse** | **6.1687** | 1.2632 | 4.497 | 3.935 | 3.353 | 1,000,000 |
| 2 fullsibs | 5.877 | 3.9238 | 2.653 | 1.339 | -0.116 | 1,000,000 |
| 1 halfsib + 1 parent (not the parent of the halfsib) | 5.5361 | 2.4912 | 3.028 | 2.056 | 0.9969 | 1,000,000 |
| 1 uncle + 1 parent (they are not related) | 5.5344 | 2.4926 | 3.028 | 2.047 | 0.9628 | 1,000,000 |
| 1 grandchildren + 1 child (they are uncle-nephew) | 4.6249 | 1.6739 | 2.623 | 1.885 | 1.084 | 1,000,000 |
| **1 parent / 1 child** | 4.086 | 1.1195 | 2.484 | 1.915 | 1.3155 | 1,000,000 |
| 1 halfsib + 1 fullsib | 3.9493 | 3.7025 | 0.8514 | -0.3731 | -1.719 | 1,000,000 |
| 1 fullsib | 3.4193 | 3.6201 | 0.3731 | -0.7899 | -2.05 | 1,000,000 |
| 2 uncles (they are not related) | 1.9935 | 2.0261 | -0.2634 | -1.168 | -2.2525 | 10,000 |
| 2 grandchildren (who are cousins) | 1.707 | 1.5767 | -0.3177 | -1.1385 | -2.0365 | 50,000 |
| 2 halfsibs (two halfsibs are also halfsibs) | 1.6348 | 1.3162 | -0.2141 | -0.9612 | -1.8105 | 1,000,000 |
| 2 halfsibs (two halfsibs are fullsibs) | 1.4454 | 1.1333 | -0.2844 | -1.034 | -1.901 | 1,000,000 |
| 2 grandchildren (who are fullsibs) | 1.4449 | 1.1318 | -0.2847 | -1.031 | -1.9115 | 1,000,000 |
| 2 uncles (who are fullsibs) | 1.4442 | 1.1325 | -0.2869 | -1.03 | -1.9075 | 1,000,000 |
| 1 grandparent/grandchild | 0.9154 | 0.8947 | -0.5804 | -1.164 | -1.79 | 1,000,000 |
| 1 uncle/nephew | 0.9149 | 0.8938 | -0.5797 | -1.16 | -1.792 | 1,000,000 |
| 1 halfsib | 0.9138 | 0.8929 | -0.5793 | -1.162 | -1.799 | 1,000,000 |
| 2 cousins (they are also cousins) | 0.4691 | 0.4605 | -0.5709 | -0.9808 | -1.4165 | 10,000 |
| 2 cousins (they are fullsibs) | 0.3661 | 0.3637 | -0.5539 | -0.8964 | -1.3425 | 25,000 |
| 1 cousin | 0.2485 | 0.2607 | -0.5054 | -0.7674 | -1.039 | 1,000,000 |

* Bold numbers (i.e., greater than 6) means informative identification.

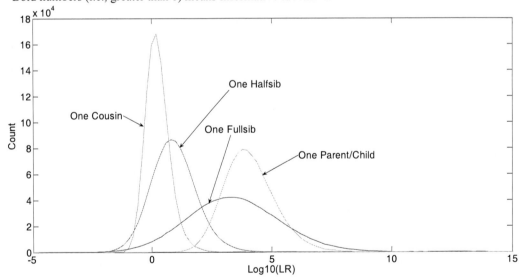

Figure 3. $Log_{10}(LR)$ distributions of single relative scenarios.

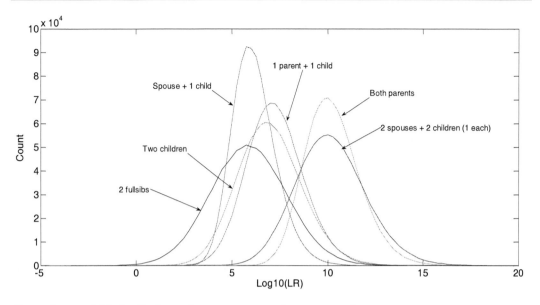

Figure 4. Log$_{10}$(LR) distributions of some common reference scenarios.

Since the data are consistent with the known power of single source relatives of various relationships, multiple reference relative pedigrees were evaluated. Again as expected, the scenarios with a higher number of closer relatives generally gave higher LRs. LRs with two children are expected to be on average 12 times greater than those for two fullsibs, which are 60 times more than those for single parents (Figure 4, Table 2). The two parents scenario gives more than 1,000 times greater LRs than one parent + one child and two children scenarios, mostly because genotypes of parents are (assumed to be) independent but genotypes of children are dependent on each other and on the missing person and parent of the missing person. The one parent + one child scenario has slightly greater average LRs and lower variance than the two children scenario. Hence, parents are more informative then children in multiple relative scenarios. This observation is consistent with the practices in paternity testing.

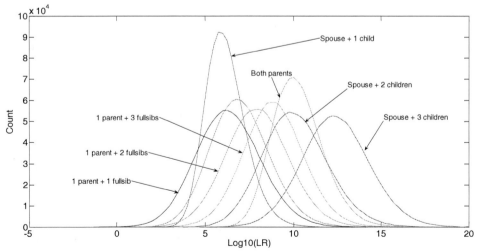

Figure 5. Log$_{10}$(LR) distributions of 1 parent + fullsibs, 1 spouse + child(ren) and both parents.

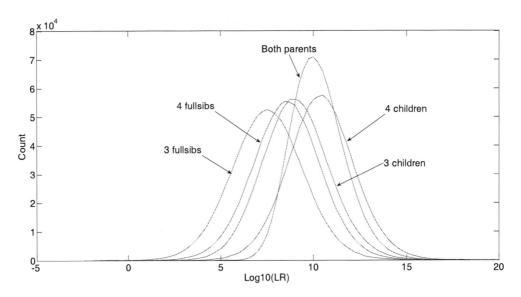

Figure 6. $Log_{10}(LR)$ distributions of high number of fullsibs and children v.s. both parents.

Spouses are typically unrelated. A LR can increase several orders of magnitude if the spouse is included in scenarios with the corresponding children as reference samples, e.g., in reconstruction cases. LRs with spouse are expected to be more than 100 times higher than those of scenarios without a spouse and if only one child is available. The LRs with a spouse could be higher with multiple children; one more child increases the LRs by two magnitudes on average with an accompanying slightly higher variance as expected (Figure 5). The scenario with two spouses + two children gives comparable LRs as the both parents scenario, although the variance is larger. The spouse + two children scenario has a similar distribution as two spouses + two children (one child for each spouse) scenario (Table 2). The average LRs of one parent + fullsib(s) scenario are apparently less than those of a spouse + children (Figure 5). The average LR of one fullsib + one child is slightly greater than one fullsib + one parent due to the closer genetic dependence between fullsib and parent. Genetic dependence can be measured by the kinship coefficient; the smaller the kinship coefficient values, the less genetic dependence there is between relationships. It would take about 7 fullsibs + one parent to obtain similar LRs on average as that of both parents, but only two children + one spouse are required to achieve similar LRs (Figure 5). Four children or 10 fullsibs can also yield comparable LRs (Figure 6).

It was interesting to notice that three fullsibs, one fullsib + one parent, one fullsib + one child and two children scenarios yielded higher LRs than one child + spouse, one common paternity testing scenario (Table 2). However, these four scenarios have much higher variance than that of one child + spouse, which leads to higher probability of false exclusions for identifications. Some scenarios' rankings are worth noting: 1) two halfsibs (two halfsibs are also halfsibs) > two halfsibs (two halfsibs are fullsibs); 2) two uncles (who are not related) > two uncles (who are fullsibs); 3) two grandchildren (who are cousins) > two grandchildren (who are fullsibs). 4) two cousins (who are also cousins) > two cousins (who are fullsibs). Since halfsibs, uncle-nephew and grandparent-grandchild have the same IBD distribution, the LR distributions of two halfsibs, uncles or grandchildren (who are fullsibs) are identical. But if the two relatives are not fullsibs, less genetic dependence between these relatives gives a higher average LR (i.e., two unrelated uncles > two grandchildren as cousin > two halfsibs as halfsib for average LR).

The same simulations as above were performed for one parent, one fullsib and one halfsib scenarios but with 15 Caucasian STRs (i.e., 13 CODIS STR + the loci D2S1338 and D19S433) (Table 3). The average LR of the one parent scenario is almost 7-fold higher with these two extra STRs, and the increment is less than 2-fold for the halfsib scenario. As already known, closer relatives will provide higher LR increments. Additional markers can provide higher LRs and more reliable identifications.

**Table 3. Means and variances of three single relative scenarios with 13 or 15 CODIS STRs (i.e. 13 core loci + D2S1338 and D19S433)**

| Scenarios | 13 CODIS STRs | | 13 CODIS + 2 STRs | |
|---|---|---|---|---|
| | Mean | Variance | Mean | Variance |
| one parent/child | 4.086 | 1.1195 | 4.9048 | 1.3348 |
| one fullsib | 3.4193 | 3.6201 | 4.0845 | 4.3641 |
| one halfsib | 0.9138 | 0.8929 | 1.1072 | 1.0835 |

## 5.3. Discussion

Choosing the most informative relatives can impact positively identification and can reduce the cost by minimizing superfluous testing. This study initially confirmed by simulation that when a single family reference samples is all that is available generally genetically closer relatives will yield higher LRs, in the order of parents > children > fullsibs > halfsibs = uncles/nephews = grandparents/grandchildren > cousins. These relationships are well-known in kinship analyses [31, 32]. However, an identification based solely using a single reference relative often may be inadequate since large proportions of LRs are small (i.e., <1,000). For instance, with a single parent, about 14.5% of LRs are less than 1,000. According to [33, 34], a minimum of 99.9% is suggested as the posterior probability (i.e., 1,000 is the minimum posterior odds threshold) for rendering an identification. In cases where there are multiple unknown persons to identify the

Posterior odds = (likelihood ratio) (prior odds)

a LR of $10^6$ is required for a one thousand missing person pool (the prior probability would be 1/1000); the prior odds will be differ depending on the number of missing persons in a particular case) [35, 36].

Table 2 shows that only both parents and 3 children + spouse have more than 99.9% of LRs greater than $10^6$. 4 children, 2 spouses + 2 children (1 each), and 2 children + spouse can yield LRs greater than $10^6$ with 99% confidence. Several more scenarios (bolded in 5th percentile column) may also be informative if the confidence level is lowered to 95% (however, false positives will increase). With both mean and variance considered, these scenarios are the most reliable for identification. Typing more markers can allow more scenarios to obtain 99% or even 99.9% of LRs greater than $10^6$. If more typing can be done, we recommend analyzing more genetic markers in concert with selecting the most informative members of a pedigree to manage the costs.

Based on the simulation results, the following guidelines are recommended in choosing relatives for missing person identification.

10. Parents are the preferred relatives and both parents of the missing person should be typed when possible. If both parents are typed, all other relatives, including fullsibs, may not be necessary.
11. Children are the second preferred relatives. Type as many children as possible or until the unknown genotype of the missing person can be reconstructed. In absence of parents, if the missing person is male, sons are preferred because of the same Y chromosome shared between father and sons; otherwise, sons and daughters are equivalent.
12. Even if a child is available, the spouse of the missing person (i.e., the father/mother of the child) should be considered for typing, if he/she is available.
13. Fullsibs are the third preferred relatives. If the missing person is male, brothers are preferred compared to sisters, because missing person and brothers share both Y chromosome and mtDNA, and it is reasonable to type less relatives with the same discrimination power due to economical reasons in some conditions; otherwise, brothers and sisters are equivalent.
14. All other distant relatives, such as grandparents/grandchildren, halfsibs, uncles/aunts and cousins, only provide limited identification capabilities based on autosomal markers, but their Y chromosomes and mtDNA can be used to increase LR or filter out false relationships.
15. Less genetic dependence between reference relatives provides a higher LR on average. This is practiced routinely for standard paternity cases where two unrelated parents are sought. But the concept can be applied to extended pedigrees as well. For example, two biologically unrelated uncles can be more informative than two related uncles.
16. With limited number of relatives, type as many as markers as possible.

## CONCLUSION

In summary, this chapter provides a descriptive approach to assist the forensic DNA community in person identification for complex forensic identity and paternity testing cases. This process evaluates the putative biological relationships of individuals by calculating and ranking pedigree LRs for multiple putative pedigrees. Adjustments for population substructure and mutation are incorporated, and LR values can be provided for any pedigree even with multiple large-step mutations.

This chapter also provides methods for calculating the pedigree likelihood based on lineage markers, in which the hypothesis of kinship is defined by a fixed relationship with the reference family. The traditional direct comparison between the haplotypes has been the hypothesis that the reference(s) and the questioned person are in the same lineage. These two hypotheses are conceptually distinguishable, although the likelihoods given them may not be significantly far apart. The pedigree likelihood usually gives more conservative results compared with the direct comparison method.

Lastly, the information content of 37 common reference pedigree scenarios were evaluated based on 13 CODIS loci to provide guidelines of choosing the appropriate relatives for reliable missing person identifications. The results confirm that first order relatives (parents and fullsibs) are the most preferred relatives to identify missing persons; fullsibs are also informative. Less genetic dependence between references provides a higher on average likelihood ratio. Distant relatives may not be helpful solely by autosomal markers. But lineage-based Y chromosome and mitochondrial DNA markers can increase the likelihood ratio or serve as filters to exclude putative relationships.

## REFERENCES

[354] Ge J, Wang T, Birdwell J D, Chakraborty R: Further remarks on: 'Paternity analysis in special fatherless cases without direct testing of alleged father' [FSI 146S (2004) S159–S161] and remarks on it [FSI 163 (2006) 158–160]. *Forensic Sci Int* 2007, 172:e6–8.

[355] Ge J, Budowle B and Chakraborty R, DNA identification by pedigree likelihood ratio accommodating population substructure and mutations, Investigative Genetics, 2010, 1:8.

[356] Ge J, Budowle B, Eisenberg A, and Chakraborty R, Pedigree likelihood ratio for lineage markers, *International Journal of Legal Medicine,* 10.1007/s00414-010-0514-9.

[357] Ge J, Budowle B, Chakraborty R. Choosing Relatives for DNA Identification of Missing Person Identification, *J Forensic Sci.* 2011 Jan;56 Suppl 1:S23-8.

[358] Elston RC, Stewart J: A general model for the genetic analysis of pedigree data. *Hum Hered* 1971, 21:523–542.

[359] National Research Council Committee on DNA Forensic Science. *An Update: the Evaluation of Forensic DNA Evidence.* Washington (DC): National Academy Press; 1996.

[360] Balding DJ, Nichols RA: DNA profile match probability calculation - How to allow for population stratification, relatedness, database selection and single bands. *Forensic Sci Int* 1994, 64:125–140.

[361] Balding DJ and Nichols RA, DNA profile match probability calculation: how to allow for population stratification, relatedness, database selection and single bands, *Forensic Science International,* 64:2-3, 1994, pp125-140.

[362] Crow JF, Kimura M: *An Introduction to Population Genetics Theory.* New York: Harper, Row, 1970: 591.

[363] AABB. Annual report summary for testing in 2006 [http://www.aabb.org/Documents/Accreditation/Parentage_Testing_Accreditation_Program/rtannrpt06.pdf]

[364] Brinkmann B, Klintschar M, Neuhuber F, Hühne J, Rolf B: Mutation rate in human microsatellites: influence of the structure and length of the tandem repeat. *Am J Hum Genet* 1998, 62:1408–1415.

[365] Budowle B, DiZinno J, Wilson M, Interpretation guidelines for mitochondrial DNA sequencing, *10<sup>th</sup> International Symposium of Human Identification,* 1999.
[366] Rolf, B., Keil, W., Brinkmann, B., Roewer, L. and Fimmers, R. (2001) Paternity testing using Y-STR haplotypes: assigning a probability for paternity in cases of mutations. *Int. J. Legal Med.* 115: 12–15.
[367] Christofides, Nicos (1975), *Graph theory: an algorithmic approach,* Academic Press, pp. 170–174.
[368] Budowle, B., Allard, M.W., Wilson, M.R. and Chakraborty, R. (2003) Forensic and mitochondrial DNA: application, debates, and foundations. *Annu. Rev. Genom. Hum. Genet.* 4: 119–141.
[369] Sigurðardóttir S, Helgason A, Gulcher JR, Stefansson K and Donnelly P, The Mutation Rate in the Human mtDNA Control Region, *American Journal of Human Genetics,* 2000, 66(5):1599-609.
[370] Nei M and Kumar S, *Molecular Evolution and Phylogenetics,* Oxford University Press, 2000, Page 35.
[371] Kimura K, A simple method for estimating evolutionary rates of base substitutions through comparative studies of nucleotide sequences, *Journal of Molecular Evolution,* Vol 16, No.2, 1980
[372] Nicolas Galtier, David Enard, Yoan Radondy, Eric Bazin, and Khalid Belkhir, Mutation hot spots in mammalian mitochondrial DNA, *Genome Res.* 2006 16: 215-222.
[373] M Stoneking, Hypervariable sites in the mtDNA control region are mutational hotspots, *Am J Hum Genet* (2000) 67: 1029-32.
[374] Neil Howell, Christy Bogolin Smejkal, D.A. Mackey, P.F. Chinnery, D.M. Turnbull and Corinna Herrnstadt, The Pedigree Rate of Sequence Divergence in the Human Mitochondrial Genome: There Is a Difference Between Phylogenetic and Pedigree Rates, *Am J Hum Genet* (2003) 72: 659-670.
[375] Sonja Meyer, Gunter Weiss, and Arndt von Haeseler, Pattern of Nucleotide Substitution and Rate Heterogeneity in the Hypervariable Regions I and II of Human mtDNA, *Genetics,* 1999, Vol. 152, 1103-1110.
[376] Budowle B, Wilson MR, DiZinno JA, Stauffer C, Fasano MA, Holland MM, Monson KL, Mitochondrial DNA regions HVI and HVII population data, *Forensic Sci Int.* 1999 Jul 12;103(1):23-35.
[377] Tully G, Bär W, Brinkmann B, Carracedo A, Gill P, Morling N, Parson W and Schneider P, Considerations by the European DNA profiling (EDNAP) group on the working practices, nomenclature and interpretation of mitochondrial DNA profiles, *Forensic Science International,* 124:1, 2001, pp83-91.
[378] Holland MM and Parsons TJ, Mitochondrial DNA sequence analysis — validation and use for forensic casework. *Forensic Sci. Rev.* 11 (1999), pp. 21–50.
[379] Roewer L, Kayser M, et al., A new method for the evaluation of matches in non-recombining genomes: application to Y-chromosomal short tandem repeat (STR) haplotypes in European males, *Forensic Sci. Int.* 114 (2000), pp. 31–43.
[380] Krawczak, M. Forensic evaluation of Y-STR haplotype matches: a comment. *Forensic Sci. Int.* 118, 114–115 (2001).
[381] Budowle B, Ge J, Aranda X, Planz J, Eisenberg A, Chakraborty R. Texas Population Substructure and Its Impact on Estimating the Rarity of Y STR Haplotypes from DNA

Evidence, Journal of Forensic Science. *Journal of forensic Science* 2009;54(5), page 1016-1021.

[382] Ge J, Budowle B, Planz JV, Eisenberg AJ, Ballantyne J, Chakraborty R. US Forensic Y Chromosome Short Tandem Repeats Database, *Leg Med,* 2010, 12(6): 289-295.

[383] Butler JM, Schoske R, Vallone PM, Redman JW, Kline MC. Allele frequencies for 15 autosomal STR loci on U.S. Caucasian, African American, and Hispanic populations. *J Forensic Sci* 2003;48(4): 908–911.

[384] Li CC, Sacks L: The derivation of joint distribution and correlation between relatives by the use of stochastic matrices. *Biometrics* 1954, 10:347–360.

[385] Thompson EA: The estimation of pairwise relationships. *Ann Hum Genet* 1975, 39:173–188.

[386] Budowle B, Bieber FR, Eisenberg AJ. Forensic aspects of mass disasters: strategic considerations for DNA based human identification. *Legal Med* 2005;7(4):230–243.

[387] Prinz M, Carracedo A, et al. DNA Commission of the International Society for Forensic Genetics (ISFG): recommendations regarding the role of forensic genetics for disaster victim identification (DVI). *Forensic Sci Int Genet* 2007;1(1): 3–12.

[388] Brenner CH. *Reuniting El Salvador families.* http://dna-view.com/ProBusqueda.htm (accessed March 16, 2009).

[389] Brenner CH, Weir BS. Issues and strategies in the identification of World Trade Center victims. *Theor Popul Biol* 2003;63(3):173–178.

In: Forensic Science
Editors: N. Yacine and R. Fellag

ISBN 978-1-61324-999-4
© 2012 Nova Science Publishers, Inc.

*Chapter 6*

# COMMINGLED ASSEMBLAGE FROM EARTHQUAKE 1755 OF LISBON: FORENSIC ANTHROPOLOGY STUDY

## *Cristiana Pereira*[1]

Professor from University of Lisbon, School of Dentistry.
Forensic Odontologist from Portuguese National Institute of Legal Medicine,
Investigator from CEAUL[a], Center of Statistic and Applications.
Investigator from CENCIFOR[b], Center of Forensic Studies.
South Branch, Lisbon, Portugal.

## ABSTRACT

In this study were analysed 1210 disarticulated teeth, 179 jaws and 65 skulls from a skeletal assemblage of commingled remains belonging to the 1755 Lisbon earthquake victims, excavated in 2004 at the Lisbon Academy of Sciences.

The main objective of this study was to contribute to the paleodemographic and paleopathological characterization of one of the world's biggest catastrophic population by forensic dental and osteological, qualitative and quantitative, methods. Morphological and anthropometric parameters from teeth and cranial bones have been considered.

To attain our purpose, we identified the teeth and jaws. The following main variables have been dealt with: paleodemography, paleopathology, age determination, minimum number of individuals, sex determination, population affinity, trauma, fire and taphonomy.

Sexing was only done on specimens identified as adults except for unidentified cranias and mandibles. There are 39 female and 49 male individuals. It suggests this population is a random sample of the living population present at the time as it is expected that the sex ration of a living population is maintained in a natural disaster context, as death rate is not biased as it is in other contexts such as war and conflict situations.

The age determination, a detailed account of the age of each individual was not possible. Instead, categorical age group were devised and quantified. The majority of individuals were adults from 35 to 50 years old. The second group was sub adults, from 7 moths *in utero* to 6 years old.

The determination of a minimum number of individuals was attempted by counting the most recurrent specimens for each population sample – teeth, jaw and crania: it is n=179.

---

[1] Corresponding author. Professora Doutora Cristiana Pereira. Tel: (+351)-218811850; Fax: (+351)-218864493; E-mail: cristiana.pereira@fmd.ul.pt. [a] http://www.ceaul.fc.ul.pt; [b] http://cencifor.org/.

By investigating the demographic profile of the sample, aspects of the structure and origin of the skeletal series are revealed. Furthermore, the next chapters will deal with pathological, traumatic and taphonomic occurrences in the skeletal sample.

The paleopathological analysis demonstrates that the overall health of the Academy skeletal sample was average for a sample of this time and place.

The presence of abnormally high frequencies of trauma in the Academy skeletal sample further strengthens the argument for the mass disaster hypothesis. Impact fractures best described as blunt force trauma on the skulls were identified in several specimens.

The taphonomic analysis provided further evidence of the main hypothesis. Burnt skulls and teeth affected by low medium and high temperatures constituted the majority of the sample, meaning these people were no doubt trapped when a fire occurred, dying from the direct cause of the fire or were already dead when flames consumed what was left of their homes, churches and palaces. Dog and rodent gnaw marks were also identified. A scenario of bodies scattered around the city for several days, with dogs scavenging whatever they can to survive may not have been far from the truth related. Staining of bones indicates bursting of blood vessels and staining by a iron-containing matter, most likely blood, as a reaction to the exposure to very high temperatures. Further staining resulted from exogenous material and soil.

With this study of the Academy skeletal sample, a contribution was made to increase the knowledge on this 1755 population. It was hypothesised that this collection was part of the victim count of the 1755 earthquake and it is suggested here that this is likely if not indeed certain. Many of pathological and taphonomical indicators suggestive of mass disaster are present in this skeletal series including random sampling, high trauma, burn marks and bite marks, high fragmentation and non-significant differences between the sexes.

However further research on the rest of the skeletal assemblage collection, post cranial sample, is necessary in order to understand the sample further.

## INTRODUCTION

This chapter is a discussion of the numerous factors that affected the composition and condition of human bone assemblages recovered from archaeological context from 1755 Earthquake of Lisbon. Circumstances of death have an impact on the human remains that we have studied. This assemblage of bone reveals the biological life history of the individuals represented from XVIII century and embodies the history of the assemblage as a culturally created entity.

The XVIII century is certainly a very history rich epoch to be studied. Earthquakes were periodical events Lisbon faced, some of which had been quite serious in view of the deaths and damage they are reported to have caused. But the destroyed area and the number of deaths in 1755 was unequally.

In the morning of all saints day, the 1$^{st}$ of November 1755, the earth shook, and the world would never be the same. One of the most terrible earthquake/tsunamis in the history of Europe struck the city of Lisbon while the people were in prayer, destroying most of the palaces and churches of the *Terreiro do Paço*, the main plaza that constituted the ruling point of Portugal's monarchy. When the aftershock's ceased and the damages counted for, the newly instituted minister of Reconstruction and Law enforcement, *Sebastião de Carvalho e Melo*, better known as the *Marquês de Pombal*, had the job of cleaning up and reconstructing the city of Lisbon in light of the other grand cities of Europe. His most famous word was delivered after being asked what to do about the disaster. He answered that "*the living must be taken care of, the dead buried and the ports closed*". With this, a great amount of victims were sunk into the river Tagus tied to destroyed ships. Several although, were left under debris and were later buried in several mass graves dug around the city in locations of previous graves to prevent the spread of diseases.

In the summer of 2004 with the renovation of the cloisters of the *Academia de Ciências de Lisboa*, the old *Convento de Jesus*, a team of archaeologists excavated and discovered hundreds of human skeletal remains on top of the old friars graves (Pereira and Antunes, 2011). The latter presented complete skeletons while the former were reduced to several layers of commingled remains (Figure 1).

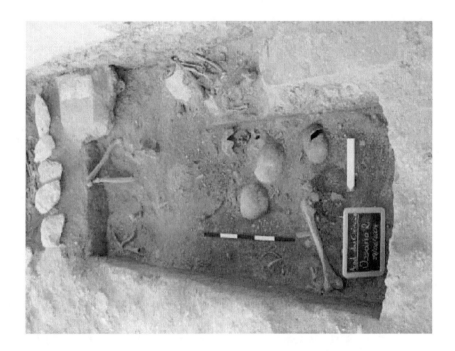

Figure 1. The top of the excavation of commingled human remains from the natural mass disaster, earthquake 1755 of Lisbon.

The sample used in this study comes from this excavations, that were carried out after suspicion arose from archaeologists that the burial site of the priests and friars from the old Convent hid a mass grave, one of the many dug up several days after the earthquake of 1755 to bury victims in order to prevent the spread of diseases, mostly plague and tuberculosis (Pereira and Antunes, 2011). The suspicions proved correct after the uncovering of thousands of commingled remains, including mixed animal and human bones, along with several archaeological artefacts that put these remains in the earthquake context. The first project consisted of a series of variables that were analysed only on the teeth isolated at the excavations. The next project was a further contribution to the study of this population and concentrates on the teeth on maxillas and mandibles, and skulls. The study consisted of a series of variables that were analysed with the goal of verifying the origin of the material relative to the 1755 earthquake. Mass disaster skeletal assemblages present a specific demographic pattern, and generally represent a random sample of the living population as time and cause is very similar among a large number of individuals. The palaeopathology of this population can indicate which conditions were present and who was affected by them. This will provide the information for comparison with typical 18$^{th}$ Century diseases. Trauma is another good indicator of mass disaster situation, the higher trauma and the more evenly distributed among sexes, the most likely the sample originated from a mass disaster. Finally, taphonomy can help to infer some of the events that resulted in the individual dying. A high presence of burn marks from heavy fires and scavenging from wild dogs and rats are also good indicators of an earthquake event, as usually fires break out and bodies left on the street are consumed by famished dogs and rats. Through these four indicators, an account of the Academia das Ciências skeletal assemblage was study (Pereira, 2010).

## ANALYSIS AND INTERPRETATION OF SKELETAL HUMAN FINDINGS

Academic defined as, "*the study of the transition of organics from biosphere into the lithosphere or geological record*" (Lyman, 1994), taphonomy originated as a subfield of paleontology (Efremov, 1940). In common sense, taphonomy is the study of "*the physical and chemical processes (induced by human, animal, or natural agents) that modify an organism after its death and through which it is incorporated into geological deposits*" (LaMotta and Schiffer, 2005).

When we study archaeological assemblages like this one, from the earthquake 1755 of Lisbon, we know they are never perfectly preserved or complete. Taphonomy provides the background by which we can investigate the multiple processes and events that cumulatively determine the content and condition of skeletal assemblages from archaeological places.

Forensic taphonomy enclose archaeological and zooarchaeological methods is an integral field of the medico-legal investigation of human remains, where the differentiation diagnosis between *ante mortem*, *peri mortem* and *post mortem* modification of human remains is scientific important (Dupras et al., 2006). Human osteology forensic books include chapters of *post mortem* modification by natural and human factors (White and Folkens, 2005), and taphonomic variables are included in laboratory manuals used for Forensic Anthropology such as *Standards for Data Collection from Human Skeletal Remains (Buikstra and Ubelaker, 1994)* and the *Guidelines to the Standards for Recovering Human Remains (Brickley and McKinley, 2004). Both used in these archaeological assemblage (mass graves) because of the importance of taphonomic investigation in the study of fragmentary and commingled skeletal assemblages where we need to distinguish between human and nonhuman factors of modification.* In practice, the study of bone modification in human skeletal assemblages is based on: recording weathering and fragmentation patterns, evidence of animal scavenging, thermal alteration, and the location and orientation of tool marks on skeletal bones.

In the analysis of human remains at the laboratory far away from field recovery, is important to remember that the alteration of bone takes place at all stages of taphonomic period of time: *ante mortem* (pre depositional stage), *peri mortem* (depositional stage), *post mortem* (post depositional and post recovery stages) (Sorg and Haglund, 2002).

The preservation of the skeleton is influenced by intrinsic factors from the bones, such as bone density, size, and shape, and by extrinsic factors, such as composition of the soil and water in the burial environment. There are two different types of measurements of preservation: completeness (the degree of fragmentation of bone) and condition (the degree of destruction of bone) (Marean, 1991).

The human taphonomy protocol from the Forms of the Museum of the Sciences Academy of Lisbon (Pereira, 2010) were designed according the Standards for Data Collection (Buikstra and Ubelaker, 1994) and Standards for Recording Human Remains (Brickley and McKinley, 2004), included those two measurements of preservation in two different forms: form 1 (completeness) and form 12 (condition). These Standards of human skeletal remains were designed for adult and immature population (skulls and lower jaws including teeth): from form 2 until 11 for adult population and from 13 until 17 for immature population, form 1 and 12 are common to the two subpopulation from these archaeological mass disaster collection from XVIII century. The completeness was recorded according to the percentage of element present and the degree of fragmentation for each adult and immature skulls and lower jaws (Pereira, 2010). From the 159 mandible adults' fragments there were 137 lower jaws: 116 with 1 fragment for lower jaw (Figure 2), 20 with 2 fragments for mandible (Figure 3) and 1 mandible with 3 fragments (Figure 4). When we registered the percentage of element present of each adult mandible: from 137 mandibles there was 70 (51, 1%) score 1 if more than 75% is present of the bone, 26 (40, 9%) score 2 when 25% to 75% is present and 11 (8%) score 3 less than 25% of the mandible jaw is present (Pereira, 2010).

Fragmentation affects the number of identifiable specimens in an assemblage, the count of elements represented and the number of individuals represented (minimum number of individuals or MNI) (Ubelaker, 2002). Several different methods are used to estimate MNI in fragmentary and comingled assemblages (Adams and Konigsberg, 2004). The MNI represented by the adult lower jaws from this collection were 137 in the 159 lower jaws fragments.

Degradation of the organic and mineral components of bone is the result of contact with microbial and chemical agents in the depositional environment – diagenesis phenomenon (Jans, 2004 and 2008). Events prior to burial will affect preservation, as an exposed body may be subject to wetting and drying, animal trampling and chewing and other events. Bone degradation takes place by two events: destruction of the collagen component by bacterial collagenase and the chemical demineralization of bone apatite (Nielsen-Marsh et al., 2000). The chemistry of ground water relative to bone and the degree of fluctuation in ground water contact with bone determine the rate of dissolution of the bone mineral. As more and more bone mineral is dissolved, pore size increases, and the bone collagen is increasingly available to microbial action. This affects the macroscopic condition of bone. Weathering, the degree of physical destruction visible on the bone, is most often recorded on a six-point scale developed by Behrensmeyer (1978) and used in Standards for Data Collection (Buikstra and Ubelaker, 1994) and adapted in our forms (Pereira, 2010). The scale starts at zero (no evidence of weathering). From stage 1 to 5, the progression of deterioration is beginning with simple longitudinal cracks until splitting of the anatomical element. It happens with the same collection from the same depositional environment from the same period of time, such this collection from 1755 earthquake of Lisbon, each bone can exhibit markedly different stages of preservation, including the weathering.

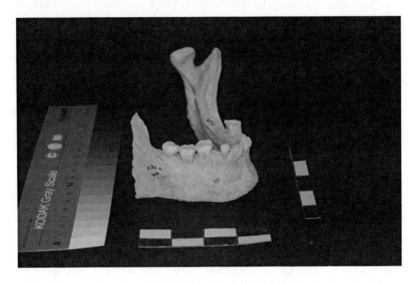

Figure 2. Lower jaw from adult male (ACL Jaw 50, ossuary 22, 45 cm to top), with 1 fragment and more than 75% present (score 1).

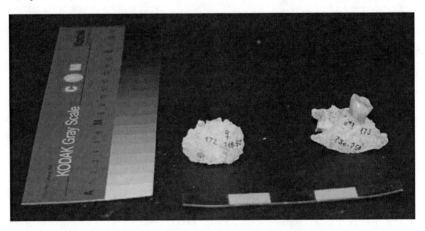

Figure 3. Lower jaw from adult (ACL Jaw fragments 172 and 173 from the same jaw, ossuary 1, 30 cm to 45 cm), with 2 fragment and less than 25% present (score 3).

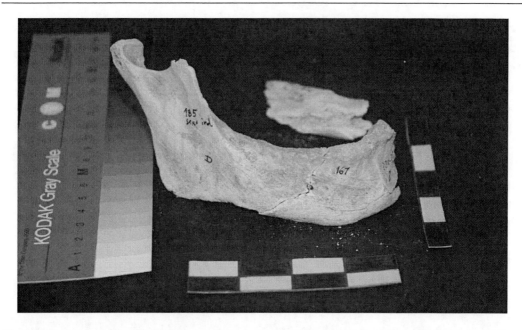

Figure 4. Lower jaw from adult (ACL Jaw fragments 167, 185 and 215 from the same jaw, ossuary 2, 30 cm to 45 cm), with 3 fragment and more than 25% and less than 75% present (score 2).

Pereira's study of earthquake 1755 of Lisbon population showed from 137 adults lower jaws, only 57 (41, 61%) had weathering (Pereira, 2010). The stages range from 1 (21, 21%) until 5 (6, 06%), (Figure 5).

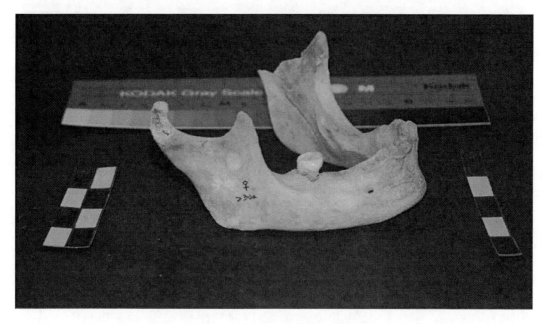

Figure 5. Lower jaw from adult (ACL Jaw 79, ossuary 22a, 15 cm to 45 cm), with weathering score 5 at external superficie of the right condyle from temporomandibular joint.

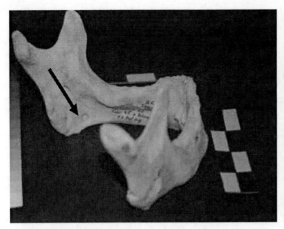 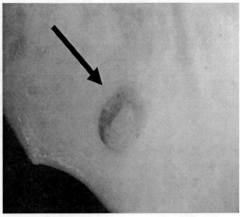

Figure 6. Lower jaw from adult (ACL Jaw 108, ossuary 22, 15 cm to 45 cm), Stafne's defect.

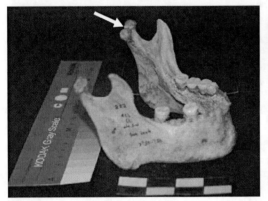 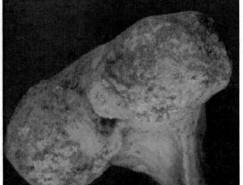

Figure 7. Lower jaw from adult (ACL Jaw 252) with congenital alteration from articular superficies temporomandibular left joint.

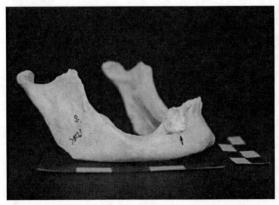 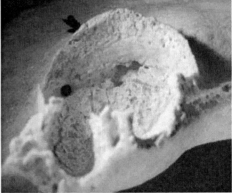

Figure 8. Lower jaw from adult (ACL 103, ossuary 33a) with a loci from inflammatory quist.

There are others factors, intrinsic factors, responsible for bone preservation such as the size, shape and density of the bone. Bone mineral is low in infants and in the elderly, the two age classes typically under-represented in skeletal assemblages. But bone density varies through life and is vulnerable to reduction during normal growth, pregnancy, illness and periods of mal nutrition. Many factors influence bone density at all stages of life, and these may influence the probability of an element's and an individual's representation in an archaeological assemblage. There are reports focuses most infants and children disappear from archaeological assemblages; however there are other reports with substantial numbers of infants and children. In the skeletal assemblage from 1755 earthquake of Lisbon (N=179), 42 (24%) lower jaws are under age 15.

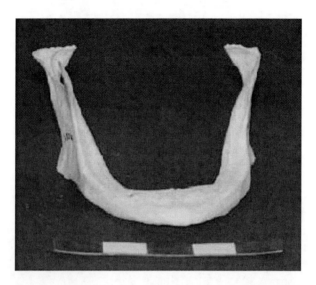

Figure 9. Lower jaw from adult (ACL 132, ossuary 33) with complete destruction of articular superficies temporomandibular joint – temporomandibular ankylosis.

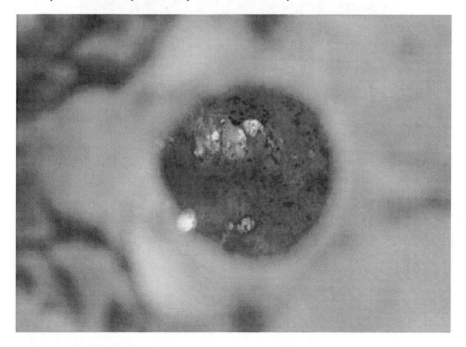

Figure 10. Adult skull (TAS 3) with lesions in inner diploe compatible with osteomyelitis (picture from inside of the skull by the occipital foramen).

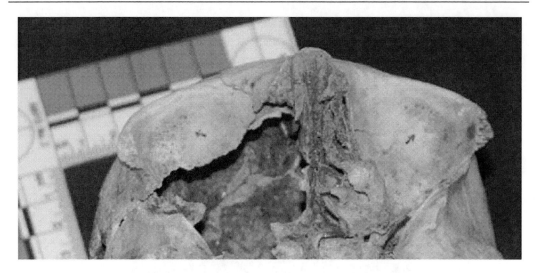

Figure 11. Adult skull (TAS 25) with lesions compatible with hyperostosis porotica/ *Cribra Orbitalia*. Porotic type of lesions was found localized mainly in the anterior parts of the orbital roof.

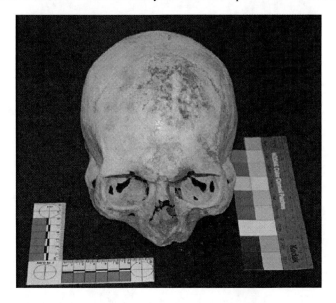

Figure 12. Adult skull (TAS 18) with lesions compatible with periostic infection by syphilis at frontal and glabella areas.

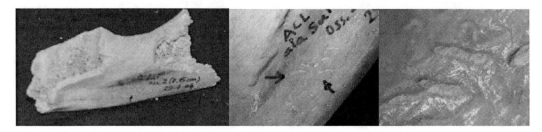

Figure 13. Fragment of mandible ACL 179, ossuary 2 with evidence of bite-marks of rodent, appearing as rows.

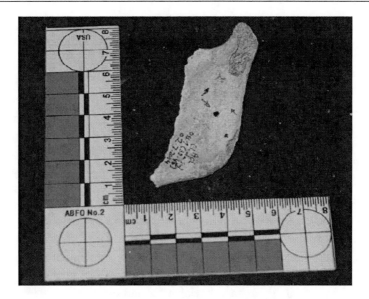

Figure 14. Fragment of mandible ACL 08 with evidence of canine puncture of a dog.

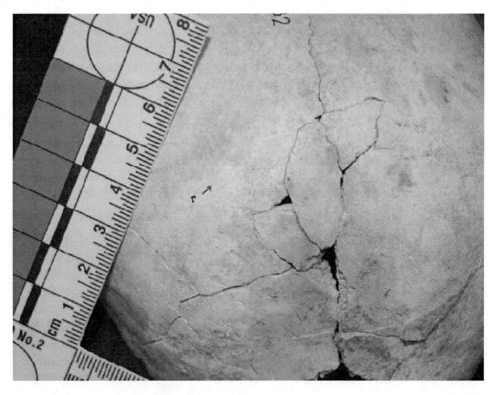

Figure 15. Adult skull (TAS 32) with evidence of linear cut mark in parietals bones, from the left to right side, it's compatible with the period of *peri mortem*, before the fire after the tsunami.

Poor preservation of skeletal assemblages difficult the ability to observe pathological conditions (Waldron, 1994) and obliterates evidence of pathological lesions even when the bone is present. There are several *post mortem* factors responsible for damage cumulatively by handling by researchers. These alterations may also include changes to the shape or surface of the bone that mimic pathology. Taphonomic changes in the skeleton can also mimic traumatic injury: *post mortem* warping, separation of sutures, and other damage to cranial bones may be interpreted as evidence of *ante mortem* or *peri mortem* cranial trauma (Crist et al., 1997). Preserved cranial features can be used for nonmetric trait analyses (Merbs, 1967). There are some pathological features well documented in this population (Figures from 6 to 12, ACL collection).

Animals are a significant source of modification to human remains before and after burial. Rodent gnaw marks are perhaps the most commonly observed animal-modification on human bones (White and Folkens, 2005). These marks are generally distinctive, appearing as rows of fine scratches or parallel sets of scratches (Figure 13). Also punctures in bone made by canines are also distinctive (Binford, 1981). In the earthquake 1755 of Lisbon skeletal assemblage, we observed two types of bite marks, one from rodent and the other one from carnivore like a dog (Figure 14).

In human skeletal assemblages, taphonomy studies try to distinguish among three broad categories of activities: violence resulting in traumatic injury and death; *peri mortem* or *post mortem* body processing for secondary burial or a particular stage of extended mortuary ritual; and body processing for consumption (cannibalism).

The first group of modification of human remains is the categories of toolmarks include cutmarks in the bone surface made by a sharp tool held perpendicularly to the bone surface; scrape marks, sets of several shallow, narrow, closely spaced marks across a bone surface; chop marks, shorter and broader than cuts; and percussion marks from hammerstones or other heavy tools or weapons used to fracture a bone (White and Folkens, 2005). The number, size, and anatomical location (and for cut and scrape marks, the orientation) of tool marks are all important, as in the exploration of what kind of tool was used: a knife, a scraper, a hammerstone, a sharp pointed weapon, or a blunt object.

The skulls and lower jaws from this skeletal assemblage present different toolmarks suggesting violence including traumatic injury or violent death, related to the following days after the earthquake and tsunami (Figures 15, 16, 17 and 18). From the 53 skulls there are 20 (38%) with patterns from toolmarks including cutmarks, hammerstones and blunt objects, which 7 (35%) skulls with evidence of fire after the violence with toolmarks.

Fractures types are important in differentiation between ancient and modern fractures. Bone in vital stage or "green" with high moisture content and intact collagen tends to fracture in a helical or curvilinear manner, whereas "dry" bone with degraded collagen or complete destruction of the organic component has more angular fracture patterns (Lovell, 1997). In the skull, depressed fractures, and radiating fracture lines occur in vital bone. The presence of healing, some degree of callus formation, new woven bone at the injury impact, is the only reliable indication of an *ante mortem* fracture. The time to initial healing, at least 3 weeks for initial callus formation (Lovell, 1997), depends on the type of fracture, location, and age of the injured person. However, stepped, longitudinal, and perpendicular fractures with acute angles and squared fracture edges indicate *post mortem* breaks in nonvital bone (Lovell, 1997).

Fractures types and the timing of traumatic injury are essential aspects of the reconstruction of bone modification in an archaeological assemblage, but more importantly, they constitute physical evidence of the existence and nature of conflict in a manner distinct from the history from the books (Walker, 2001).

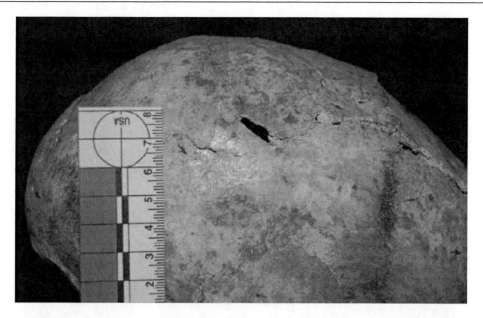

Figure 16. Adult women skull (TAS 11) with traumatic lesion by blunt instrument of parietal right bone with a fracture with internal bevel from the blunt impact and depression area with radial fractures, compatible with the period of time *peri mortem*.

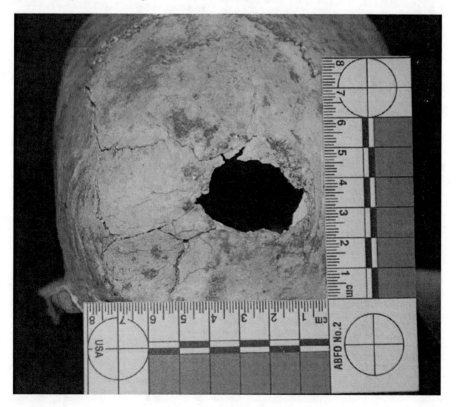

Figure 17. Adult women skull (TAS 11) with evidence of traumatic lesion by instrument compatible with a bullet in frontal area. Presence of radial fractures on the right side compatible with entrance wound with delamination, projection of the bullet from the left side tangential to the frontal bone.

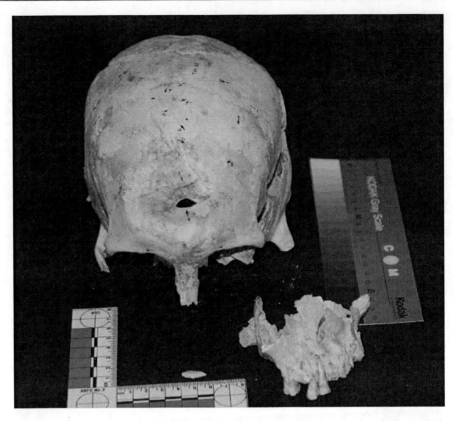

Figure 18. Adult skull (TAS 26) with multiple tool marks suggesting the violence of the circumstances of death of these population, compatible with ambient of earthquake.

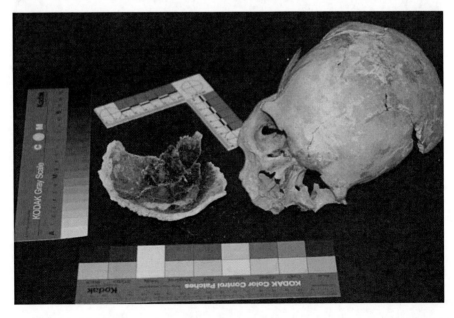

Figure 19. Adult skull (TAS 27) with evidence of fire action. In inner diploe dark color with presence of a cut mark near the occipital bone with 25,26 cm of length compatible with *peri mortem* lesion before the fire. This is the reason why the fire is in inner diploe.

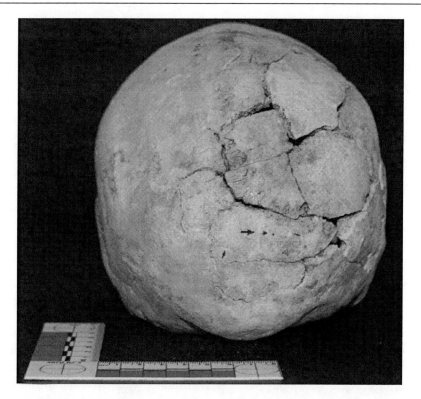

Figure 20. Adult skull (TAS 4) with evidence of fire near the death with alterations of occipital and right parietal bones with heat fractures with bone deformation during organic venting occurs.

*Peri mortem* injuries in skeletal assemblage from earthquake 1755 of Lisbon tell the story of the violent deaths with traumatic injury: 33% of the skulls had evidence of impact sites by blunt force, depressed cranial fractures, inward crushing and margins from edged weapons. All these features survive high temperatures of the fire after the earthquake. The *post mortem* evidence of fractures was present in all skulls (100%), because of the other factor (thermal alteration of human bone), with loss of organic components leaving the bones fragile and susceptible to additional erosion or fracturing from heat, any impact occurring as part of the fire scene, or the influence of extinguishment and recovery methods. In many instances these *post mortem* artefacts are recognizable, but the danger lies with their ability to either mimic or obscure antecedent traumatic features.

Heat changes the structure of bone mineral crystals (Lyman, 1994) and analysis of heat-related skeletal trauma must begin by understanding the anatomy of the outside protective layers of the cranial bones, skin, muscle and fat. Especially the differential thicknesses and anatomical distributions of soft tissue structures determine how, where, and at what point bone becomes exposed. Beginning with superficial burns to skin, thermal destruction systematically reduces soft tissue layers and bone by pyrolyzing all organic materials. Once the soft tissue undergo dehydration, contraction, and charring with loss of tissue mass, the bone is exposed and initiates a sequence of color alterations that signifies stages of organic pyrolysis rather than an indicator of temperature. Thermal alteration is recorded as change in color and texture of bone (Figure 19). Color ranges from ivory or yellow to brown, reddish brown, black, gray-blue, and white (calcined) (Lyman, 1994). The color of thermally altered bone generally corresponds to the temperature of the heat source (Shipman et al., 1985), but color change is also dependent on the state of the bone when burned (Lyman, 1994). Textural changes range from exfoliation and longitudinal cracking that mimics weathering to warping and cracking in a checkerboard pattern (checking). Studies of the differential response of bone to thermal alteration when fleshed, defleshed but still vital, and nonvital (dry), seem to result in inconsistent findings (Correia, 1997). However, some studies suggest that bone burned when dry is not subject to the same kind of warping and longitudinal splitting characteristic of vital bone (Buikstra and Swegle, 1989). Color difference between the external surface and broken edges can reveal whether the bone was whole or already broken when burned.

Delamination is the most common heat-related fracture type observed in the skull. This presents in the external table as small tensile surface cracks and areas where the outer table shrinks, separates, and exposes the underlying diploe. In several cases, delamination produced externally bevelled features mimicking ballistic or blunt trauma complete with full thickness linear fractures and associated fragmentation. Delamination can occur during the fire with gradual fragmentation from thermal destruction, while cooling after the fire, or may be induced by any external force or *post mortem* handling of fragile calcined remains during extinguishment, recovery, transport and analysis.

Advanced calcinated and impacts from the surrounding dynamic fire environment may also produce full thickness fractures involving the inner table. Best observed in calcined bone, any complete defect during the early stages of burning often has margins outlined in deep black from the pressurized venting of organic materials within the vault. The presence of typified curved tissue-regression fractures in cranial bones are a signature of burning direction along the bone, where retractions of bulky tissue and periosteum permanently watermark bone with a series of semicircular arcs as exposed bone reacts to heat (Figures 20 to 22).

Another feature observed in cranium by the heath is the "exploded skull" (Figure 23). This appearance is due to external events and the brittle mechanical properties of the thermally altered bone create that appearance. Heat affects the inorganic mineral component through deformation, shrinkage, fracturing, and fragmentation. The most common example of this is seen in delamination, where the outer table separates from the inner table and diploe, leaving fragments to fall and litter below the skull. While fragile enough to fracture from their own weight, destruction of calcined bone increases when external forces are applied. The collapse of building materials onto the body can cause further mechanical fractures, evidence appeared in some skulls from the skeletal assemblage of earthquake 1755 of Lisbon (Pereira, 2010).

The common features of traumatic injuries are easily evaluated during most stages of burning. Any compromise in skin integrity prematurely exposes bone to thermal destruction, not normally observed. The sites of penetration, cut marks, or lacerations open early and focus damage much like the effects of advanced decomposition around a *peri mortem* injury. This was observed in this skeletal assemblage with effects of heat on the blunt, sharp, and ballistic trauma in cranial bone. Common to both ballistic and blunt force injuries, skin lacerations prematurely and focally opened from rapid shrinkage of elastic skin over cranial bone. Accelerated exposure of traumatized areas of entrance, exit, or impact sites prematurely initiates the process of organic degradation to bone seen in stages of color changes earlier than in exposure of non-traumatizes areas.

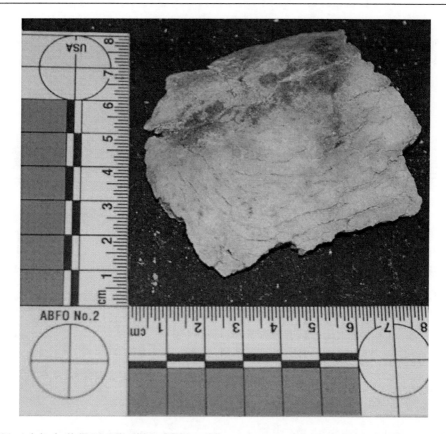

Figure 21. Adult skull (TAS 29) with evidence of fire action: curved tissue regression fractures (pulls away from fire), the importance of diagnosis of the presence of soft tissues. Superficies of protection, showing the soft tissue pulls away from the fire showing the direction of the fire.

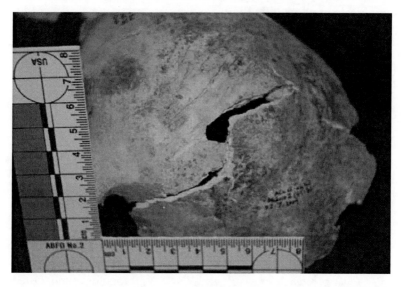

Figure 22. Adult skull (TAS 30) with evidence of fire action: deformation of bone like tension / shrinking due to the heat.

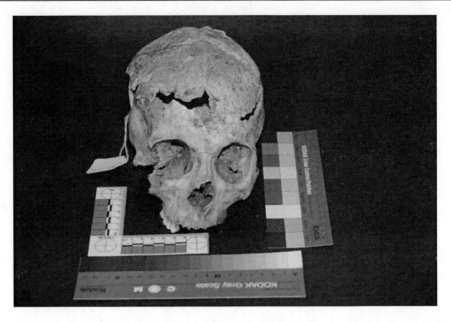

Figure 23. Adult skull (TAS 10) with evidence of fire action. The appearance of "exploded skull" an arrested phase of thermal destruction to soft and hard tissue.

## CONCLUSION

The goal of this chapter has been to demonstrate that each archaeological assemblage of human remains is unique, invaluable resource but not one to be studied in isolation. Context is important, minimally the point that you locate the assemblage in space and time. Skeletal assemblages are created and modified in many ways from the time of their deposition until the day they are studied, and that history is recorded in the assemblage composition and the taphonomic profile. Taphonomy restores the link between the site formation processes and the laboratory analysis of the human skeleton. We will certainly maximize our understanding of the past if we study the entire history of skeletal assemblage.

## REFERENCES

Adams BJ, Konigsberg LW. 2004. Estimation of the most likely number of individuals from commingled human skeletal remains. *Am J Phys Anthropol* 125:138-151.

Behrensmeyer AK. 1978. Taphonomic and ecologic information from bone weathering. P*aleobiology* 4:150-162.

Binford LR. 1981. *Bones: Ancient Men and Modern Myths.* New York: Academic Press.

Brickley M, McKinley Jl. 2004. *Guidelines to the Standards for Recording Human Remains. Institute for Field Archaeologists Paper N.º 7.* Anthropology and Osteoarchaeology, Institute for Field Archaeologists, and the Department of Archaeology, University of Southampton.

Buikstra JE, Swegle M. 1989. Bone modification due to burning: experimental evidence. In: Bonnichson R, Sorg MH, editors. *Bone Modification*. Orono: University of Maine Center for the study of the first Americans. pp. 247-258.

Buikstra JE, Ubelaker D. 1994. *Standards for Data Collection from Human Skeletal Remains. Arkansas Archeological Survey Research Series N.º* 44. Fayetteville: Arkansas Archeological Survey.

Correia PMM. 1997. Fire modification of bone: a review from the literature. In: Haglund WD, Sorg MH, editors. *Forensic Taphonomy: The Postmortem Fate of Human Remains*. Boca Raton, Fla.: CRC Press. pp.275-294.

Crist TAJ, Washburn A, Park H, Hood I, Hickey MA. 1997. *Cranial bone displacement as a taphonomic process in potential child abuse cases*. In Haglund WD, Sorg MH, editors. Forensic Taphonomy: The Postmortem Fate of Humans Remains. Boca Raton, FLA.: CRC Press.pp.319-336.

Dupras T, Schultz JJ, Wheeler SM, Williams LJ. 2006. *Forensic Recovery of Humans Remains: Archaeological Approaches*. Boca Raton, Fla.: Taylor and Francis.

Efremov IA. 1940. Taphonomy: a new branch of paleontology. *Pan- American Geol* 74:81-93.

Jans MME, Nielsen-Marsh CM, Smith CI, Collins MJ, Kars H. 2004. Characterization of microbial attack on archaeological bone. *J Archaeol Sci* 31:87-95.

Jans MME. 2008. Microbial bioerosion of bone – a rewien. In Wisshak M, Tapanile L, editors. *Current developments in bioerosion*. Springe.pp.397-413.

LaMotta V, Schiffer M. 2005. Archaeological formation processes. In: Renfrew C, Bahn P, editors. *Archaeology: The Key Concepts*. London: Routledge.pp.121-127.

Lovell NC. 1997. Trauma analysis in paleopathology. *Yearbook*.

Lyman RL. 1994. *Vertebrate Taphonomy*. New York: Cambridge University Press.

Marean CW. 1991. Measuring the post-depositional destruction of bone in archaeological assemblages. *J Archaeol Sci* 18:677-694.

Merbs CF. 1967. Cremated human remains from Point of Pines, Arizona. *Am Antiquity* 32:498-506.

Nielsen-Marsh C, Gernaey A, Turner-Walker G, Hedges R, Pike A, Collins M. 2000. The chemical degradation of bone. In: Cox M, Mays S, editors. *Human Osteology in Archaeology and Forensic Science*. London: Greenwich Medical Media. pp.439-454.

Pereira C. 2010. *Contribuição para a Identificação Demográfica de uma População Catastrófica por Parâmetros Dentários – População não Identificada relacionada com o Terramoto de Lisboa de 1755*. Tese de doutoramento. Faculdade de Medicina: Universidade de Lisboa.

Pereira C, Antunes MT. 2011.Vítimas do Terramoto de 1755 no Convento de Jesus (Academia das Ciências de Lisboa) – Identificação demográfica por parâmetros dentários. In: Memórias da Academia das Ciências de Lisboa – Classe de Ciências. Tomo XLIII,Volume II, Lisboa 2006/2007. Imprensa Nacional – Casa da moeda. pp. 389-421.

Shipman P, Walker A, Bichell D. 1985. *The Human Skeleton*. Cambridge: Harvard University Press.

Sorg MH, Haglund WD. 2002. Advancing forensic taphonomy: purpose, theory, and process. In: Haglund WD, Sorg MH, editors. *Advances in Forensic Taphonomy: Method, Theory, and Archaeological Perpectives*. Boca Raton, Fla.: CRC Press. pp. 4-29.

Ubelaker DH. 2002. Approaches to the study of commingling in human skeletal biology. In: Haglund WD, Sorg MH, editors. *Advances in Forensic Taphonomy: Method, Theory and Archaeological Perspectives.* Boca Raton, Fla: CRC Press.pp.331-354.

Waldron T. 1994. *Counting the Dead: The Epidemiology of Skeletal Populations.* New York: John Wiley & Sons.

Walker PL. 2001. A bioarchaeological perspective on the history of violence. *Ann Rev of Anthropol* 30:573-596.

White TD, Folkens PA. 2005. The Human Bone Manual. New York: Academic Press.

In: Forensic Science
Editors: N. Yacine and R. Fellag

ISBN 978-1-61324-999-4
© 2012 Nova Science Publishers, Inc.

*Chapter 7*

# FORENSIC DNA DATABASES IN EUROPE: ETHICAL CHALLENGES

### *Luciana Caenazzo[a] and Kris Dierickx[b]*

[a]Department of Environmental Medicine and Public Health, Legal Medicine, University of Padua
[b]Katholieke Universiteit Leuven, Faculty of Medicine, Centre for Biomedical Ethics and Law, Leuven, Belgium

### ABSTRACT

Advances in DNA technology and the discovery of DNA polymorphisms have facilitated the creation of DNA databases of individuals for the purpose of criminal investigation. Therefore, a considerable range of possibilities have been opened up for criminal investigations, and if we compare the DNA profiles of biological evidence found at the crime scene, with the DNA profiles in the database, we can identify the possible perpetrator of the crime. Logically, as the number of citizens whose DNA has been analysed and included in a database increases, the probability of locating suspects also becomes greater. It became obvious that the value of a DNA database is directly related to the number of records that it contains. Depending on legislation in the country, samples and profiles may be stored permanently or for a limited time, routinely searched for matches with crime scene samples and used for familial searching.

Some European countries have just legislated, or are drafting laws, with the aim of regulating databases for criminal purposes, with appropriate laws.

The reason for the different regulations surrounding a biobank designed for medical research and a biobank designed for forensic investigation is that there are, obviously, different purposes in the balance between individual rights and justice interests.

Forensic DNA databases can be useful in criminal investigations to identify socially dangerous individuals. However, it is important to ensure that the application of Forensic DNA databases does not contrast with individual civil rights and society liberties.

---

[1] Corresponding author. Professora Doutora Cristiana Pereira. Tel: (+351)-218811850; Fax: (+351)-218864493; E-mail: cristiana.pereira@fmd.ul.pt. [a] http://www.ceaul.fc.ul.pt; [b] http://cencifor.org/.

Although the laws that regulate the institution of forensic DNA databases in the EU are basically similar, the Member States can still make different choices regarding the management of their national forensic DNA database.

The aim of our paper is to evaluate and discuss, from an ethical point of view, some issues concerning the EU forensic DNA database management and which imply specific ethical attention and demand explicit policy choices that are collection of the DNA samples, minor's profiles inclusion and problems related to sample storage.

The provisions regarding these issues are different among the European Countries and even if in those countries where legal provisions have been established, not everything is completely resolved and some legal implementations that take in account an ethical perspective still seem to be necessary.

## INTRODUCTION

Today, Short Tandem Repeat (STR) typing methods are widely used for human identity testing applications including forensic DNA analysis. What makes DNA interesting from the viewpoint of forensic science is that the strings of nucleotides show variations, either in sequence or in length, that make it possible to discriminate between individuals.

A genetic profile is constructed from short tandem repeats (STRs), stretches of DNA containing core repeat units of between two and seven nucleotides in length that are tandemly repeated from approximately a half dozen to several dozen time. Although the human genome contains thousands upon thousands of STR markers, only a small core set of loci have been selected for use in forensic DNA and human identity testing. Commercial kits are now available to generate DNA profiles containing these core STR loci [1]. The actual technology allows forensic scientists to determine how many repeats of the STR sequence are actually present in a biological sample, the combination of the STRs analyzed is unique for every individual that they have become essential for forensic purposes. Commercially available kits, which provide all reagents ready-to-use, simplify generation of STR profiles and provide results on a uniform set of core STR loci to make it possible for national and international sharing of criminal DNA profiles [2].

The subsequent possibility to construct digital representations of profiles and store them in continuously searchable computerised databases has made possible a vastly expanded role for DNA profiling in many criminal investigations, and if one compares the genetic profile of biological evidence found at the crime scene, with the profiles in the database, he can identify the possible perpetrator of the crime.

A forensic DNA database stores genetic profiles obtained from crime scene stains, crime suspects and/or convicted offenders. These genetic profiles consist of a unique set of numbers that can only be used for identification purposes, as they do not contain any information on the genetic structure of an individual.

The complete process for STR typing includes sample collection, DNA extraction, DNA quantitation, PCR amplification of multiple STR loci, STR allele separation and typing and profile interpretation. Then, the profile must be entered into the database, compared with the other genetic profiles, and the statistical significance of a match (if observed) must be reported; otherwise, the elimination from the database has to be considered, according to the provisions of the law of each specific EU States.

Some European countries have just legislated, or are drafting laws, with the aim of regulating databases for criminal purposes, with appropriate laws.

Depending on the Country legislation, in a forensic DNA database samples and profiles may be stored permanently or for a limited time, routinely searched for matches with crime scene samples and used for familial searching. Furthermore, some biobanks may include all convicted offenders in their database or only those who have committed some particular offence like murder or rape. Others also include suspects of certain offences or, as the UK National DNA database (NDNAD), from anyone arrested by the police in connection with a recordable offense [3].

The underlying principles of the different forensic DNA databases in the EU are practically the same, but the Member States can still make different choices regarding the management of their particular National forensic DNA database [3].

Of course, the reason for the necessity of different regulations surrounding a biobank designed for medical research and a biobank designed for forensic investigation is that there are different purposes in the balancing between individual rights and justice interests.

Logically, as the number of citizens whose DNA has been analysed and included in a database increases, the probability of locating suspects also becomes greater. It became obvious that the value of a DNA database is directly related to the number of records that it contains.

Though forensic DNA databases represent an important tool in criminal investigations, allowing the identification of suspected or convicted individuals, it is important to consider that this investigation method should be in proportion with the protection of individual civil rights and liberties of society at large [4-5].

Our aim is to evaluate and discuss, from an ethical point of view, some issues concerning the EU forensic DNA database management and which imply specific ethical attention and demand explicit policy choices that are collection of the DNA samples, minor's profiles inclusion and problems related to sample storage.

The provisions regarding these issues are different among the European Countries and even if in those countries where legal provisions have been established, not everything is completely resolved and some legal implementations that take in account an ethical perspective still seem to be necessary. Even if the resolution of this matter is not possible with this contribution, we will however seek to highlight the complexity of the ethical issues related to these problems that are often encountered when innovative technologies become available.

## THE COLLECTION OF THE DNA SAMPLES

The genetic profiles are determined in DNA samples collected from crime scene stains, bodies of crime suspects and bodies of convicted offenders.

The crime scene stains constitute the least problematic topic of the three because, in collecting them, law enforcement officers do not have to physically deal with persons. In most Member States they can therefore, without many restrictions, collect DNA samples from the crime scenes they are investigating.

One ethical problem however could arise from considering that the collected DNA could also belong to innocent persons, especially when DNA stains are collected from a public place: it is questioned whether the collection and use of biological traces unintentionally left by individuals in public places ("abandoned" DNA) can be considered as licit. This technique is commonly applied whenever investigators need physical evidence connecting a suspect to a crime scene, and it might lead to the possibility of constructing illegal and informal DNA databases in possession of the authorities.

From an ethical point of view, the collection of DNA samples from a person's body can be regarded as a violation of one's privacy. The most severe kind of privacy violation is considered to be the intrusion into the bodily integrity.

In medical and clinical research practices, the potentially problematic nature of this issue is usually anticipated by informed consent.

Otherwise, in the context of criminal investigation, informed consent doesn't always seem to be necessary, because the individual whose sample is collected represents a threat to the safety of society, thus justifying the physical act of taking a DNA sample. Furthermore, according to most EU Member States, this procedure is only minimally intrusive and it is performed in accordance with standard medical practices, so it cannot be considered as a violation of the right to physical integrity.

In the EU forensic database legislations, we can observe a difference in the treatment of crime suspects and of convicted offenders, as suspects are supposed to be treated as innocent as long as they are not convicted.

Therefore, in most Member States a specific permission form the Court is needed to collect a DNA sample from a suspect (e.g. Italy, Germany and Belgium). However, the refusal from the suspect to undergo the procedure would make him more suspicious, so one does not really have a choice than to comply.

In Italy, refusing to give the sample implies that the Judge can command the coercive collection (sample may be taken by Court order forcibly, if necessary), in France the refusal to allow the taking of a biological sample is punished by a year's imprisonment and by a fine of 15000€ [6].

In contrast, in most Member States, samples can be coercively collected from convicted offenders without many restrictions, as they are considered to be under the custody of the State and holding diminished rights, making coercive sampling legitimate.

Another possible ethical issue specifically related to genetic profiles and not present in other forensic identifiers, is that each individual partly shares his/her genetic profile with the biological relatives. This means that the police also holds (albeit incomplete) information on people who have not been involved in any kind of offence. In fact, when a full DNA profile, obtained from a crime scene, has not matched an existing profile on the DNA forensic database, some countries apply the "familial searching" procedure, which is a searching method based on knowledge about the probability of matches between the STR markers of two members of the same family as opposed to the probability of matches between these markers when the individuals compared are unrelated.

Familial searching, applied to identify the genetic profiles of relatives of an unknown offender stored in a database, utilizes the increased likelihood of similarity between the DNA profiles of those who have a direct genetic relationship in order to identify a parent, child or sibling of an individual whose profile is available for searching. Familial searching therefore refers not to the social arrangement of families but to the genetic relationships between individuals – a distinction which is important for investigative as well as ethical reasons regarding information that police can obtain in an indirect way [7]. There are some issues regarding the use of this search investigation procedure, arising from both the searching of profiles on the forensic database and the subsequent investigative directives that involve a list of individuals derived from such a search. Forensic investigations may reveal a genetic link between individuals (previously unknown by one or both parties) and make such information known to them for the first time, or the absence of genetic links which participants previously assumed to have existed. There is also the question of whether this kind of procedure violates privacy and confidentiality of individual whose biological material was originally collected for example as part of an earlier intelligence-led mass screen and if it constitutes a disproportionate interference with privacy rights of individuals involved [8].

The use of this particular procedure will bring the police into contact with a number of individuals who have not been prosecuted for a recordable offense, who have no criminal record, and who are subjected to interview only because they are genetically related to someone whose profile is on the database [7]. Furthermore, it is reported [9] that privacy advocates argue that familial searching may increase discrimination and racial disparities. Statistically, certain groups (e.g. racial, ethnic, social class, etc.) are more likely to be arrested and/or prosecuted, and therefore these same groups are more likely to have submitted a DNA sample for storage in a database. Due to their higher representation in DNA databases, families belonging to a certain demographic may be unfairly scrutinized. This disparity is not peculiar of DNA forensic databases and in order to resolve the problem the entire justice system would probably need to be renewed, not just the process of familial searching.

## MINOR'S PROFILES INCLUSION

Another important issue regarding the collection of DNA samples is whether DNA sampling of minors should be allowed, considering the fact that this category is usually regarded as a vulnerable group and in need of special protection and consideration in research, in other areas of law and in daily life.

In the Italian forensic database, for example, for the provisions of the Law85/2009 [10], children are included because they have committed an offence, otherwise their profiles are used for familial matching, to identify missing persons, unknown bodies or part of them.

Genetic profiles of children are now included in the Italian forensic database without previous ethical or legal debate regarding the criteria of their inclusion, the storage and the removal of records, because by law they are allowed to be included therein, considering them simply and enough well-represented by their legal representatives.

Although it seems reasonable to take profiles for serious offences and keep them for a limited time, it would be appropriate to store them in a separate part of the database considering children as yielding persons capable of 'growing out' of criminal behavior.

This point further serves to highlight the basic principle of most European DNA databases that the interests of security of society overcome the individual right of giving informed consent, even in cases when the individual belongs to a group that is considered vulnerable [11-12].

In the EU forensic database survey, samples from minors are treated similarly to those from adults. Among European countries, only Germany has specific provisions regarding minors. The profiles of minors are checked every five years, and must be removed when retaining them in the system seems no longer necessary [6]. In the Portuguese legislation, the National Council of Ethics for Life Sciences (CNECV) on the draft bill regarding the DNA profile database issued the following recommendations: *"... the right of minors and incapacitated persons were deemed worthy of special protection. Only in exceptional cases, such for identification of victims or missing person s, should these DNA profiles be obtained"* [13].

## SAMPLE RETENTION

Generally, forensic DNA databases store DNA profiles derived from several sources: unidentified crime scene stains, crime suspects, convicted offenders and sometimes missing persons.

Most countries also store the DNA samples from which the DNA profiles were derived with the purposes of quality control, test result disputes and technology updates. However, this procedure raises important ethical issues which must be taken into account: in fact, in contrast with the DNA profiles, the DNA samples themselves are considered to contain highly personal genetic information on the individuals from which they were taken. In particular, the storage of samples could constitute a privacy rights violation, also considering the fact that some individuals are subjected to forced and non-consensual sampling of their genetic material, which could lead to future secondary use of the sample itself.

We must consider that genetic analyses on DNA from biological samples constitute a special kind of information: they can predict future medical conditions, discover whether someone is genetically predisposed to develop specific disorder, reveal information on the health status of relatives and be used for discrimination purposes. Furthermore, there could be an interest in certain other uses of these samples besides DNA profiling for identification purposes as for example research regarding genetic predispositions to violent behaviour [14-15].

Sample storage for forensic purposes does not seem to be strictly necessary, because in case of doubt relatively to quality control or test result disputes, the DNA sample can be obtained from the individual by means of the collection of a new sample. Furthermore, regarding the issue of the necessity to keep the samples in order to upgrade the corresponding profile in case of the advent of new technology, we believe, in according to Van Camp [14], that it is not a valid justification: although in case of a radical change in technology the sample itself is the only possibility to upgrade the result, it must be considered that evolution in technology has no end, therefore this issue will never be definitively solved.

Legislators must provide, in the legislation regarding whether or not to allow the storage of DNA samples in their databases, a balance between opposing standpoints previously illustrated. In fact, most Countries have added particular provisions on data protection into their forensic DNA laws, but in most cases only the DNA profiles are the object of interest, not the DNA samples from which the profiles are obtained.

In the EU States members there are significant differences regarding the criteria of storage and keeping of the reference samples. There are countries which distinguish between suspect and convicts regarding the treatment of samples, which must be destroyed in case of acquittal; in contrast, samples of convicted offenders are maintained for a number of years after the sentence has passed, or in relation to the age of the offenders (Czech Republic France, The Netherlands, Italy et al.). Denmark and Latvia do not take this difference into account and they retain all samples for a certain period of time. In Countries as Germany Belgium, Lithuania and Sweden samples must be destroyed as soon as possible, completely precluding any possible secondary use of the samples [14].

## Conclusion

Forensic DNA databases are of great value for society, being one of the most effective forensic identification tools currently available, and countries have a great interest in creating and maintaining them. However, this investigation method, that requires legislative authorisation, financial support and judicial endorsement, could be used against individual civil rights and liberties of society at large. These particular aspects regarding forensic DNA databases, should both be considered and mediated.

The provisions regarding collection of the DNA samples, minor's profiles inclusion and problems related to sample storage in forensic DNA databases, are different among the European Countries, and even if in those countries where legal provisions have been established, not everything is completely resolved and some legal implementations that take in account an ethical perspective still seem to be necessary.

This goal is attainable via the creation of responsible forensic DNA database policies, characterized by a reasonable balance between the purpose of crime detection and the respect of fundamental individual rights.

A major apprehension is that police officers will abuse and misuse the gained information to harass and prosecute innocent people, however legislators and involved personnel are working together to create procedures and policies that will help to verify that the obtained information will not be discharged without careful evaluation.

Different strategies can be utilized to consult the communities including education sessions, interviews, surveys, focus groups, deliberative democracy and public discussion meetings. These types of approaches will lead to better understanding of the public's needs and concerns regarding these aspects.

Guidelines for collection of the DNA samples, minor's profiles inclusion and use and retention of DNA samples should be well defined, shared by all parties involved (police, database custodians, prosecution etc.). Any disputes or problems regarding samples and profiles should only be decided by court, qualified to consider all relevant aspects.

Proper protection of human rights could be achieved in databases by establishing appropriate provisions on their use and manage. It seems that the vast majority of the population in democratic countries is normally willing to cooperate with the police, especially when investigations of severe crimes are concerned. Clear definitions and transparent behaviour of law enforcement agencies will reassure individuals in giving up their privacy rights to some extent for the sake of the common good.

Building this faith in the public opinion will assure that privacy rights and society welfare will not contradict but rather complement each other.

Regulation of management of DNA databases for forensic purposes require specific provisions regarding the collection of the DNA samples, minor's profiles inclusion and sample storage. As the EU Member States national policies regarding these issues are different and sometimes even non-existent, a unified legislative framework on the European level could perhaps offer the most effective safeguard of individual genetic privacy in these contexts.

## REFERENCES

[390] Butler J.M. Genetics and genomics of core STR loci used in human identity testing. *J Forensic Sci.* (2006). 51:253-265.

[391] Butler J. M. Short tandem repeat typing technologies used in human identity testing. *BioTechniques* (2007).43:Sii-Sv.

[392] Van Camp N., Dierickx K. "National Forensic DNA Databases in the EU", *European Ethical-Legal Papers N°9,* Leuven, 2007.

[393] Patyn, A., Dierickx, K. Forensic DNA databases: genetic testing as a societal choice. *J Med Ethics*, (2010) 36: 319-20.

[394] Van Camp, N., Dierickx, K. The expansion of forensic DNA databases and police sampling powers in the post 9/11 era: ethical considerations on genetic privacy. *Ethical Perspectives: Journal of the European Ethics Network,* (2007) 14:237-268.

[395] Duguet A., Rial-Sebbag E., Lacore M., Cambon-Thomsen A. Forensic DNA Analysis and Biobank in France in: Dierickx, K., Ed., Borry, P. (2009). New challenges for biobanks. Ethics, law and governance. Antwerpen/Oxford: Intersentia pg 203.

[396] Williams R, Johnson P. Inclusiveness, effectiveness and intrusiveness: issues in the developing uses of DNA profiling in support of criminal investigations. *J Law Med Ethics.* (2006) 34:234-47.

[397] http://www.btp.police.uk/PDF/FOI_policies_intelligenceledDNAscreening_Policy.pdf

[398] Gershaw CJ, Schweighardt AJ, Rourke LC, Wallace MM, Forensic utilization of familial searches in DNA databases. Forensic Science International: *Genetics* (2011) 5:16–20.

[399] Italian Parliament. Adesione della Repubblica italiana al Trattato concluso il 27 maggio 2005 tra il Regno del Belgio, la Repubblica federale di Germania, il Regno di Spagna, la Repubblica francese, il Granducato di Lussemburgo, il Regno dei Paesi Bassi e la Repubblica d'Austria, relativo all'approfondimento della cooperazione transfrontaliera, in particolare allo scopo di contrastare il terrorismo, la criminalità transfrontaliera e la migrazione illegale (Trattato di Prum). 2009 June. http://www.camera.it/parlam/leggi/09085l.htm.

[400] Tozzo P, Pegoraro R, Caenazzo L. Biobanks for non-clinical purposes and the new law on forensic biobanks: does the Italian context protect the rights of minors? *J Med Ethics.* 2010 (12):775-778.

[401] Levitt M., Tomasini F. Bar-coded children: an exploration of issues around the inclusion of children on the England and Wales National DNA database. *Genomics and Criminal Justice* (2006) 2 (1) 41–56.

[402] Aguas C., Carvalho S. DNA Databases and Biobanks: The Portuguese Legal and Ethical Framework in: Dierickx, K., Ed., Borry, P. (2009). New challenges for biobanks. Ethics, law and governance. Antwerpen/Oxford: Intersentia. pg 218-219.

[403] Van Camp, N., Dierickx, K. The retention of forensic DNA samples: a socio-ethical evaluation of current practices in the EU. *J Med Ethics*, 2008 (34):606-610.

[404] Levitt M. Forensic databases: benefits and ethical and social costs. *Br. Med. Bull.* (2007) 83:235-248.

In: Forensic Science
Editors: N. Yacine and R. Fellag

ISBN 978-1-61324-999-4
© 2012 Nova Science Publishers, Inc.

*Chapter 8*

# LIP PRINTS: PAST, PRESENT AND FUTURE

### *Ana Castelló[1]\*, Fernando Verdú[2]†*

[1]University of Valencia EG, Facultad de Medicina, U. D. Medicina Legal, Av/ Blasco Ibañez, n°15, 46010 Valencia, Spain
[2]University of Valencia EG, Address: Facultad de Medicina, U. D. Medicina Legal, Av/ Blasco Ibañez, n°15, 46010 Valencia, Spain

### ABSTRAC

Unquestionably fingerprints are evidences of great value in forensic investigation. Moreover, they are the most known and studied. Nevertheless other prints: palmar, plantar, those of ear or lip prints, also can be useful. The work reviews the possibilities of the lip prints to contribute to solve a criminal event. The way followed for different investigators who have dedicated themselves to study them is revised. Also the methods necessary to find them and to reveal them are described. After knowing its potential it is possible to conclude that lip prints will be an interesting evidence for the criminal investigation, whenever they are evaluated of the suitable form and with the prudence that is demanded in Forensic Sciences.

## 1. INTRODUCTION

There is no doubt that, even today, fingerprints continue to be one of the most valuable clues in criminal investigation. In contrast, other types of prints, such as palm, sole, ear and lip prints, encounter serious difficulties when it comes to being accepted as evidence in a court case.

This can be explained by looking back at history. The former, fingerprints, have been studied now for many years ago. Research has been carried out on them and consequently data has been published that scientifically shows that they are unique and immutable [1].

---
\* Biochemist Ph D.Sci, Professor of Legal Medicine; Telephone/Fax:+34 963864165; E-mail: Ana.Castello@uv.es.
† MD, PhD., Professor of Legal Medicine; Telephone: +34 963864165 +34 96864820; Fax: +34963864165; E-mail: Fernando.Verdu@uv.es.
[1] Corresponding author. Professora Doutora Cristiana Pereira. Tel: (+351)-218811850; Fax: (+351)-218864493; E-mail: cristiana.pereira@fmd.ul.pt. [a] http://www.ceaul.fc.ul.pt; [b] http://cencifor.org/.

Moreover, advances in the means of image processing enable information to be obtained on fingerprints that at first seemed to be of little use. Information technology also provides the opportunity to create databases that enable quick and effective comparisons.

Not only can fingerprints lead to identification through a lophoscopic study, but DNA may also be obtained from the epithelial cells that remain on them [2].

Furthermore, they may provide even more information: in 2008, several studies were published in which exogenous material found on fingerprints was analysed. Traces of explosives, drugs or any substance with which the perpetrator of a crime has come into contact can be obtained and examined so as to determine what is called "the chemical fingerprint", so adding very interesting information to the investigation [3,4,5].

Forensic interest in fingerprints is, therefore, quite evident, but what about other types of prints? It would appear to be logical that there is no reason why palm, sole, lip or ear prints should be any less useful. However, to be accepted as such, studies have to be published that prove their individuality and immutability. In the meantime they are used only as a support to the investigation and only occasionally are regarded as valid evidence.

In the following paragraphs we are going to review the history of one of the previously mentioned clues, that of lip prints, and report on the work that has been carried out on them and the information available to date.

## 2. Lip Prints. Background

Anthropologists were the first to observe and describe the presence of grooves in human lips [6]. However, it was Edmond Locard who suggested that they would be interesting for identification purposes [7]. Nevertheless, his thesis was aimed more at the morphological observation of the lips, rather than at the study of the *pattern* that the lip grooves formed on a backing material.

Curiously, it was not a forensic scientist who first saw the identification potential of lip grooves, but a lawyer and writer, Erle Stanley Gardner. His most famous character, Perry Mason, in *The Case of the Crimson Kiss* [8], uses the print left by some lips on the victim's forehead to demonstrate the innocence of his client and, at the same time, to implicate the victim's so-called friend and companion. The intervention of a forensic fingerprint expert, on this occasion examining the lip print, turns out to be decisive in solving the case.

Following this initial idea reality overtook fiction, as is so often the case, and, in 1950, LeMoyne Snyder claimed, in his *Homicide Investigation,* that the value of lip prints for identification purposes were comparable to those of fingerprints [9].

As a consequence of his work, he was asked to advise on a case of someone who had been run over that the Los Angeles police force were investigating. A lip print belonging to the victim, found on the chassis of the car, showed without any doubt that contact had taken place between the vehicle and the victim.

From then on, various research groups began to determine the real value of lip prints in resolving criminal cases. Consequently, Martín Santos proposed an initial lip print classification system that consisted of grouping together the grooves and lines into simple and compound ones. Each category was then subdivided into other more specific ones [10].

In the same year, Professor Kazuo Suzuki and his team studied prints obtained from lips bearing lipstick. By doing so, they showed that the differences between prints made by different lips were clearly observable [11].

To confirm these results, the prints of members of various Japanese families were used. Their experiment shows that, although there may be similar features, it is possible to differentiate one from another [12] and so they proposed a new classification system of five groups, the first being in turn subdivided into two [13].

In the studies they undertook on the prints of twins, they came to the same conclusions. Here, they compared the prints of brothers or sisters and also those corresponding to their parents. Moreover, the experiment was repeated after three years to check possible variability over time. The data indicated the immutability of the prints.

Following these initial works, other researchers devoted their efforts to corroborating the individual and unalterable nature of lip prints [14,15].

Some years later, in 1975, Professor Suzuki's team published an interesting article in which he described how the lip print was used in the investigation of two criminal cases [16]. In one of them, when comparing the print found with one taken from the suspect, some similarities were observed, but it could not be concluded that they were the same. At the end of the investigation it was discovered that it was the brother of the individual arrested who had been the perpetrator of the crime. This fact, say the authors of the work, reaffirms the individual nature of lip prints.

These first cases were followed by others of an equally interesting nature, such as that described in the article entitled *Lip print identification* in *Identification News* [17,18] where a person was identified by the lip print left on the back of a photograph.

Also worthy of note was the investigation carried out by the FBI with the aim of solving a series of bank robberies, committed by someone who at first was regarded as a skilled and slippery operator. One day, however, he made a mistake: on fleeing, he ran into a glass door and left a lip mark there.

Although a woman was being looked for, the perpetrator of the crimes turned out to be a man disguised so to avoid being identified. His lip print coincided with that obtained from the glass door and this evidence was used to prosecute him.

It should be stressed, however, that this type of evidence has to be used prudently and never as the only evidence in an accusation. Lip prints can only be considered as just another contribution to the investigation which, combined with all the rest of the information, may lead to the judicial truth.

One example of an unfortunate application of prints as evidence can be found in the *El pueblo vs. Davis* case. The facts were as follows:

During an investigation into a homicide a lip print was found on an adhesive tape. The accusation against Lavelle L. Davis, who was tried and sentenced to 45 years in prison in 1997, was built up around this clue. Since then he has appealed against this sentence several times and in 2006, a judge ordered a retrial. As a result Davis has been pardoned and freed.

This story is just one example of the inappropriate use of Forensic Sciences. A single clue is not enough to sustain a criminal case. Not even almighty DNA would be sufficient on its own to prove the innocence or guilt of a suspect. It is the body of evidence (both from the laboratory and documentary and witnesses' testimonies) that lead as near as possible to the truth.

While the suitability of lip prints as evidence was being discussed in various circles, other researchers proposed new classification systems. Those of Afchar-Bayat [19] and Jose M. Domínguez [20] are particularly worthy of mention.

## 3. LATENT LIP PRINTS

Using the above described procedures, lip prints may be studied and, through comparison with undoubted ones, contribute to the identification of the participants in a criminal event.

However, developments in cosmetic products have complicated research into this type of clue. At the end of the last century so-called "permanent lipsticks" came onto the market. These, according to the manufacturers, do not leave a mark, or at least do not leave a visible mark, but... a latent one?

This was the question that the members of the "Medical Ethics and Forensic Sciences Research Group" at the Faculty of Medicine in Valencia asked themselves. Having posed the question, a line of research was begun, the results of which are as follows:

In principle, it is logical to think that lips made-up with permanent lipstick will leave an invisible or latent mark on coming into contact with any surface. So, applying what is already known about fingerprints, and with the help of the appropriate reagents, it should be possible to reveal lip prints.

The first step in the work plan consisted of checking whether the products that were used on fingerprints were effective also for lip prints.

The results indicated that the reagents for fingerprints are not very effective for this other type of print. In fact it was not possible to reveal them with any degree of quality unless they were very recent and on non-porous surfaces [21].

This inability, it was decided, could probably be explained by the different chemical composition of the two types of print. It was, therefore, necessary to look for new products capable of "revealing" these prints.

The working hypothesis was established that, although the integral components of the different permanent lipsticks varied depending on the manufacturer, all of them contained moisturising products. Various reagents were then selected that had an affinity with fats, among them those called lysochromes.

This term describes a group of compounds that is noted for their capacity to react with fats so forming a coloured product. They are also very sensitive and detect even the minimum amount of the print in question.

Experiments carried out with three of them - Sudan III, Oil-Red-O and Sudan Black – showed their effectiveness in treating lip prints. Used directly on the print, in powder form or prepared in a solution, they managed to reveal both recent and old prints on all types of surfaces (porous and non-porous). Of the three, Sudan Black proved to be the most effective [22,23].

Having found a valid work tool, several drawbacks had at first to be overcome, such as those due to the characteristics of the surface on which the print has been made. Lysochromes are undoubtedly sensitive and effective but sometimes what is revealed may not be discernable due to the problem of the contrast between the reagent colour (the black of Sudan

Black or red of Sudan III and Oil-Red-O) and the backing on which the print is made. To solve this problem, fluorescent reagents were used.

Once again and returning to the first stage of the research, luminescent developers were first tested on fingerprints. They were then used on 60-day old lip prints on serviettes providing quality results [24].

In further studies, the capacity of another chemioluminescent reagent, Nile Red, was assessed. This is frequently used in histopathology for observing fats. The results were spectacular: minimum amounts of reagents managed to reveal prints of up to 750 days old [25,26,27].

On analysing all this data, it was deduced that the lysochromes and fluorescent reagents could be used to reveal latent lip prints on a large number of surfaces, but would they be useful on human skin? Clearly, this is an especially problematic surface as it contains the same organic elements that prints produce. Using the same elements to detect prints would interfere in their development. As an added problem, prints on skin are not expected to last long.

Effective procedures have been designed for fingerprints, so much so that DNA can even be extracted from cellular remains found on them [28,29].

However, research into the case of lip prints, has scarcely begun.

To date, the first works published conclude that lysochromes – specifically Sudan Black– are valid for working on this complicated surface.

The results that luminescent reagents provide, however, are interesting. Contrary to what was found on different types of materials, fluorescent powders are more effective for fingerprints than Nile Red on human skin [30,31].

Revealing lip prints on human skin is, therefore, without any doubt an interesting line of research which needs to be developed further.

## 4. LIP PRINTS VS. FINGERPRINTS

Once the means has been found for obtaining the lip print, it is necessary to devote the time required to determining its consistency as evidence. So that they may accepted as such, their individuality and immutability has to be shown. Different authors have worked on these issues, providing information that supports the hypothesis that prints are unique and unvarying [32,33]. Theoretically, therefore, they would be valid for identification purposes following a cheiloscopic study [34].

However, can they provide more information? In the introduction the "triple identification capability" of fingerprints was referred to. Can lip prints do the same?

Firstly, it is accepted that finger prints are unique and immutable. Studies have been undertaken on lip prints that reach the same conclusion: they are different for each individual and unalterable.

However, there is a difference between the two types of prints: the existence of databases. Lophoscopic studies, with the aid of information technology, have on occasions managed to assign a fingerprint to an individual. This possibility does not exist in the case of lip prints. Identification can only be achieved by comparison between an undoubted sample and the one in question.

As regards DNA, the two types of prints have the same individualising potential. In the same way that genetic material is extracted from fingerprints, lip prints can also retain traces of epithelial cells from which to obtain a profile. Furthermore, according to what has so far been published, the best revealer of this type of vestige - Sudan Black- does not interfere in genetic analysis [35].

The capacity of prints to retain exogenous material remains to be assessed. Here, lip prints are ahead of fingerprints, as work was undertaken some time ago to determine the composition of lipsticks. In 1980 an article was published proposing the use of high pressure liquid chromotography as an appropriate means for discovering the components of the problem sample [36]. Later other procedures were suggested, such as a combination between thin layer chromotography and gases [37] or analysis by neutron activation.

To conclude, lip prints will provide interesting clues for criminal investigation as long as they are evaluated in an appropriate way and with the caution demanded by Forensic Sciences. The teachings of professor Locard should not be forgotten when he warned that: *"Physical evidence cannot be wrong, it cannot perjure itself, it cannot be wholly absent. Only human failure to find it, study and understand it, can diminish its value."*

## 5. REFERENCES

[405] Cole Simon A. *Suspect Identities: A History of Fingerprinting and Criminal Identification,* Harvard University Press, EEUU, 2002.

[406] Van Ooschot RAH, Jones MK. DNA fingerprints from fingerprints. *Nature* 1997;387:767.

[407] West M J, Went M J. The spectroscopic detection of exogenous material in fingerprints after development with powders and recovery with adhesive lifters. *Forensic Sci Int.* 2008;174(1):1-5.

[408] West M J, Went M J. The spectroscopic detection of drugs of abuse in fingerprints after development with powders and recovery with adhesive lifters. *Spectrochim Acta A Mol Biomol Spectrosc.* 2009;71(5):1984-1988.

[409] Ng PH, Walker S, Tahtouh M, Reedy B. Detection of illicit substances in fingerprints by infrared spectral imaging. *Anal Bioanal Chem.* 2009 Aug;394(8):2039-2048.

[410] Kasprazak J. Possibilities of cheiloscopy. *Forensic Sci Int.* 1990;46:145-151.

[411] Locard E. *Manual de técnica policíaca* 1ª ed., José Montesó, Barcelona, 1934.

[412] Stanley G E. *The Case of the Crimson Kiss,* 1948.

[413] Snyder L. *Homicide Investigation* 3ª ed, Thomas, Springfield, 1977.

[414] Santos M. Queiloscopy, A supplementary stomatological means of identification, *Int. Microform J. Leg. Med.* 1976;2:66.

[415] Suzuki K, Suzuki H, Tsuchihashi A. *On the female lips and rouge.* Shikwa Gakuho 1967;67:471.

[416] Suzuki K, Tsuchihashi Y. Personal identification by means of lip prints *J Forens Med* 1970;17:52-57.

[417] Suzuki K, Tsuchihashi Y. A new attempt of personal identification by means of lip prints *Can Soc Forens Sci J* 1971;4:154-158.

[418] Hirth L. et al. Lip prints - variability and genetics. *Human Genetik.* 1975;30:47-62.

[419] Augustine J, Barpande S R, Tupkari J V. Cheiloscopy as an adjunct to forensic identification: a study of 600 individuals. *J Forensic Odontostomatol* 2008;27:44-52.

[420] Suzuki K, Tsuchihashi Y. Two criminal cases of lip print *Acta Criminol Japan* 1975;41:61-64.

[421] Uma Maheswari T N. *Lip prints,* Medical University, Chennai, 2005. www.tnmmu.ac.in/dis/24024103.pdf

[422] Kenneth J. *Lip print identification Identification News* 1978 ; 5-6.

[423] Afchar-Bayar M. Determination de l'identitè par les empreintes des lévres chez les femmes de Iran, *Societé de Mèdicine Legale* 1978 ;589–592.

[424] Dominguez J M, Romero J L, Capilla J M. Aportación al estudio de las huellas labiales. *Rev. Esp. Med. Legal* 1975 ;2(5) :25–32.

[425] Seguí M A, Feucht M M, Ponce A C, Pascual F, Persistent lipsticks and their lip prints: new hidden evidence at the crime scene. *Forensic Sci. Int.* 2000;112:41–47.

[426] Castelló A, Alvarez M, Miguel M, Verdú F. Long-lasting lipsticks and latent prints. Forensic Science Communications [online], April 2002. http://www.fbi.gov/hq/lab/fsc/backissu/Apr2002/verd.html

[427] www.tesisenxarxa.net/TESIS_UV/AVAILABLE/TDX-0613105-130234//negre.pdf (accessed)

[428] Castelló A. et al. Revelado de huellas labiales invisibles con reactivos fluorescentes. *Cuad. med. forense.* 2003;34:43-47.

[429] Castelló A, Alvarez M, Verdú F. Use of fluorescent dyes for developing latent lip prints. *Coloration Technology* 2004;120(4):184-187.

[430] Castelló A, Alvarez M, Verdú F. Luminous lip-prints as criminal evidence. *Forensic Sci Int.* 2005;155:185-187.

[431] Castelló A, Verdú F. Development of latent lip prints on multicoloured surfaces. A problem resolved using fluorescent dyes. *Indian Internet Journal of Forensic Medicine & Toxicology.* 2006;4(2) http://www.icfmt.org/index2.htm

[432] Trapecar M, Balazic J. Fingerprint recovery from human skin surfaces. *Sci Justice.* 2007 Nov;47(3):136-140.

[433] Färber D, Seul A, Weisser HJ, Bohnert M. Recovery of latent fingerprints and DNA on human skin. *J Forensic Sci.* 2010 Nov;55(6):1457-1461.

[434] Navarro E, Castelló A, López JA, Verdú F. Criminalystic: Effectiveness of lysochromes on the developing of invisible lipstick-contaminated lipmarks on human skin. A preliminary study . *Forensic Sci Int.* 2006;58:9-13.

[435] Navarro E, Castelló A, López JA, Verdú F. More about the developing of invisible lipstick-contaminated lipmarks on human skin: the usefulness of fluorescent dyes . *Journal of Forensic and Legal Medicine.* 2007;14:340-342.

[436] Sivapathasundharam B, Prakash PA, Sivakumar G. Lip prints (cheiloscopy*). Indian J Dent Res.* 2001;12(4):234-237.

[437] Coward R C. The stability of lip pattern characteristics over time. *J Forensic Odontostomatol.* 2007;25(2):40-56.

[438] Morais Caldas I, Magalhães T, Afonso A. Establishing identity using cheiloscopy and palatoscopy. *Forensic Sci. Int.* 2007;165:1–9.

[439] Castelló A, Alvarez M, Verdú F. Just lip prints? No: there could be something else, *FASEB J.* 2004;18:615–616.

[440] Reuland D J, Trinler W A. A comparison of lipstick smears by high performance liquid chromatography. *J Forensic Sci Soc.* 1980;20(2):111-120.
[441] Russell L W, Welch A E. Analysis of lip sticks. *Forensic Sci Int.* 1984;25:105-116.

In: Forensic Science
Editors: N. Yacine and R. Fellag

ISBN 978-1-61324-999-4
© 2012 Nova Science Publishers, Inc.

*Chapter 9*

# THE USE OF MICROMANIPULATION WITH ON CHIP LV-PCR SYSTEM TO ISOLATE CELLS FROM BIOLOGICAL MIXTURES

### *Caixia Li[a,b], Lan Hu[a,b,*], Anquan Ji[a,b], Junping Han[a,b]*
[a]Institute of Forensic Science, Ministry of Public Security, Beijing 100038, China
[b]Key Laboratory of Forensic Genetics, Ministry of Public Security, Beijing 100038, China

### ABSTRACT

Cell separation method proved to be an effective solution for biological mixtures in forensic science. Many of the current platforms adopted laser capture microdissection (LCM) system. Here micromanipulation method was combined with on-chip low volume PCR (LV-PCR) to select and detect single cells. The micromanipulation platform is more economical compared with the LCM system. Three fresh oral epithelial cells could be completely genotyped by two STR kits. Sixty parallel single cell LV-PCRs were performed using Identifiler®; 13 complete profiles (21.7%) were obtained. Seventy single cells were typed by MiniFiler®, showing 48.6% full profiles. The method was successfully utilized in a fatal rape case, where swabs from the victim's nipples were analyzed. Mucosal cells with an intact nucleus were captured by micro capillary resulting in amplification of the suspect's DNA profile, while mixed DNA profile was obtained by routine method. These results showed great promise for biological mixtures.

**Keywords:** Mixture sample; Mucosal cell; Micromanipulation; LV-PCR

---

[*] Corresponding author. Dr. Lan Hu. Tel: (86)-10-66269503; Fax: (86)-10-66269503; E-mail: hulan328@yahoo.com licaixia@tsinghua.org.cn.
[1] Corresponding author. Professora Doutora Cristiana Pereira. Tel: (+351)-218811850; Fax: (+351)-218864493; E-mail: cristiana.pereira@fmd.ul.pt. [a] http://www.ceaul.fc.ul.pt; [b] http://cencifor.org/.

## 1. INTRODUCTION

DNA genotyping plays an important role in forensic science nowadays, but biological mixtures are problematic and quite challenging for successful detection. In order to solve the problem, cell separation method was employed and proved to be effective [1, 2]. Compared with a mixed DNA profile, generation of a single-person DNA profile greatly enhances the value of a DNA sample for use as evidence against a perpetrator. Laser capture microdissection (LCM) is a commonly used method to isolate specific cells from mixtures [3-6]. Micromanipulation which is usually used in IVF (*in vitro* fertilization) therapy and PGD (preimplantation genetic diagnosis) was introduced into forensic science for oral epithelial cell isolation by Findlay, *et al* [7]. The micromanipulation platform is more economical compared with techniques yielding similar precision, such as laser capture microdissection (LCM). Here we have combined micromanipulation with 1.5-μL of on-chip LV-PCR system to isolate and detect specific cells. The system was successfully utilized in mucosal cells isolation from casework specimens.

## 2. CASE BACKGROUND

In April 2010, a weaving bag was found in a garden, in which a female corpse was packed. Different kinds of biological evidences were collected. The suspect's DNA was found in two specimens: nipple swabs and fingernails. But mixed profiles of male/female were obtained for both specimens by routine method. Then the nipple swabs were re-analyzed by micromanipulation cell separation method.

## 3. MATERIALS AND METHODS

### 3.1. Routine DNA Detection Method

The sample was treated with MagAttract® DNA Mini M48 kit (Qiagen, Germany) to extract DNA following the manufacturer's guidelines. The equivalent of 1 ng DNA was amplified using the AmpFlSTRs Identifiler® kit (Applied Biosystems, Foster City, CA) following the manufacturer's specifications. Positive control (AmpFLSTR® Control DNA 9947A, Applied Biosystems, 0.1 ng/μL) and negative control (no DNA template) DNA amplifications were performed.

One microliter of amplified DNA was denatured in 10 μL of loading buffer and applied to a 3130 XL Genetic Analyzer (Applied Biosystems), followed by data analysis using Genemapper ID V3.2.1 software (Applied Biosystems).

### 3.2. Sample Preparation for Micromanipulation

Fresh buccal swabs were collected from healthy volunteers and used for sensitivity study. The sample was incubated in TNE buffer (10 mM Tris-HCL, pH 8.0; 10 mM NaCl; 0.1 mM

EDTA) at 37°C for 20 minutes. After centrifugation at 9000×g for 3 min and removal of the supernatant, the cell pellet was re-suspended in 30 μL of TNE buffer. Then 1 μL of gentian violet solution (0.05 g/mL) was added to the cell suspension to achieve good visual identification of cells. After staining for 5 minutes, the solution was pipetted onto a microscope slide.

Micromanipulation was performed under inverted microscope (Olympus, Japan) with Transfer Man NK2 micromanipulator (Eppendorf, Germany). Sterile glass capillaries (Eppendorf) with an inner diameter of 80 μm were employed to transfer cells. The AG480F AmpliGrid® slide (Advalytix AG, Germany) was used as a collection platform for cell deposition and on-chip LV-PCR.

## 3.3. Cell Lysis and On-chip LV-PCR

For cell lysis, 0.75 μL of Proteinase K (0.4 mg/mL) was added to each reaction position, and covered with 5 μL of mineral oil (Advalytix AG). After incubation for 40 min at 56 °C and 10 min at 99 °C, 0.75 μl of PCR master mix of Identifiler® or (and) MiniFiler® (Applied Biosystem) was added. PCR conditions were as follows: 95°C for 11 minutes; 28 cycles of 94°C for 20 seconds, 59°C for 1.25 minutes and 72°C for 1.25 minutes, followed by 60°C for 45 minutes. Positive controls (AmpFLSTR® Control DNA 9947A, 0.1 ng / μL) and negative controls (no DNA template) were applied to each AmpliGrid slide. PCR products (total of 1.5 μL) were transferred to 10 μL of loading buffer. Electrophoresis was performed exactly as described in section 3.1.

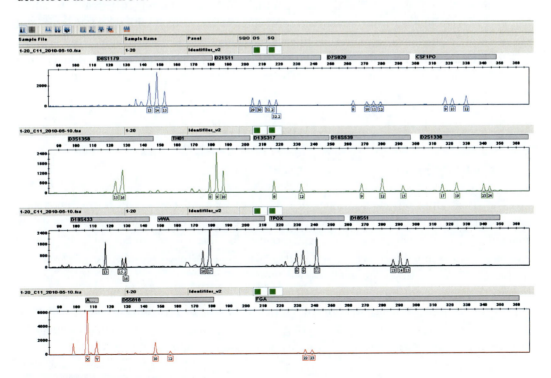

Figure 1. Mixed DNA profile obtained by routine method.

Five replicates of the experiment were conducted for casework samples, consisting of three cells each. Consensus DNA profiles were generated from alleles that were triplicated in the five replicate PCR reactions.

## 4. RESULTS

### 4.1. Sensitivity Study

Three fresh buccal cells could be completely genotyped by both Identifiler® and MiniFiler® kits. Sixty parallel single cell LVPCRs were performed using Identifiler®, 13 complete allelic profiles (21.7%) and 13 profiles of 13~15 loci were obtained. Seventy single cells were typed by MiniFiler®, showing 48.6% full profiles and 18.6% profiles of 6~8 loci. The results are listed in Table 1.

### 4.2. Casework Sample Analysis

Mixed DNA profile of male/female was obtained for the nipple swabs and fingernails by routine method. The mixed profile includes STR alleles of both the victim and the suspect (Figure 1). Then the nipple swabs were re-analyzed by micromanipulation and LV-PCR method for possible male mucosal cell separation and detection. Three cells with intact nuclei were captured and detected, and five replicates were conducted. Alternatively, DNA genotypes were obtained from a single person, which is concordant with the DNA profile of the suspect. Detailed genotyping results of each of the five replicates are summarized in Table 2. The consensus DNA profile is listed in the last column. One of the electrophoresis profiles of the five replicates is shown in Figure 2. The cell capture process is shown in Figure 3.

## 5. DISCUSSION

### 5.1. Sensitivity Study

The sensitivity study demonstrates that the micromanipulation-LV-PCR combination is highly sensitive for single cell assay. Even a single cell can be genotyped completely sometimes (21.7%), which showed great promise for forensic mixtures and trace sample analysis. Even with the high sensitivity, allelic dropout and allelic drop-in were still observed in Tables 1 and 2. Replicate analyses were necessitated to get a reliable profile [8-10]. Casework samples are difficult to detect compared with fresh cells, because of the DNA degradation and the influence of different carrier materials, thereby three or more cells need to be captured; but too many cells may bring the mixed profile problem again. So we usually capture three cells for each of the replicates, and recover a composite DNA profile.

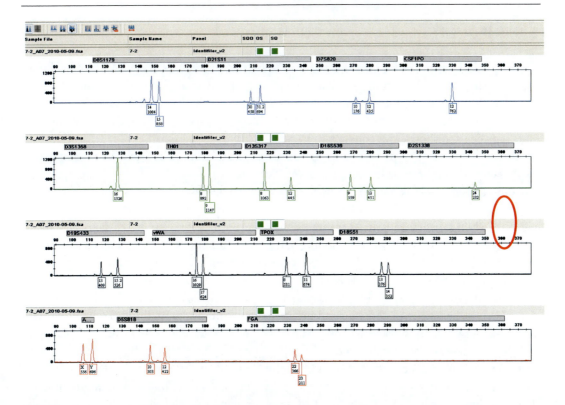

Figure 2. One of the electrophoresis profiles obtained by cell separation method (Red circles indicate allele dropout. Allele call and peak height are shown under each peak).

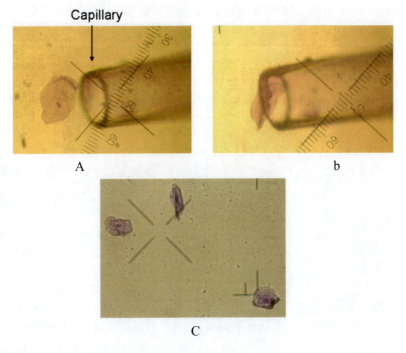

Figure 3. Mucosa cell isolation and collection by micromanipulation. A, Identification of cells with intact nuclei; B, capture of cells with a microcapillary; C, transfer of cells to a low-volume PCR slide.

## 2. Specific Cell Separation from Cell Mixtures

In sexual assault cases, skin surface swabs from sites such as the face and nipple can provide saliva samples from the assailant. Swabbing a large area of the victim's skin surface, however, can yield a mixed profile of cells from both the victim and perpetrator. Unfortunately, such a mixed profile of cells can often be of limited use, unless mathematical and statistical methods are conducted to separate the mixed profile [11, 12]. Here we employed cell separation method as an alternative. Besides skin cells from the victim, a skin swab taken during a rape investigation may contain cells derived from the perpetrator. Isolation of cells such as mucosal cells from a sample including skin cells can be performed based upon cell morphology and size. For instance, skin surface cells usually have no nucleus, while mucosa cells have an intact nucleus. Further, oral epithelial cells (diameter, mean±SD, 107.7±15.3 µm) are relatively larger than nipple skin surface cells (diameter, mean±SD, 57.2±10.9 µm). Together, these discrepancies allow for simple separation by micromanipulation under a microscope.

Complicating cell separation, however, is the frequent occurrence of cell folding and deformity on the carrier materials, resulting in difficulty in differentiating cells by either size or morphology. Here, we selected only cells with an intact nucleus and obtained the DNA profile of a male perpetrator that is consistent with the suspect. A report by Schulz, et al. [13] identified a new technique that can additionally be used to discriminate between skin and mucosal cells, using cytoskeleton analysis. As our method utilized only morphological analysis, incorporation of clearly defined tests to identify cell type would increase the reliability of micromanipulation. We expect that a combined approach will yield more precise results.

In addition to analysis of swabs from a victim's skin surface, micromanipulation and LV-PCR can also be applied to other biological mixtures. One such example includes the isolation of vaginal cells from penis swabs of sexual assailants. Furthermore, we have successfully employed the method in another fatal casework sample, in which a suspect's mucosa cells were separated from a victim's blood-immersed cigarette butt. Figure 4 shows the specimen picture and the mucosa cells presented on it. Sperm cell isolation can also be carried out in this platform, but it is time-consuming and labor-intensive owing to the small size of spermatozoa.

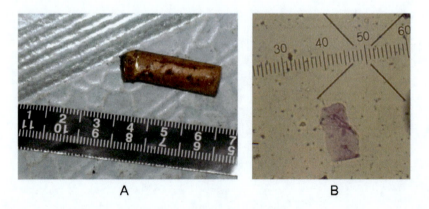

Figure 4. Blood-immersed cigarette butt (A) and mucosal cell presented on it (B).

## 3. CHARACTERISTICS OF THE PLATFORM

Successful capture of an intact cell is the key to the experiment. Replicate experiments are also necessitated to get reliable profiles. The micromanipulation platform is composed of two parts: an inverted microscope and a micromanipulator. The cost of this platform is much lower than that of cell isolation by laser capture microdissection (LCM). The primary drawback compared to LCM is that micromanipulation is less automated. Further, extensive training is necessary to become an experienced manipulator.

The on-chip LV-PCR provides high sensitivity to the whole method. However, it is not perfect in the present state. Gas bubbles in the reaction reagents during manual operation are encountered sometimes for the Ampligrid slide; bubbles may grow during the denaturation steps and finally burst to destroy the reaction spot or merging with the adjacent spots. The problem may be minimized to some degree by the use of a pipette for small volumes (0.1–2.5 µL).

In addition, increased sensitivity is accompanied by increased risk of contamination. The most important thing is to avoid contamination by laboratory setup and quality control of reagents [14].

## 6. CONCLUSION

We have developed a cell separation platform by the combination of micromanipulation with 1.5-µL of on-chip LV-PCR system. The platform is highly sensitive that three fresh oral epithelial cells can be fully genotyped by two forensic STR kits. Furthermore, the combination was successfully applied to mucosal cells' isolation from cell mixed specimens of real caseworks, which proved to be an efficient and economical solution to address the biological mixture problem.

## REFERENCES

[442] Bauer M., Thalheimer A., Patzelt D. (2002). Paternity testing after pregnancy termination using laser microdissection of chorionic villi. *Int J Legal Med*, 116, 39-42.

[443] Di Martino D., Giuffrè G., Staiti N., Simone A., Todaro P., Saravo L. (2004). Laser microdissection and DNA typing of cells from single hair follicles. *Forensic Sci. Int.*, 146S, 155-157.

[444] Elliott K., Hill D.S., Lambert C., Burroughes T.R., Gill P. (2003). Use of laser microdissection greatly impoves the recovery of DNA from sperm on microscope slides. *Forensic Sci. Int.*, 137, 28-36.

[445] Sanders C.T., Sanchez N., Ballantyne J., Peterson D.A. (2006). Laser microdissection separation of pure spermatozoa from epithelial cells for short tandem repeat analysis. *J. Forensic Sci.*, 51, 748-757.

[446] Anslinger K., Bayer B., Mack B., Eisenmenger W. (2007). Sex-specific fluorescent labelling of cells for laser microdissection and DNA profiling. *Int. J. Legal Med.*, 121, 54-56.

[447] Vandewoestyne M., Van H.D., Van N.F., Deforce D. (2009). Automatic detection of spermatozoa for laser capture microdissection. *Int. J. Legal Med.,* 123, 169-175.
[448] Findlay I., Taylor A., Quirke P., Frazier R., Urquhart A. (1997). DNA fingerprinting from single cells. *Nature,* 389, 555-556.
[449] Gill P., Whitaker J., Flaxman C., Brown N., Buckleton J. (2000). An investigation of the rigor of interpretation rules for STRs derived from less than 100pg of DNA. *Forensic Sci. Int.,* 112, 17-40.
[450] Budowle B., Eisenberg A.J., van Daal A. (2009). Validity of low copy number typing and applications to forensic science. *Croat Med. J.* 50, 207-217.
[451] Li C.X., Qi B., Ji A.Q., Xu X.L., Hu L. (2009). The combination of single cell micromanipulation with LV-PCR system and its application in forensic science. *Forensic Sci. Int. Genet.,* S2, 516-517.
[452] Clayton T.M., Whitaker J.P., Sparkes R., Gill P. (1998). Analysis and interpretation of mixed forensic stains using DNA STR profiling. *Forensic Sci Int.,* 91, 55-70.
[453] Bill M., Gill P., Curran J., Clayton T., Pinchin R., Healy M. Buckleton J. (2005). PENDULUM--a guideline-based approach to the interpretation of STR mixtures. *Forensic Sci Int.,* 148, 181-189.
[454] Schulz M.M., Buschner M.G., Leidig R., Wehner H.D., Fritz P., Häbig K., Bonin M., Schütz M., Shiozawa T., Wehner F. (2010). A new approach to the investigation of sexual offenses-cytoskeleton analysis reveals the origin of cells found on forensic swabs. *J Forensic Sci.,* 55, 492-498.
[455] Caragine T., Mikulasovich R., Tamariz J., Bajda E., Sebestyen J., Baum H., Prinz M. (2009). Validation of testing and interpretation protocols for low template DNA samples using AmpFlSTR® Identifiler®. *Croat Med. J.,* 50, 250-267.

# INDEX

## A

Abraham, 39
absorption spectra, 108
abuse, 54, 175, 184
access, 35
accounting, viii, 60, 63, 64, 71, 76, 77
acetic acid, 116, 118, 119
acid, 26, 32, 113, 119
active oxygen, 114, 117, 121
adaptation, 12
adaptations, 96
adenosine, 88
adjustment, 89, 132
adults, x, 149, 153, 155, 173
adverse effects, 117
aesthetic, 12
affective disorder, 87, 100, 105
age, x, 11, 106, 111, 115, 121, 123, 124, 127, 149, 156, 160, 174
agencies, 175
aggression, 110
alanine, 27
albinism, 87, 90, 93, 100, 101, 102, 103, 104, 105
algorithm, ix, 130, 131, 137
allele, 26, 30, 33, 47, 49, 62, 68, 69, 72, 73, 74, 83, 89, 90, 91, 92, 95, 96, 98, 99, 102, 104, 106, 131, 132, 133, 134, 139, 170, 191
amine, 113
amines, 125
ammonium, 28
amphibians, 51
anatomy, 18, 163
ancestors, 65
ankylosis, 157
annealing, 28, 31
anthropology, vii, 18
antibody, 109, 120
antigen, 109, 120

antioxidant, 115, 126
Argentina, 59, 63, 64, 65, 66, 67, 73, 78, 79, 80, 81, 82
arginine, 89
arrest, 18
ascorbic acid, 114, 118
Asia, 75
assault, 39, 43, 192
assessment, 15, 64, 69, 81
attribution, 24
authentication, 52
authenticity, 25, 45
authorities, 172
autosomal recessive, 101, 102
avian, 103

## B

background radiation, 25
bacteria, 25, 41
banks, 96
base, 2, 5, 11, 12, 25, 37, 54, 93, 112, 118, 137, 139, 146
beef, 54
Beijing, 187
Belgium, 169, 172, 175
benefits, 177
bias, 67, 92
biodiversity, 51
biological samples, ix, 24, 53, 107, 174
biomarkers, 124, 127
biosphere, 152
biosynthesis, 89
birds, 2, 50, 51
body fluid, 25, 109, 126
Bolivia, 65
bonding, 27
bonds, 25, 27
Bosnia, 29, 42

bounds, 62
Brazil, 65, 85
breeding, 52
brothers, 144, 181
buccal swabs, ix, 25, 130, 188
burn, x, 150, 152

# C

calcium, 92, 94, 100
cancer, 93, 95
capillary, xi, 2, 30, 119, 187
carnivores, 12
case study, 15, 16, 39
catalyst, 112
catalytic activity, 25, 92
catastrophes, ix, 130
categorization, 97
cation, 41, 102
cattle, 8, 35, 48, 49, 54
cell surface, 88, 93, 98
challenges, 55, 101, 176
charring, 163
chemical, 20, 25, 26, 42, 87, 108, 111, 114, 115, 120, 152, 153, 167, 180, 182
chemical degradation, 167
chemiluminescence, 125, 126
child abuse, 167
childhood, 87
children, 140, 141, 142, 143, 144, 157, 173, 176
chloroform, 24, 29
chorionic villi, 193
chromatography, 26, 29
chromosome, 48, 61, 81, 82, 88, 89, 90, 91, 92, 93, 100, 122, 123
cities, 65, 66, 67, 69, 151
citizens, xi, 67, 169, 171
civil rights, 169, 171, 175
classes, 17, 99, 156
classification, 97, 98, 104, 180, 181, 182
cleaning, 32, 113, 114, 117, 151
cleavage, 25, 92
climates, 12
cloning, 40
clothing, 16, 25, 39, 44, 111
clustering, 68, 75
clusters, 68, 71, 72, 75, 76, 77, 79
coding, 32, 34, 36, 52, 54, 74, 90, 94
collagen, 29, 43, 153, 160
colonization, 82
color, 2, 7, 9, 11, 13, 18, 19, 20, 21, 22, 37, 38, 55, 56, 86, 87, 88, 89, 90, 91, 92, 93, 95, 97, 98, 99, 100, 101, 102, 103, 104, 105, 106, 162, 163, 164

commercial, 31, 35, 68, 113
common sense, 152
communities, 50, 175
community, 35, 78, 86, 95, 145
compatibility, 37
competition, 25
complement, 34, 134, 175
complex interactions, 26
complexity, 61, 86, 131, 134, 135, 136, 139, 171
composition, 34, 62, 63, 78, 79, 80, 150, 153, 166, 182, 184
compounds, 25, 26, 27, 114, 116, 182
computation, 134, 136
computer, 81, 97
computer software, 97
conductivity, 30
confidentiality, 173
conflict, x, 61, 149, 160
connective tissue, 2
consensus, 31, 190
conservation, 111
constituents, 25
construction, 38
consumption, 43, 160
contaminant, 29, 113, 114
contamination, 17, 24, 28, 29, 30, 31, 32, 44, 117, 121, 193
contour, 66, 72, 77, 110
controversial, 105
convergence, 110
cooling, 12, 164
cooperation, viii, 59
correlation, 132, 147
correlations, 98
cortex, 5, 7, 18, 19, 21, 22
cortisol, 124
cosmetic, 21, 182
cost, 138, 143, 193
cotton, 16, 112, 116, 117
covering, 5
cracks, 108, 154, 164
cranium, 164
crimes, 14, 35, 175, 181
criminal behavior, 173
criminal investigations, ix, xi, 35, 107, 169, 170, 171, 176
criminals, 99
Croatia, 29, 42
crocodile, 50
crown, 5
crystals, 108, 118, 119, 120, 163
cultural influence, 83
culture, 21, 78, 89, 91

cuticle, 2, 5, 7, 13, 18, 19, 22
cycles, 28, 30, 189
cycling, 10, 28
cysteine, 88
cytochrome, 36, 50, 51, 53, 54
cytoplasm, 27, 87
cytoskeleton, 192, 194
Czech Republic, 174

# D

damages, 19, 150
danger, 163
data analysis, 188
data set, viii, 59, 61, 67
database, xi, 35, 36, 47, 68, 75, 95, 138, 146, 169, 170, 171, 172, 173, 175, 176
database management, 170, 171
death rate, x, 149
deaths, 150, 163
decay, 16, 40
decomposition, 21, 115, 164
decontamination, 17, 32
Deer, 49
defects, 22
deformation, 163, 164, 165
degradation, 27, 29, 36, 38, 46, 113, 117, 121, 123, 153, 164, 190
dehydration, 163
democracy, 175
demographic change, 63
denaturation, 193
dendritic cell, 7, 87
Denmark, 97, 175
deoxyribonucleic acid, 40
deoxyribose, 25
deposition, 127, 166, 189
deposits, 14, 152
depressed fracture, 160
depression, 161
depth, 122
derivatives, 115, 118, 119, 120, 122
dermis, 12, 27, 87
destruction, 153, 157, 160, 164, 167
detectable, 113
detection, 26, 30, 41, 42, 57, 79, 92, 104, 105, 125, 175, 184, 188, 190, 194
detergents, 114, 117, 121
deviation, 70, 71
diabetes, 91
differential diagnosis, 109
diffusion, 123
direct observation, 119

directives, 173
disaster, x, 33, 34, 147, 150, 151, 152, 153
discontinuity, 46, 81
discrimination, 24, 33, 144, 173, 174
diseases, 21, 22, 55, 93, 151
disequilibrium, 90, 91
disintegrin, 92
disorder, 21, 174
displacement, 167
distilled water, 114, 116
distribution, viii, 7, 13, 38, 41, 60, 61, 62, 63, 64, 68, 69, 70, 71, 72, 74, 76, 77, 78, 79, 83, 99, 109, 111, 114, 138, 139, 142, 143, 147
divergence, 88
diversity, 7, 53, 83, 86, 104
doctors, 121, 125
dogs, x, 13, 35, 47, 53, 150, 152
donors, 67, 106
draft, 174
drawing, 16
drugs, 180, 184
drying, 6, 113, 125, 153
dyes, 20, 21, 25, 27, 29, 185

# E

earthworms, 51
East Asia, 54, 88, 92, 96, 99, 103
ecology, 60, 82
editors, 167, 168
education, 175
El Salvador, 147
electrophoresis, 27, 30, 41, 190, 191
elongation, 6, 25, 37
emission, 113
enamel, 113
encoding, 88, 90, 91, 92, 100
endangered species, 50
endothelial cells, 93, 106
energy, 69
enforcement, 151
England, 176
enlargement, 2, 21
environment, viii, 21, 26, 31, 60, 87, 88, 153, 164
environmental conditions, 15, 20
environmental factors, 99
enzyme, 24, 93, 115, 122
enzymes, viii, 36, 85, 87, 92, 116, 122
epidemiology, 80
epidermis, 12, 27, 87
epithelial cells, xi, 2, 123, 180, 184, 187, 192, 193
erosion, 11, 163
ethanol, 24, 26, 28

ethical issues, 95, 171, 174
ethnic background, 67
ethnicity, viii, 85, 94
etiology, 105, 109
EU, 169, 170, 171, 172, 173, 174, 175, 176
Europe, v, 3, 60, 81, 82, 83, 87, 102, 150, 169
evidence, vii, ix, x, xi, 1, 2, 14, 15, 16, 17, 21, 23, 30, 31, 35, 37, 39, 46, 52, 60, 88, 92, 93, 94, 95, 96, 99, 103, 107, 108, 111, 112, 121, 124, 125, 130, 150, 153, 158, 159, 160, 161, 162, 163, 164, 165, 166, 167, 169, 170, 172, 179, 180, 181, 182, 183, 184, 185, 188
evolution, 34, 46, 49, 50, 53, 57, 86, 89, 95, 96, 99, 101, 103, 106, 174
examinations, 47, 98
excavations, 151
exclusion, 46
exercise, 54
exons, 88, 89, 90, 91, 92, 93
experimental condition, 116
explosives, 180
exposure, x, 12, 20, 32, 87, 95, 150, 164
external environment, 5
extraction, 24, 26, 28, 31, 40, 43, 49, 68, 122, 170
extracts, 28, 42, 43

# F

faith, 175
false negative, 114, 117, 123
false positive, ix, 45, 107, 113, 114, 117, 121, 144
families, 34, 65, 131, 132, 147, 172, 173, 181
family members, 130, 131, 132, 135
farms, 54
fat, 2, 163
fauna, 51
FBI, 181
fear, 3
feces, 25
fertilization, 34, 188
fetus, 2
fiber, 2, 5, 7, 11, 17, 22
fibers, vii, 1, 7, 12, 14, 16, 17, 18
filiform, 6
filters, 145
filtration, 30, 32
financial, 175
financial support, 175
fingerprints, xi, 14, 24, 39, 94, 114, 179, 180, 182, 183, 184, 185
fires, 152
fishing, 54
fixation, 86

flame, 119
flocculation, 42
fluid, ix, 6, 107
fluorescence, 19, 100, 122
focus groups, 175
follicle, 2, 3, 4, 6, 7, 9, 10, 11, 12, 13, 21
follicles, 3, 12, 13
food, 25, 52
food products, 52
foramen, 157
force, x, 150, 163, 164, 180
Ford, 53, 97, 100
formamide, 30
formation, 10, 91, 111, 119, 160, 166, 167
formula, 113, 133
foundations, 146
fractures, x, 22, 150, 160, 161, 163, 164, 165
fragments, 21, 31, 34, 38, 42, 68, 153, 154, 155, 164
France, 14, 45, 46, 172, 175, 176
free radicals, 25
frequency distribution, 62, 72, 73
freshwater, 50

# G

gel, 27, 29, 41, 119
genus, 51
geography, 81, 82, 83
Germany, 44, 59, 82, 172, 173, 175, 188, 189
gland, 3
glucose, 118
glutamate, 89
glycine, 113
goose, 12
governance, 176
grants, 47
granules, 5, 7, 8, 21, 27, 97
graph, 135, 137
grass, 69
Greece, 92
Greeks, 92
grouping, 69, 78, 180
guidance, 114, 138
guidelines, ix, 31, 105, 130, 144, 145, 146, 188
guilt, 18, 181

# H

haplotypes, viii, 60, 61, 62, 63, 68, 75, 76, 77, 78, 79, 80, 81, 82, 135, 137, 145, 146, 147
hardness, 110
healing, 160

health, x, 95, 150, 174
health status, 174
hearing loss, 87, 99
height, 110, 191
heme, 40
hemoglobin, 25, 108, 111, 113, 118, 119, 120, 121, 122, 124, 127
heterogeneity, 61, 63, 80
heterozygote, 31
Hispanic population, 147
histidine, 89
histology, 18
historical data, 77
history, viii, 59, 63, 80, 81, 96, 108, 150, 160, 166, 168, 179, 180
HLA, 40
homes, x, 150
homicide, 43, 53, 108, 181
hormone, 27, 56, 94, 101
hormones, 4, 87
host, 51, 102
hot spots, 146
hotspots, 34, 45, 137, 146
hybridization, 41, 94
hydrogen, 25, 108, 112, 115, 116
hydrogen peroxide, 25, 108, 112, 115, 116
hydrolysis, 40
hypothesis, x, 27, 33, 86, 102, 130, 135, 145, 150, 182, 183

# I

IBD, 139, 143
Iceland, 94
ideal, 29
illicit substances, 184
image, 97, 98, 105, 180
image analysis, 97, 98, 105
imagination, 115
immigrants, 65, 75
immigration, 63, 64, 65, 68, 77, 78, 80
immunity, 94, 104
impregnation, 111
imprisonment, 172
in situ hybridization, 100
in utero, x, 149
in vitro, 38, 89, 106, 188
incidence, 110
independence, 137
indexing, 52
indirect measure, 88
individual rights, 169, 171, 175
individuality, 180, 183

infancy, 38
infants, 21, 156
infection, 126, 158
inferences, 95
inflammation, 93
information technology, 110, 183
informed consent, 172, 173
inheritance, 102
inhibition, 26, 27, 28, 29, 42, 125
inhibitor, 26, 28, 40, 41, 42, 43, 47, 101, 122
inhibitor molecules, 28
injuries, 163, 164
injury, iv, 160, 163, 164
innocence, 180, 181
insects, 12, 30
insertion, 137
insulation, 3, 12
integration, 49, 79
integrity, 164, 172
intelligence, 38, 173
interference, 27, 62, 113, 117, 125, 173
intermediaries, 14, 15
internal controls, 26
intervention, 180
introns, 32, 36
iodine, 117
ion-exchange, 26
ions, 30
Iran, 185
iris, 55, 87, 91, 93, 95, 97, 99, 100, 102, 103, 104, 105
iron, x, 111, 150
irradiation, 32
isolation, 4, 24, 42, 78, 118, 166, 188, 191, 192, 193
issues, xi, 31, 35, 44, 170, 171, 172, 175, 176, 183
Italy, 1, 172, 175

# J

Japan, 45, 185, 189
justification, 174

# K

keratin, 5, 12, 24
keratinocytes, 2, 12, 27, 104
kinship, ix, 130, 134, 135, 139, 143, 144, 145

# L

landscape, 81, 82, 83

larvae, 36
Latin America, 75
Latvia, 175
law enforcement, 24, 171, 175
laws, 110, 169, 170, 174
lead, 86, 95, 96, 108, 123, 172, 174, 175, 180, 181
legislation, xi, 169, 171, 173, 174
Lepidoptera, 51
lesions, 25, 157, 158, 159
liberation, 115
life cycle, 14
light, 6, 9, 17, 18, 21, 86, 87, 88, 89, 96, 97, 103, 105, 111, 114, 115, 151
lipids, 2, 39
liquid chromatography, 123, 127, 186
liquids, 32, 117
Lithuania, 175
localization, 89, 99
loci, 32, 33, 36, 41, 44, 47, 48, 49, 52, 55, 61, 68, 69, 71, 72, 73, 74, 79, 80, 82, 83, 88, 91, 94, 95, 96, 98, 99, 101, 102, 131, 134, 135, 136, 137, 139, 143, 145, 147, 156, 170, 176, 190
locus, 30, 48, 54, 56, 63, 68, 70, 71, 73, 78, 79, 102, 103, 104, 105, 131, 132, 134, 135, 136, 139
luciferase, 39
luminescence, 109, 111, 113, 114, 119, 122
lying, 5
lysis, 24, 27, 28, 122, 189

# M

macromolecules, 28
magnetic particles, 57
magnitude, 142
majority, x, 3, 19, 32, 65, 67, 79, 92, 136, 139, 149, 150, 175
malignant melanoma, 86, 90, 100
man, 99, 181
management, 169, 171, 175
mandible, 153, 158, 159
manipulation, 28
mapping, 48, 49, 93, 104
mass, ix, x, 29, 33, 34, 42, 94, 122, 129, 147, 150, 151, 152, 153, 163, 173
materials, 2, 14, 15, 110, 114, 163, 164, 183, 190, 192
maternal lineage, 34
matrix, 2, 10, 88
matter, iv, x, 2, 24, 41, 150, 171
measurement, 105
measurements, 88, 97, 104, 105, 153
mechanical properties, 164
media, 112

medicine, 38
Mediterranean, 3
medulla, 5, 7, 8, 9, 13, 18, 19, 20, 22
melanin, viii, 5, 7, 25, 27, 38, 42, 85, 87, 88, 89, 90, 91, 92, 93, 94, 97, 98, 99, 102
melanoblasts, 92
melanocyte stimulating hormone, 56, 98, 100, 105
melanoma, 56, 90, 91, 98, 99, 100, 103
melatonin, 124
melting, 28
melting temperature, 28
membership, 11, 69, 71
membranes, 121
memory, 23
Mesopotamia, 65
metal ion, 25
metal ions, 25
methanol, 119
methodology, 23, 89
$Mg^{2+}$, 25, 26
mice, 91
microorganisms, 26, 42
microsatellites, 48, 49, 61, 146
microscope, 5, 9, 22, 23, 97, 117, 118, 119, 189, 192, 193
microscopy, vii, 1, 5, 18, 19, 97
Middle East, 75
migrants, 65
migration, 94
military, ix, 65, 129
minors, 173, 176
misuse, 175
mitochondria, vii, 1, 33, 34, 36, 45, 49
mitochondrial DNA, ix, 33, 45, 46, 49, 50, 51, 52, 53, 54, 81, 130, 145, 146, 147
modelling, 105
models, 110, 134, 135, 137
modifications, 20, 25
moisture, 160
moisture content, 160
molecular biology, 60, 94
molecules, 24, 25, 27, 28, 29, 32, 36, 38, 49, 57, 88, 99
morphogenesis, 10
morphology, 2, 19, 20, 21, 38, 51, 57, 102, 192
mosaic, 34
mucosa, 192
multi-ethnic, 78, 80
murder, 18, 171
muscles, 3, 12
mutant, 103

# N

natural disaster, x, 149
natural selection, 86, 93, 96
necrosis, 92
neovascularization, 106
nerve, 12
neuroblastoma, 99
neurodegeneration, 93
neutral, 40, 61, 96
Nile, 183
nodes, 22, 132
nuclear family, 132
nuclei, 6, 24, 190, 191
nucleic acid, 25, 41
nucleotide sequence, 146
nucleotides, 37, 135, 137, 170
nucleus, vii, xi, 1, 5, 24, 29, 33, 118, 120, 187, 192
nutrition, 157

# O

obesity, 91, 101
objective criteria, 98
obstacles, 12
offenders, 170, 171, 172, 174
oocyte, 34
optical fiber, 38
organ, 2, 24
organelles, 27
organism, 26, 35, 120, 152
organs, 12
osteology, 152
osteomyelitis, 157
oxidation, 88, 108, 109, 111, 112, 115
oxygen, 108, 111, 112, 115, 121, 125, 127
oxyhemoglobin, 124, 127

# P

paints, 113
paleontology, 152, 167
parallel, xi, 160, 187, 190
parentage, 46, 47, 48
parenthood, 94
parents, ix, 130, 131, 133, 139, 140, 141, 142, 143, 144, 145, 181
participants, 97, 173, 182
pathology, 160
pedigree, ix, 130, 131, 133, 134, 135, 136, 137, 138, 139, 144, 145, 146
penis, 192
peptide, 87
percentile, 144
periosteum, 164
peritonitis, 102
permission, 172
peroxide, 25, 115
peroxide radical, 25
Peru, 65
phenol, 24, 29
phenolic compounds, 25
phenolphthalein, 109, 115, 116, 117
phenotype, 38, 56, 86, 89, 97, 98, 99, 100, 102, 103, 105
phenotypes, viii, 85, 88, 93, 94, 95, 99, 103
phosphate, 25
photographs, 97
physical characteristics, viii, 85
physics, 110
physiological mechanisms, viii, 85
pigmentation, vii, viii, 4, 13, 19, 55, 56, 85, 86, 87, 88, 89, 90, 91, 92, 93, 94, 95, 96, 97, 98, 99, 100, 101, 102, 103, 104, 105
plants, 52, 86
platform, xi, 61, 187, 188, 189, 192, 193
PM, 53, 55, 101, 102, 104, 147
Poland, 82
polarized light microscopy, 19
police, 14, 86, 95, 171, 172, 173, 175, 176, 180
policy, 170, 171
policy choice, 170, 171
polyacrylamide, 27
polyunsaturated fat, 101
polyunsaturated fatty acids, 101
pools, 110
porosity, 110
Portugal, 149, 150
positive correlation, 96
potassium, 92, 100
Prader-Willi syndrome, 104
prayer, 150
precipitation, 26, 42
predators, 3, 12, 47
pregnancy, 2, 156, 193
preparation, 25, 112, 113, 120
preschoolers, 99
preservation, 43, 153, 156, 159
prevention, 38
primate, 102
principles, 171
probability, xi, 15, 31, 33, 46, 47, 62, 71, 130, 131, 132, 133, 134, 135, 136, 138, 139, 143, 144, 146, 157, 169, 171, 172
prognosis, 38

project, 68, 152
protection, 12, 86, 90, 95, 117, 165, 171, 173, 174, 175
proteinase, 24, 29
proteins, 26, 88, 90, 93, 101, 102, 111, 122
proteolysis, 93
proteolytic enzyme, 92
puberty, 4
pubis, 9
public health, 55
public opinion, 175
pulp, 113
purification, 28, 41, 122
PVP, 27, 40
pyrolysis, 163
pyrophosphate, 38, 57

## Q

quality control, 174, 193
quantification, 23, 30, 55, 79, 102, 105
query, 63, 71
quinacrine, 122
quinone, 27

## R

radiation, 86, 87, 90, 96
radicals, 25
rape, xi, 14, 171, 187, 192
reaction time, 87
reactions, 26, 31, 113, 117, 190
reagents, 25, 28, 32, 109, 111, 112, 116, 117, 118, 119, 122, 126, 170, 182, 183, 193
real time, 126
reality, 180
receptors, 12, 93, 104
recognition, 99
recombination, 36, 49, 68
recommendations, iv, 147, 174
reconstruction, 108, 114, 124, 127, 142, 160
recovery, 15, 17, 33, 153, 163, 164, 184, 185, 193
red blood cells, 121
refractive index, 23
regionalization, 69
regression, 164, 165
regulations, 169, 171
relatives, ix, 34, 42, 130, 131, 135, 138, 139, 141, 143, 144, 145, 147, 172, 174
relaxation, 86, 96
relevance, viii, 85
reliability, ix, 37, 85, 192

repellent, 4
replication, 36, 57
researchers, 16, 29, 35, 112, 113, 116, 121, 159, 181, 182
residues, 25, 40
resilience, 5
resolution, viii, 41, 43, 47, 60, 79, 81, 171
resources, ix, 130, 139
response, 87, 164
restriction fragment length polymorphis, 24, 50
restrictions, viii, 59, 61, 67, 171, 172
retina, 91
retrovirus, 42
RH factor, 109
ribosomal RNA, 36, 52
rights, iv, 172, 173, 174, 175, 176
rings, 21
risk, 30, 89, 95, 98, 99, 101, 103, 193
RNA, 36, 90, 121, 124, 127
robberies, 181
rodents, 5
root, vii, 1, 2, 5, 6, 10, 13, 17, 18, 21, 22, 24, 33, 34, 35, 38, 70, 71
roots, 13, 21, 33, 35
routes, 65
rules, 44, 194
rural population, 65
Russia, 45, 81

## S

safety, 125, 172
saliva, 41, 47, 49, 109, 121, 126, 127, 192
salmon, 29, 43, 54
scanning electron microscopy, 19
science, vii, xi, 1, 24, 25, 170, 187, 188, 194
scope, 16, 61, 79
sebum, 2
secrete, 2
security, 35, 173
sediments, 41
self-assessment, 97
semen, 14, 109, 121
sensitivity, 26, 28, 30, 43, 112, 113, 114, 117, 119, 120, 121, 188, 190, 193
sequencing, vii, 1, 35, 36, 38, 45, 46, 49, 50, 53, 57, 146
serum, 26, 28, 42
serum albumin, 26, 28, 42
services, iv
settlements, 65
sex, x, 2, 9, 11, 48, 50, 94, 123, 127, 149
sex chromosome, 123

sex hormones, 94
sex ratio, x, 149
sexual dimorphism, 2
sexual intercourse, 39
shade, 9
shape, 5, 6, 8, 11, 13, 18, 19, 21, 72, 110, 118, 119, 120, 153, 156, 159
sheep, 103
showing, xi, 3, 34, 63, 68, 72, 74, 79, 94, 165, 187, 190
shyness, 87
sibling, 130, 172
siblings, ix, 130
signal transduction, 100
signals, 12, 87, 93
signs, 96, 114
silica, 25, 29, 43, 119
simulation, 143, 144
simulations, 139, 140, 143
single-nucleotide polymorphism, 88, 99
siRNA, 98
skeletal remains, 29, 30, 35, 40, 43, 45, 46, 49, 115, 126, 151, 153, 166
skeleton, 153, 160, 166
skin, viii, 2, 3, 7, 11, 12, 24, 27, 30, 55, 56, 85, 86, 87, 88, 89, 90, 91, 92, 95, 96, 97, 98, 99, 101, 102, 103, 104, 105, 163, 164, 183, 185, 192
skin cancer, 89, 98, 103
SNP, 36, 53, 54, 55, 90, 91, 92, 95, 96, 98, 99, 104, 134
social class, 173
social costs, 177
social life, 2
society, 169, 171, 172, 173, 175
sodium, 28, 32, 92, 100, 112, 118
sodium hydroxide, 28, 112, 118
software, 61, 68, 134, 188
solubility, 120
solution, vii, xi, 28, 40, 112, 113, 114, 182, 187, 189, 193
somatic cell, 34
South Africa, 51
South America, 41, 43, 66, 75, 78
South Asia, 88, 92, 104
South Korea, 50
Southeast Asia, 51
Spain, 65, 107, 179
spatial frequency, 61, 62, 64
spatial information, 60, 61
species, vii, 1, 4, 7, 22, 29, 35, 36, 43, 48, 49, 50, 51, 52, 53, 54, 118, 120
specifications, 188
spectrophotometry, 97, 105

spectroscopy, 104, 121
sperm, 26, 34, 45, 193
spermatogenesis, 93
spin, 29, 43
spindle, 5
squamous cell, 86
squamous cell carcinoma, 86
stability, 185
stabilization, viii, 85, 87
standardization, 47, 49
stars, 27
state, 21, 33, 46, 67, 68, 111, 116, 121, 124, 164, 193
states, 14
statistics, viii, 59, 60, 61, 79
stereomicroscope, 19
sterile, 24, 31, 112
stimulant, 87
storage, 170, 171, 173, 174, 175
stratification, 63, 146
strictures, 22
stroma, 87
STRs, ix, 33, 35, 44, 95, 123, 130, 136, 138, 139, 143, 170, 194
structural characteristics, 19, 38
structural protein, 12
structure, x, 2, 5, 9, 14, 17, 18, 19, 22, 23, 38, 40, 60, 63, 65, 69, 79, 80, 81, 82, 83, 105, 135, 146, 150, 163, 170
subgroups, 100
substitution, 29, 137
substitutions, 45, 146
substrate, 38, 99
substrates, 89
success rate, 29, 45
sucrose, 118
Sudan, 182, 183, 184
suicide, 108, 109
sulfate, 28
Sun, 51, 52
suppression, 90, 91
susceptibility, 91, 95, 99
sweat, 12
Sweden, 175
swelling, 22
sympathetic nervous system, 3
syndrome, 102
synthesis, viii, 27, 40, 85, 86, 87, 90, 91, 94, 96, 101
syphilis, 158

# T

tandem repeats, 95, 170
tannins, 25

taphonomy, x, 149, 152, 153, 160, 167
target, 24, 25, 26, 28, 43, 90
taxonomy, 51
techniques, vii, 1, 18, 28, 36, 38, 108, 109, 113, 118, 119, 122, 124, 188
technologies, 38, 40, 171, 176
technology, ix, xi, 24, 36, 129, 169, 170, 174, 180
teeth, ix, x, 33, 34, 36, 45, 49, 149, 150, 152, 153
temperature, 9, 12, 28, 123, 124, 163
tension, 69, 82, 165
territory, 64, 65, 73, 78, 80
terrorism, ix, 130
testing, vii, 1, 30, 31, 32, 35, 44, 47, 48, 54, 67, 93, 94, 142, 143, 145, 146, 170, 176, 193, 194
texture, 110, 163
therapy, 188
thermal destruction, 163, 164, 166
thermoregulation, 4
time use, 18
tincture, 108, 118
tissue, vii, 1, 6, 17, 21, 43, 115, 163, 164, 165, 166
tones, 9
tooth, 49
TP53, 94
trade, 35
traditions, 78
trafficking, 101, 106
training, vii, 1, 35, 37, 193
traits, 18, 19, 22, 23, 38, 86, 92, 97, 98
trajectory, 96, 110
transcription, 88, 100
transcripts, 90
transformation, 4, 69
transition mutation, 138
transmission, 131, 133, 134, 135, 136, 137, 138
transport, viii, 85, 87, 93, 94, 102, 105, 121, 164
transportation, 88, 111
transversion mutation, 138
trauma, x, 22, 149, 150, 152, 160, 163, 164
treatment, 21, 28, 40, 42, 113, 116, 119, 172, 174
tuberculosis, 151
tumors, 91
Turks, 65
turtle, 50
twins, 56, 98, 181
tyrosine, 88

## U

UK, 50, 171
uniform, 13, 111, 170
United, 40, 41
United States, 40, 41

unstable compounds, 96
upholstery, 14, 108, 122
urban, 61, 65, 80, 83
urban population, 80
urea, 25
USA, 17, 39, 40, 44, 49, 50, 51, 53, 57, 68, 81, 90, 100, 103, 126, 129
UV, 12, 32, 86, 124, 185
UV irradiation, 32
UV radiation, 12, 86

## V

vacuum, 17
Valencia, 105, 106, 107, 113, 179, 182
validation, 41, 46, 47, 126, 147
variables, x, 14, 15, 16, 36, 149, 152
variations, 11, 45, 57, 89, 91, 170
vegetables, 113
vehicles, 113, 125
vertebrates, 52, 53
victims, ix, 129, 147, 149, 151, 174
Vietnam, 40, 45
violence, 108, 160, 162, 168
violent behaviour, 174
violent crime, 14
vision, 2
visual acuity, 87
visualization, 60, 61
vitamin D, 86, 94, 96

## W

Wales, 176
war, ix, x, 45, 129, 149
Washington, 40, 146
wastewater, 115, 126
water, 4, 5, 24, 28, 38, 112, 120, 153
weapons, 109, 160, 163
wear, 16
welfare, 175
wells, 38
West Africa, 96
Western Europe, 75, 90
wetting, 153
white blood cells, 118, 120, 122
wilderness, 65
wildlife, 35, 49, 50, 51
Wisconsin, 44, 45, 68
witnesses, 14, 39, 181
wood, 117
wool, 4, 12, 16

workers, 26
World Trade Center, 147
worldwide, viii, 59, 63, 68, 75, 77, 79, 80, 88

## Y

Y chromosome, ix, 95, 122, 123, 130, 144, 145
yield, 27, 28, 30, 43, 112, 143, 144, 192